Karl A. LeBlanc

Editor

Laparoscopic and Robotic Incisional Hernia Repair

Current Considerations

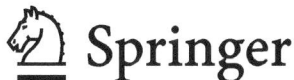

Springer

Editor
Karl A. LeBlanc
Surgeons Group of Baton Rouge
Our Lady of the Lake Physicians Group
Baton Rouge, LA
USA

ISBN 978-3-030-08087-7   ISBN 978-3-319-90737-6   (eBook)
https://doi.org/10.1007/978-3-319-90737-6

Printed on acid-free paper

This Springer imprint is published by the registered company Springer Nature Switzerland AG
The registered company address is: Gewerbestrasse 11, 6330 Cham, Switzerland

Laparoscopic and Robotic Incisional Hernia Repair

To my wife and best friend, Zinda. Your support and affection throughout my career has allowed me to do what I love and love what I do.

The laparoscopic repair of incisional hernias continues to grow. There are a number of changes that have occurred since the first procedure in 1991. The multiplicity of meshes has provided the surgeon many different materials with which to choose. There have been adaptions of different devices that are attached to the products to make the insertion and/or fixation easier than in the past. The fixation of these prostheses continues to undergo further refinement as new devices are introduced.

As with any common procedure in the armamentarium of the surgeon, there have been and continue to be areas of discussion or controversy. The limits and benefits of the procedure are an area of constant debate. It is generally agreed that the reduction in infectious complications is consistent. Newer areas of conversation are the need to close the fascial defect in all cases and the location of the mesh itself. Historically the intraperitoneal location was accepted but this is now being challenged and the placement in the preperitoneal space is gaining in popularity. The short- and long-term benefits of this opinion will require more time.

The most significant change to the laparoscopic approach has been the use of the surgical robot. This device has allowed the surgeon to close the defect more easily and more effectively. Additionally, it provides a platform to more easily perform the preperitoneal dissection and the posterior component separation. There has been a very rapid growth of this modality in the repair of all hernias. It is hoped that the adoption of this technology does not result in the lack of attention to the important tenets of the ventral and incisional hernia repair.

Laparoscopic and Robotic Incisional Hernia Repair—Current Considerations has brought some of the current thought leaders together to author the chapters to detail the art and science of this operation. I have specifically selected the topics of the chapters to provide sound advice and recommendations to the practicing surgeon. It is meant to be a resource for both the seasoned laparoscopic surgeon and the novice. I do hope that we have achieved this goal.

Baton Rouge, LA   Karl A. LeBlanc

Acknowledgments

I wish to extend my sincere gratitude to all of the authors that have taken the time and effort to contribute to this work. Without their support, this would not have become the textbook that I strived to achieve.

I do want to also thank Springer Medical Publishers for allowing me the ability of making this book a reality and providing Elise Paxson as my Developmental Editor. She has been invaluable to the development and production of this excellent textbook.

Contents

Contributors

James Avruch, MD Department of General Surgery, St. Elizabeth Medical Center, Boston, MA, USA

Igor Belyansky, MD, FACS Department of Surgery, Anne Arundel Medical Center, Annapolis, MD, USA

Jonathan D. Bouchez, MD Department of Surgery, Carolinas Medical Center, Atrium Health, Charlotte, NC, USA

Deepa V. Cherla, MD Department of Surgery, University of Texas Health Science Center at Houston, Houston, TX, USA

Basking Ridge, LA, USA

David Earle, MD, FACS Tufts University School of Medicine, Boston, MA, USA

Philip E. George, MD Department of Surgery, Mount Sinai Hospital of New York, Icahn School of Medicine, New York, NY, USA

Ciara R. Huntington, MD Department of Surgery, Carolinas Medical Center, Atrium Health, Charlotte, NC, USA

Desmond T.K. Huynh, MD Cedars-Sinai Medical Center, Los Angeles, CA, USA

David A. Iannitti, MD, FACS Division of Hepatobiliary and Pancreatic Surgery, Carolinas Medical Center, Atrium Health, Charlotte, NC, USA

Brian P. Jacob, MD Department of Surgery, Mount Sinai Hospital of New York, Icahn School of Medicine, New York, NY, USA

Shyam S. Jayaraman, MD Department of Surgery, Anne Arundel Medical Center, Annapolis, MD, USA

Ryan M. Juza, MD Division of Minimally Invasive and Bariatric Surgery, Department of Surgery, Penn State Hershey Medical Center, Hershey, PA, USA

Omar Yusef Kudsi, MD, MBA, FACS Department of Surgery, Good Samaritan Medical Center, Tufts University School of Medicine, Brockton, MA, USA

Karl A. LeBlanc, MD, MBA, FACS, FASMBS Surgeons Group of Baton Rouge, Our Lady of the Lake Physician Group, Clinical Professor, Surgery, Louisiana State University Health Sciences Center, Baton Rouge, LA, USA

Mike K. Liang, MD Department of Surgery, University of Texas Health Science Center at Houston, Houston, TX, USA

Jerome R. Lyn-Sue, MD, FACS Division of Minimally Invasive and Bariatric Surgery, Department of Surgery, Penn State Hershey Medical Center, Hershey, PA, USA

Vashisht Madabhushi, MD University of Kentucky, Lexington, KY, USA

Robert G. Martindale, MD, PhD Oregon Health and Science University, Portland, OR, USA

Yuri W. Novitsky, MD Department of Surgery, Columbia University Medical Center, New York, NY, USA

Sean B. Orenstein, MD Oregon Health and Science University, Portland, OR, USA

Eric M. Pauli, MD, FACS, FASGE Division of Minimally Invasive and Bariatric Surgery, Department of Surgery, Penn State Hershey Medical Center, Hershey, PA, USA

Clayton C. Petro, MD Department of Surgery, Cleveland Clinic, Cleveland, OH, USA

J. Scott Roth, MD, FACS University of Kentucky, Lexington, KY, USA

Zachary Sanford, MD Department of Surgery, Anne Arundel Medical Center, Annapolis, MD, USA

Shirin Towfigh, MD Beverly Hills Hernia Center, Beverly Hills, CA, USA

Benjamin Tran, BS Department of Surgery, Mount Sinai Hospital of New York, Icahn School of Medicine, New York, NY, USA

J. Tyler Watson, MD Our Lady of the Lake Regional Medical Center, Baton Rouge, LA, USA

H. Reza Zahiri, DO Department of Surgery, Anne Arundel Medical Center, Annapolis, MD, USA

Abbreviations

A

ACD   Anterior component separation
AHSQC   Americas Hernia Society Quality Collaborative
ASHP   American Society of Health-System Pharmacists
AWR   Abdominal wall reconstruction

B

BMI   Body mass index

C

CI   95% confidence interval
cPTFE   Condensed polytetrafluoroethylene
CRP   C-reactive protein
CS   Components separation

D

DHA   Docosahexaenoic acid

E

EPA   Eicosapentaenoic acid
ePTFE   Expanded polytetrafluoroethylene
ERAS   Enhanced recovery after surgery
ESR   Erythrocyte sedimentation rate
eTEP   Enhanced-view totally extraperitoneal

H

HbA1C   Glycosylated hemoglobin

I

IDSA   Infectious Diseases Society of America
IFU   Instructions for use
IPOM   Intraperitoneal onlay mesh
IS   Incentive spirometry
ISI   Intuitive Surgical, Inc.

L

LVHR   Laparoscopic ventral hernia repair

M

mic   Minimum inhibitory concentration
MIS   Minimally invasive surgery
MRSA   Methicillin-resistant *Staphylococcus aureus*
MSSA   Methicillin-sensitive *S. aureus*

N

NPO   *nil per os*
NSAID   Nonsteroidal anti-inflammatory drug
NSQIP   National Surgical Quality Improvement Program

O

OR   Odds ratio

P

PC   Patient cart
PCA   Patient-controlled analgesia
PCS   Posterior component separation
PCU   Poly-carbonate-urethane
PDLLA   Poly(D,L)–lactide
PEEK   Polyetheretherketone
PGCL   Poly(glycolide-cocaprolactone)

POL   Polyester
PP   Polypropylenepolyester
PTFE   Polytetrafluoroethylene
PUR   Polyurethane
PVDF   Polyvinylidene fluoride

R

RASD   Robotic-assisted surgical device
RCT   Randomized controlled trial
rRMR   Robotic retromuscular repair
RTM   Reconstructive Tissue Matrix
rTAR   Robotic transversus abdominis release
rVHR   Robotic ventral hernia repair
VHR   Ventral hernia repair

S

SC   Surgeon console
SCD   Sequential compression device
SHEA   Society for Healthcare Epidemiology of America
SIS   Surgical Infection Society
SPM   Specialized proresolving molecules
SSI   Surgical site infection

T

TAP   Transversus abdominis plane
TAPP   Transabdominal preperitoneal
TAR   Transversus abdominis release
TID   Thrice daily

V

VC   Vision cart

Karl A. LeBlanc

Introduction

The minimally invasive surgical repair of ventral and incisional hernias has its roots in the retromuscular repair promoted by Rives and Stoppa many years ago [1, 2]. This repair placed mesh between the peritoneum and the rectus muscles via an open approach. Transfascial sutures fixed the prosthetic in place. The long-term results were favorable. This repair continues to be used in the appropriate situations. With the advent of laparoscopic surgery in the late 1980s and early 1990s, the early believers in this technology adopted these methods to the repair of inguinal and incisional hernias. Interestingly the first known mention of a repair of any hernia laparoscopically was attributed to Dr. P. Fletcher at the University of the West Indies in 1979 [3].

The purpose of this textbook is to provide the current methods as recommended by the thought leaders of these repairs. The various options laparoscopically and robotically assisted are presented in the chapters. We have also tried to focus on the pre-, intra-, and postoperative care of these patients. The surgeon should have knowledge of all of the aspects of the care of these patients. We have tried to provide this information.

Laparoscopic Repair

The first successful repair of an incisional hernia using the laparoscopic method was by this author in 1991. The tenets of the procedure mimicked those of the Rives-Stoppa repair. A small series of patients was reported in 1993 [4]. Since this initial report there has been a slow but steady increase in the utilization of this methodology to repair these hernias. It is now commonplace to repair midline hernias as well as those located in the other regions of the abdominal cavity laparoscopically.

The development and growth of the laparoscopic incisional and ventral hernia repair fueled concomitant development of a large variety of prosthetic materials specifically designed for placement of mesh into the abdominal cavity with contact with the intestine. These are called the tissue-separating meshes. "Improved" products have replaced many of these materials over the years but several of them are still available. This is extensively reviewed in Chap. 5, "Implants Used for Hernioplasty."

As with any surgical field, there has been and continues to be areas of controversy. The first controversy revolved around the clinical benefit of the laparoscopic approach to the repair of these hernias. This technique does provide bene-

K. A. LeBlanc
Surgeons Group of Baton Rouge,Our Lady of the
Lake Physician Group, Clinical Professor, Surgery,
Louisiana State University Health Sciences Center,
Baton Rouge, LA, USA

© Springer International Publishing AG, part of Springer Nature 2018
K. A. LeBlanc (ed.), *Laparoscopic and Robotic Incisional Hernia Repair*,
https://doi.org/10.1007/978-3-319-90737-6_1

fit especially in the reduction in infection [5–10]. Other controversies have included the need and/or benefit of closure of the fascial defect. Most recently, the concern of the placement of any mesh material against the intestine has resulted in techniques to place the prosthetic material in the preperitoneal space. These are discussed in the various chapters of this textbook.

Current Surgical Robot Repair

The first surgical robot resulted from combining a few computer technologies to result in the founding of Intuitive Surgical, Inc. (ISI) based in Sunnyvale, CA, in 1995. The first prototype of their surgical robot was called Lenny (derived from Leonardo da Vinci). After successful feasibility demonstration, the Mona (derived from the Mona Lisa) was the second prototype. It was the first prototype to be used in human testing. Further refinements led to the development of the da Vinci® Standard surgical system. These initial robots had only three arms and were initially marketed and sold in Europe in 1999. They achieved FDA clearance in the United States in 2000 for general surgical applications. Clearance for thoracic and urological procedures followed 1 year later. The fourth arm was added to the system in 2003.

Continued refinements resulted in the release of the da Vinci S® product in 2006 (Fig. 1.1). The arms were lighter and smaller with improved visualization with high-definition video. In 2009, the da Vinci Si® was released (Fig. 1.2). This continued on the improvements for the surgeon console, among others, as well as higher resolution 3D magnification. This was also introduced with the available integration of a second surgeon console to allowing operators to use the system in unison. This required a "passing off" of the controls between consoles enhancing surgeon training and collaboration.

The more compact da Vinci Xi® system was introduced in 2014 (Fig. 1.3). This system has enhanced abilities to more easily dock the robot and other significant enhancements such as the ability to place the trocars closer together. Double docking (placement of trocars on the opposite of the abdo-

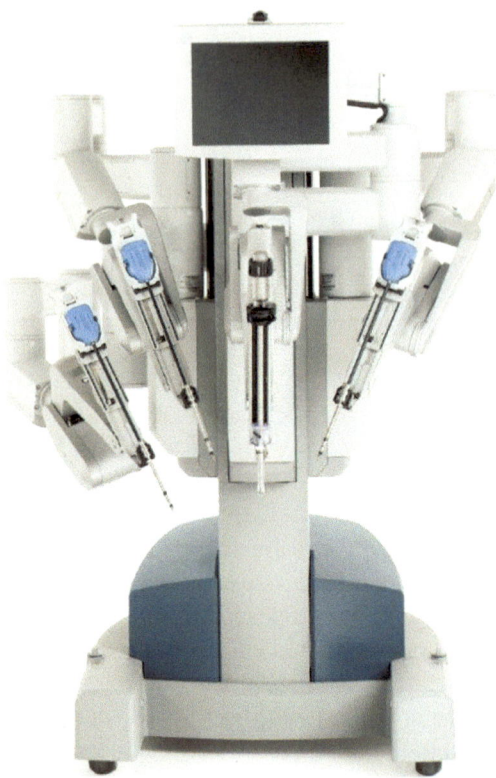

Fig. 1.1 S patient cart

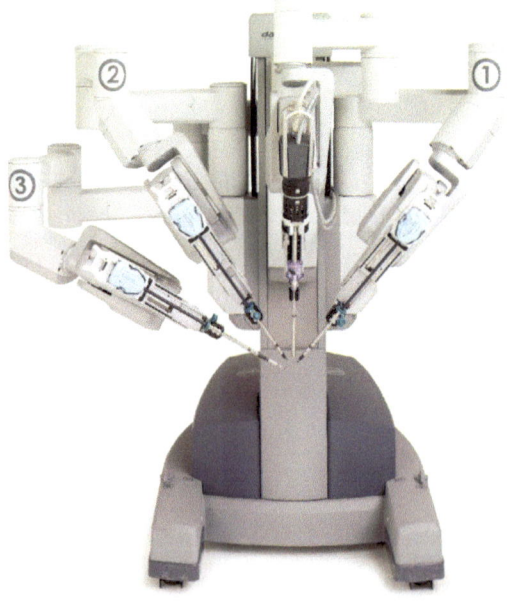

Fig. 1.2 Si patient cart

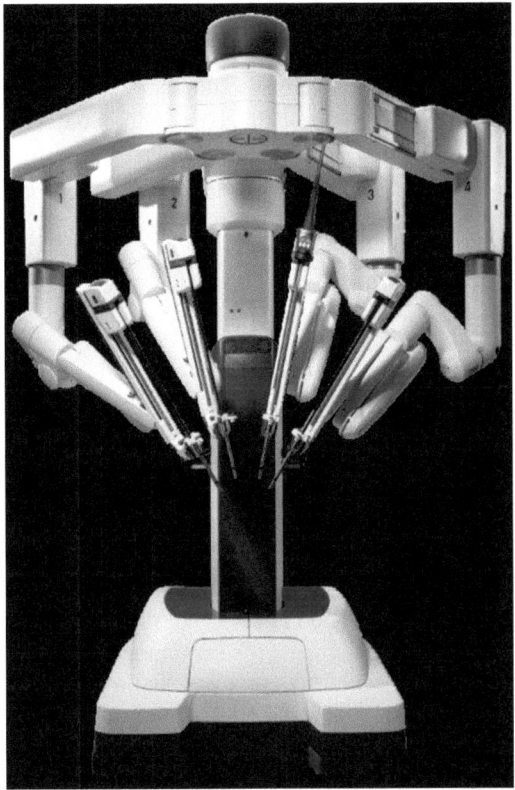

Fig. 1.3 Xi patient cart

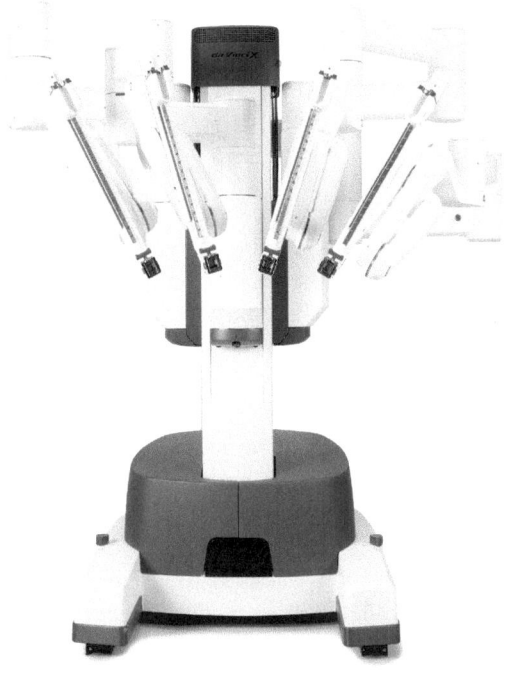

Fig. 1.4 X patient cart

men) no longer required the movement of entire robot as the boom could be rotated in position. Additionally, instruments and the camera could be interchanged between trocars, making multi-quadrant abdominal surgery much more feasible. This system has an available integrated operative table, TruSystem™ 7000dV (Trumpf Medezin Systeme, Saalfeld, Germany) that allows its motion to coincide with the robot via direct computer communication. This allows repositioning of the operating table while maintaining the anatomical orientation of the patient relative to the arms of the robot.

Just released in 2017 was the 5th generation of robot, the da Vinci X® (Fig. 1.4). This system mimics the da Vinci Xi® platform in many ways such as the thinner, enhanced arms, laser guidance, 3DHD vision, and the second surgeon console. There are a few sacrifices in the ease of deployment and docking but the goal is to create a price point for emerging markets. All of the above products have received the CE and FDA

510(k) clearances. However, the Standard and da Vinci S® systems are discontinued and are no longer supported by the company. All three of the currently supported products feature dual surgeon consoles, laser technology for fluorescent imaging, and single-site operative capability.

The robotic platform to perform surgery has been used in the urological and gynecological arenas for many years. The potential value of the robot-assisted repair was explored as early as 2003 [11]. In this porcine model it was shown that the intracorporeal suturing of a mesh to the posterior fascia was feasible. A small French study involving 11 patients was the first report of mesh fixation with suturing with the robot in humans [12]. It appeared that this method might not be associated with the chronic postoperative pain that is seen in the laparoscopic method. Another later study of 13 patients also showed that this was feasible with good results [13]. In that study, there was one recurrence, but no patient experienced chronic suture pain. In 2014, the FDA approved the repair of hernias using the ISI Si robot. Since then there has been tremendous growth in the utilization of the da Vinci systems for hernia repair. This is particularly evident in the repair of incisional and ventral hernias of all types due to the articulation of the wrists allowing easier intra-abdominal suturing than laparoscopic instrumentation.

Although not released at the time of this writing, the da Vinci SP® single-port system may be introduced after the publication of this textbook (Fig. 1.5). It will allow the introduction of articulated instruments and the camera through a single port that requires a diameter of approximately 2.5 cm. It cannot be known of this will be beneficial in the repair of incisional hernias at this time, but one could speculate that surgeons will endeavor to adapt these methods to benefit their patients.

The only other surgical robot approved for use in the United States is the Senhance™ system by TransEnterix, Inc. (Morrisville, NC, USA). Unlike the current generations of the ISI robots, this robot provides haptic feedback and eye tracking of the surgeon (Fig. 1.6). This allows the surgeon to move his or her eyes and the camera movements correspond to their movements. Additionally, it does not require the use of a specific optical system and each arm has a separate "cart" rather than all arms on one cart as does the da Vinci systems. It does not have the degrees of movement of the da Vinci systems and more mimics traditional laparoscopic instruments without a wrist.

Future Surgical Robotic Systems

Due to the very large market and potential for financial success, there are several other companies that are actively engaged in the development of newer systems that could allow repair of ventral (and other) hernias. It is not really known if all will be easily used for hernia repair. Each, it would seem, will seek to differentiate themselves in many different ways whether it be enhanced capabilities or pricing. Most likely, the next one to market will be the SPORT surgical system by Titan Medical, Inc. (Toronto, Canada) (Fig. 1.7). It is a single-port system with multi-articulating instruments. It is not currently available for sale.

Little is known about the other companies that are in various stages of development. Cambridge Medical Robotics, Ltd. (Cambridge, England) has a working prototype of the Versius (Fig. 1.8). Each arm of the robot has three joints similar to the human arm and is on individual carts that allow the position to be similar to a standard laparoscopic procedure.

Other companies that are known at the time of the writing of this chapter are listed in Table 1.1. It is unknown if any of these robots will allow use in the repair of hernias. The reader is referred to the Internet for future offerings from these companies.

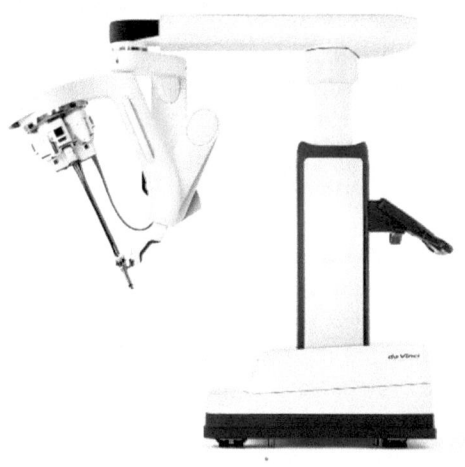

Fig. 1.5 SP patient cart (The da Vinci SP® is still in development, is not 510(k) cleared, and the safety and effectiveness of the product has not been established. The technology is not currently for sale in the US)

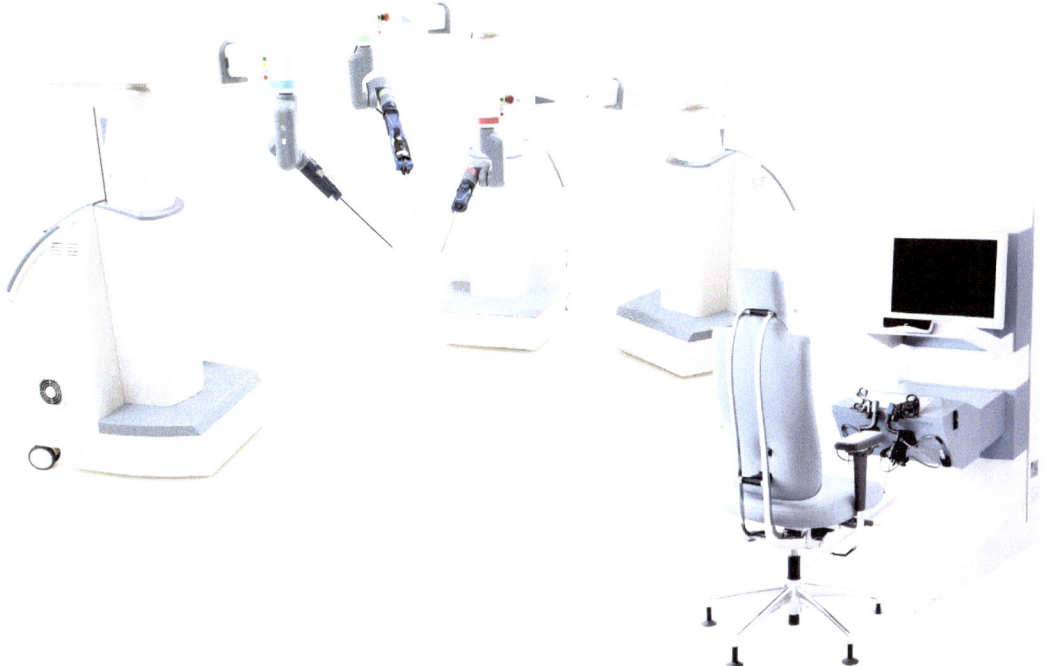

Fig. 1.6 Senhance system

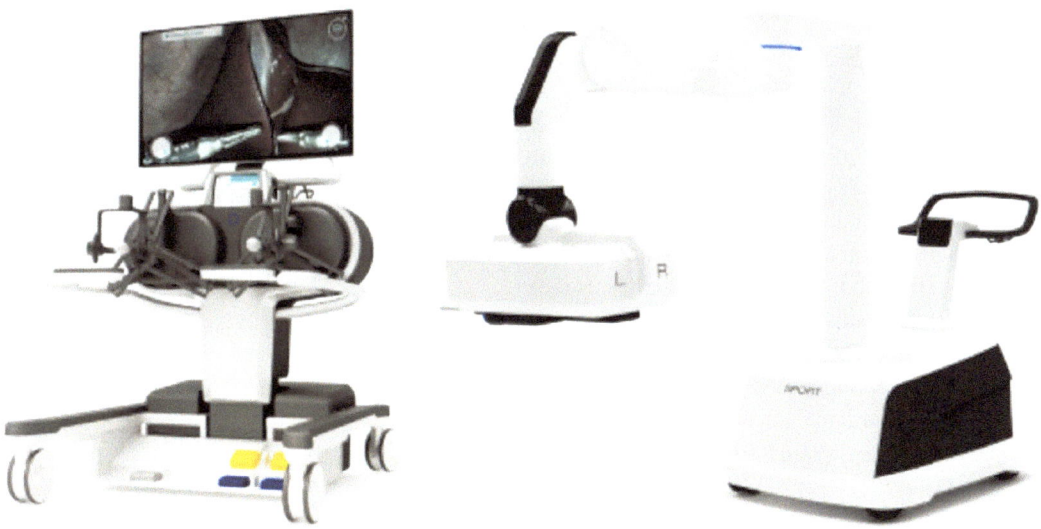

Fig. 1.7 Titan SPORT system

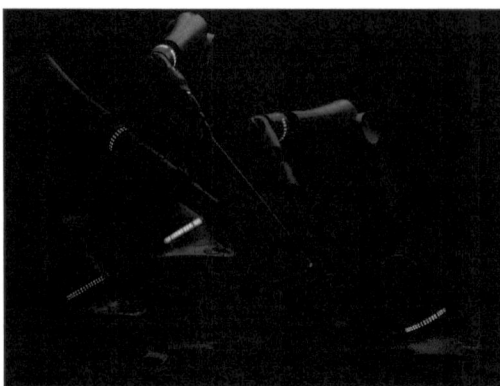

Fig. 1.8 Versius (this company-provided photo is intentionally dark)

Table 1.1 Known surgical robotic companies

Company	Location
Auris	San Carlos, CA, USA
Avatera Medical	Jena, Germany
Medtronic, Inc.	Minneapolis, MN, USA
Meere	South Korea
Micro Medical Instruments	Calci, Italy
Verb Surgical, Inc.	Mountain View, CA, USA

Conclusion

The laparoscopic approach to the repair of incisional and ventral hernias continues to be refined and improved. The continual development of newer mesh products indicates the response of industry to the ongoing needs of the surgeons and their patients. The introduction of the robot to repair these hernias is seen as another advancement. The current and future offerings in this technology appear to signal the continued adoption of this method of repair. Surgeons interested in the future of hernia surgery should follow these developments closely.

References

1. Rives JJ, Flament JB, Delattre JF, et al. La chirurgie moderne des hernies de l'aine. Cah Med. 1982;7:13.
2. Stoppa RE. The treatment of complicated groin and incisional hernias. World J Surg. 1989;13(5):545–54.
3. Ger R. The management of certain abdominal herniae by intra-abdominal closure of the neck of the sac. Ann R Coll Surg Engl. 1982;64:342–4.
4. LeBlanc KA, Booth WV. Laparoscopic repair of incisional abdominal hernias using expanded polytetrafluroethylene: preliminary findings. Surg Laparosc Endosc. 1993;3(1):39–41.
5. Itani KMF, Hur K, Kim LT, Anthony T, Berger DH, Reda D, Neumayer L, Veterans Affairs Ventral Incisional Hernia Investigators. Comparison of laparoscopic and open repair with mesh for the treatment of ventral incisional hernia: a randomized trial. Arch Surg. 2010;145(4):322–8.
6. Sauerland S, Walgenbach M, Habermalz B, et al. Laparoscopic versus open surgical techniques for ventral or incisional hernia repair. Cochrane Database Syst Rev. 2011;3:CD007781.
7. Zhang Y, Zhou H, Chai Y, al e. Laparoscopic versus open incisional and ventral hernia repair: a systematic review and meta-analysis. World J Surg. 2014;38(9):2233–40.
8. Al Chalabi H, Larkin J, Mehigan B, McCormick P. A systematic review of laparoscopic versus open abdominal incisional hernia repair with meta-analysis of randomized controlled trials. Int J Surg. 2015;20:65–74.
9. Arita NA, Nguyen MT, Nguyen DH, et al. Laparoscopic repair reduces incidence of surgical site infections for all ventral hernias. Surg Endosc. 2015;29(7):1769–80.
10. Savitch SL, Shah PC. Closing the gap between the laparoscopic and open approaches to abdominal wall hernia repair: a trend and outcomes analysis of the ACS-NSQIP database. Surg Endosc. 2016;30(8):3267–78.
11. Schluender S, Conrad J, Divino CM, Gurland B. Robot-assisted laparoscopic repair of ventral hernia with intracorporeal suturing. Surg Endosc. 2003;17(9):1391–5.
12. Tayar C, Karoui M, Cherqui D, Fagniez PL. Robot-assisted laparoscopic mesh repair of incisional hernias with exclusive inracorporeal suturing: a pilot study. Surg Endosc. 2007;21(10):1786–9.
13. Allison N, Tieu K, Snyder B, Pignazzi A, Wilson E. Technical feasibility of robot-assisted ventral hernia repair. World J Surg. 2012;36(2):447–52.

Deepa V. Cherla and Mike K. Liang

Introduction

Ventral incisional hernias are abdominal wall fascial defects secondary to incisions as opposed to primary ventral hernias that are congenital or spontaneous in etiology (e.g., umbilical hernia) [1]. Although much of the evidence behind the management of patients and treatment of these two diseases is similar, there are important differences. Most striking are the differences in surgical outcomes. For example, high-quality studies demonstrate the long-term hernia recurrence rate of ventral incisional hernias to be 30–70% while for primary ventral hernias to be 5–30% over the course of 5–10 years [2–5]. These differences in absolute risk affect decision-making by shifting the balance of risk and benefit. This chapter will focus on ventral incisional hernias and only briefly discuss the nuances of the care of patients with primary ventral hernias.

Patients with ventral incisional hernias often present with medical history and physical exam findings that affect surgical decision-making [6,

7]. Options for the patient and clinician include nonoperative management or surgical repair [6–12]. The choice of treatment can change over time as presentation and comorbidities evolve. Once the decision for surgical repair is made, the process of selecting open, laparoscopic, or robotic repair is affected by multiple factors including surgeon skill/experience, patient history, and hernia type [7].

Minimally invasive ventral hernia repair has been shown to decrease rates of surgical site infection and hospital length of stay compared to open repair; yet, less than one-third of all ventral hernia repairs are performed using a minimally invasive surgical technique [13–19]. Not all cases may be amenable to a minimally invasive approach and not all surgeons may feel comfortable performing a minimally invasive repair, particularly in complex settings. Some of the barriers to adoption of laparoscopic ventral hernia repair may be able to be overcome by utilizing a robotic platform. The robotic approach is increasingly being used for ventral hernia repair in the United States of America (USA) [20]. In 2014, 25% of USA hospitals had at least one robotic surgical platform and worldwide 570,000 robotic assisted surgical procedures were performed [21]. Much of this demand may be driven by industry, patients, and surgeons who may perceive robotic surgery to be associated with less pain, shorter hospital stays, and faster recovery [22, 23].

D. V. Cherla (✉)
Department of Surgery, University of Texas Health Science Center at Houston, Houston, TX, USA

Basking Ridge, NJ, USA

M. K. Liang
Department of Surgery, University of Texas Health Science Center at Houston, Houston, TX, USA
e-mail: mike.liang@uth.tmc.edu

© Springer International Publishing AG, part of Springer Nature 2018
K. A. LeBlanc (ed.), *Laparoscopic and Robotic Incisional Hernia Repair*,
https://doi.org/10.1007/978-3-319-90737-6_2

Patient Clinical History

A patient's clinical history is important in decision-making between the nonoperative and surgical treatment options for a ventral incisional hernia. Factors that affect the outcomes include not only surgical technique but also patient factors. Potentially modifiable patient risk factors associated with surgical complications include obesity, medical comorbidities, and smoking.

Obesity and Obesity-Related Comorbidities

Obesity and obesity-related comorbidities such as diabetes mellitus are an epidemic in the USA and other developed nations. Currently, it is estimated that two-thirds of adults in the USA are overweight (body mass index [BMI] ≥ 25 kg/m^2) or obese (BMI ≥ 30 kg/m^2) [24, 25]. The mean BMI of patients with ventral hernias typically hovers around 33 kg/m^2 [26–30]. In an analysis of the American College of Surgeons National Surgery Quality Improvement Project, 67% of patients undergoing laparoscopic ventral hernia repair were obese [26, 27]. Following ventral hernia repair, obese patients are at an increased risk of prolonged hospital length of stay, reoperation, hospital readmission, surgical site infection, and hernia recurrence [6, 7, 26–30]. While it is widely accepted that elective surgery in patients with BMI greater than or equal to 50 kg/m^2 is at prohibitive risk for hernia recurrence and complications, a growing body of evidence suggests that even among patients with a BMI of 40–50 kg/m^2, outcomes are poor, with high wound complications and hernia recurrence [6, 7, 31–33]. Some surgeons believe that elective ventral hernia repair should only routinely be undertaken among patients with BMI less than 40 kg/m^2 [6, 7]. Clearly, this is not always feasible but signifies the importance of obesity as a risk factor.

In addition, obesity is associated with related medical problems such as diabetes mellitus, which affect wound healing and increase the risk of wound complications. Outcomes of patients with well-controlled as opposed to poorly controlled diabetes are vastly different following abdominal surgery. These patients are at twofold increased odds (odds ratio [OR] 1.95–2.32, 95% confidence interval [CI] 1.11–4.82) of suffering from a major complication or infectious complications [6, 7, 34, 35]. Elective ventral hernia repair is not recommended in patients with a glycosylated hemoglobin (HbA1C) higher than 8.0%, and individualized preoperative interventions, including diet modification and glucose control plans are recommended for individuals with HbA1C between 6.5 and 8.0% [6, 7].

Among comorbid patients where it is safe to delay elective ventral hernia repair, preoperative medical interventions such as counseling, physical conditioning, and weight loss programs (prehabilitation) including surgical interventions such as weight loss surgery can be initially offered [36–38]. While no studies have evaluated this issue specifically in patients with ventral hernias, among patients with other surgical diseases, these programs have been shown to be effective in achieving weight loss [36–38]. It is unclear if the effectiveness of these programs to achieve weight loss and improve physical conditioning can be translated to patients with ventral hernias. Exercise and diet have potential unique challenges in patients with hernias related to underlying poor patient physical function and the risk of exercise exacerbating hernia-related symptoms and signs. Another option includes weight loss surgery, which is the only sustainable method for prolonged weight loss, but may not be appropriate for all patients [6, 7]. The safety and feasibility of weight loss surgery before or in conjunction with ventral hernia repair is unknown. Currently, ventral hernia repair among patients with BMI greater than 30 kg/m^2 should (ideally) not be recommended without individualized preoperative intervention (this may include counseling, diet, physical fitness programs, or weight loss procedure). There is an ongoing trial assessing the impact of a preoperative exercise and weight loss program on outcomes after VHR [39].

Once it has been decided that a comorbid patient will be scheduled for elective ventral hernia repair, the choice of surgical approach must be determined. Because of the increased risk of wound complications in comorbid patients, there has been great interest in the role of minimally invasive ventral hernia repair in this population. In studies of the National Surgical Quality Improvement Program [26, 27, 29] the effect of laparoscopy on reducing complications in ventral hernia repair was greater in obese patients than for nonobese patients. Furthermore, the hospital length of stay was significantly decreased in patients with a BMI greater than 30 kg/m². These benefits of minimally invasive surgery are also seen among patients with diabetes when evaluating national databases [40].

Minimally invasive repair of ventral hernias is feasible and often provides the best surgical option for diabetic or obese patients requiring surgery [13–16]. Scant published research exists concerning robotic incisional hernia repair in obese or diabetic individuals; however, surgeons report that the robotic platform may make the surgery technically and physically easier for the surgeon to perform [21–23].

Tobacco Use

Smoking affects ventral hernia outcomes through the development of lung disease, coughing, and its impact on wound healing. Current smokers have an increased risk for surgical site infections and hernia recurrence following ventral hernia repair, as supported by large database studies (Table 2.1) [41–46]. Subsequently, many hernia experts currently do not recommend elective ventral hernia repair for patients who are current smokers or who are utilizing tobacco products, such as chewing tobacco, cigars, and pipe-smokers [6, 7, 41–46]. Nicotine testing is reasonable to perform, but may be reserved for patients who report quitting smoking yet for whom physicians maintain high clinical suspicion of tobacco use [6, 7]. Patients should abstain from smoking for at least 1 month prior to elective repair, as randomized controlled trials have demonstrated that smoking cessation for 4 weeks or more prior to surgery improves outcomes (Table 2.1) [47–50].

Table 2.1 Smoking and surgery

Study	Year	Population	N	Primary outcome	OR (95% CI)
Large cohort studies and effect of smoking on outcomes of ventral hernia repair					
Danzig et al. [41]	2016	NSQIP	3730	Repeat VHR at 1 year	1.70 (1.08–2.70)
		VHR			
Kaoutzanis et al. [42]	2015	NSQIP	28,269	Wound infection	1.46 (1.13–1.88)
		VHR			
Fischer et al. [43]	2014	NSQIP	1974	Complications	1.41 (1.04–1.91)
		VHR with Panniculectomy			
Lovecchio et al. [44]	2013	NSQIP	17,211	Readmission	1.30 (1.05–1.62)
		VHR			
Swenson et al. [45]	2008	VHR with mesh	506	Mesh infection	2.18 (1.09–4.36)
Finan et al. [46]	2005	VHR	1505	SSI	2.46 (1.33–4.57)
Randomized controlled trials on effect of preoperative smoking cessation					
Thomsen et al. [47]	2010	Breast cancer	130	All complications	1.00 (0.75–1.33)
Lindstrom et al. [48]	2008	Inguinal hernia	117	All complications	0.51 (0.27–0.97)
		Umbilical hernia			
		Cholecystectomy			
		Joint prosthesis			
Sorensen et al. [49]	2007	Inguinal hernia	189	Wound infection	1.43 (0.51–5.03)
		Incisional hernia			
Moller et al. [50]	2002	Orthopedic	108	All complications	0.34 (0.19–0.64)

NSQIP national surgical quality improvement program, *VHR* ventral hernia repair, *SSI* surgical site infection, *OR* odds ratio

The magnitude of benefits seen with minimally invasive surgery in patients with comorbidities such as obesity and diabetes are not seen with smokers [51]. This is likely because many of the poor outcomes associated with smoking are not just related to wound healing but include respiratory complications such as pneumonia or higher rates of postoperative intubation [51]. Thus, even with the use of minimally invasive techniques, elective ventral hernia repair is not recommended in current smokers.

Surgical History

Adhesions can significantly affect the complexity of a ventral hernia repair and make a minimally invasive approach formidable. Patients with multiple prior open abdominal surgeries, prior lysis of adhesions for small bowel obstruction, prior mesh placement, or prior intra-abdominal inflammatory process (i.e., intestinal perforation or major abdominal trauma), may require an extensive lysis of adhesions during ventral hernia repair. This may or may not be feasible through a minimally invasive approach [13–16].

While a minimally invasive lysis of adhesions can be safely performed by experienced surgeons, the risk of enterotomy or missed enterotomy represents a high-stakes complication [13–16]. Recognizing when to convert to open prior to causing an enterotomy is crucial; this threshold depends on individual surgeon skill and judgment to optimize the proportion of cases that can be safely performed with a minimally invasive technique while avoiding missed enterotomies. Inexperienced surgeons have reported extremely high rates of missed and recognized bowel injuries [52–54]. Patients who suffer an enterotomy during laparoscopic ventral hernia repair are four times as likely to suffer complications, including mesh infection and enterocutaneous fistula [55–58]. Even if the enterotomy can be repaired with minimally invasive techniques, synthetic mesh placed in the intraperitoneal space is at increased risk of mesh infection and complications. Thus, these patients may need to be converted to open (increased risk for wound

complication), have a repair with utilizing a highly infection resilient mesh (biologic or bioprosthetic), or perform an even more complex repair with preperitoneal or retromuscular mesh placement (see section below on contamination [55–58].

Among the most serious complication for ventral hernia repair is a missed enterotomy [55–58]. Intestinal injuries can occur either as an unrecognized full thickness bowel injury or a partial thickness injury such as a thermal injury that then evolves into a full thickness injury. Patients may present with fever, leukocytosis, tachycardia, or even sepsis due to substantial intra-abdominal contamination. In this setting the repair should be considered "failed" and any intraperitoneal synthetic mesh needs to be removed. These patients are at increased risk of major complications including enterocutaneous fistula and death [55–58].

High-quality data on the safety, efficacy, and effectiveness of robotic surgery with lysis of adhesions do not exist. Some surgeons contend that robotics facilitates technically superior adhesiolysis to laparoscopic approaches through wristed instruments, three-dimensional video imaging systems that provide improved views of complex anatomical relationships, and improved instrument manipulation and ergonomics [59–61]. The robotic platform may allow surgeons to perform a minimally invasive, complex lysis of adhesions that otherwise be more difficult using a pure laparoscopic approach. However, other surgeons argue that the robot remains limited for complex lysis of adhesions. For example, if extensive adhesions exist throughout the abdomen, some surgeons recommend that adhesiolysis be performed laparoscopically prior to docking the robot since the robotic platform is better suited for working in a targeted area not involving more than two abdominal quadrants [22, 59–61]. Some of these limitations are lessened with the newest generation of robotic platforms that allows for true multi-quadrant surgery [22, 59–61]. A multi-institutional retrospective review of 368 patients showed that surgeons performing a ventral or incisional robotic hernia repair converted to open in only 0.8% of cases, most frequently due to dense adhesions [62]. Rates of conversion for laparoscopic to open incisional hernia repair, in contrast, range from 0 to 12% [13–16].

While minimally invasive ventral hernia repair has substantially improved short-term outcomes compared to open surgery, surgeons should use their best judgment based upon their skill and experience as to when to utilize minimally invasive approaches and when convert to open to minimize the risk of enterotomy and missed enterotomy. A robotic platform may have a role for some surgeons to perform a minimally invasive lysis of adhesions in a safer fashion in select patients.

Hernia Characteristics

Important hernia-related considerations that affect the decision between robotic, laparoscopic, and open ventral hernia repair include the hernia size and the ability to achieve primary fascial closure, hernia location, and the presence of contamination. In addition, the nuances of treating primary ventral hernias as opposed to ventral incisional hernia will be reviewed.

Defect Size

The European Hernia Society has defined ventral incisional hernias as small (<4 cm in width), medium (4–10 cm in width), and large (>10 cm width) [1]. An additional category regardless of defect size is loss of domain where substantial intra-abdominal contents chronically reside outside of the abdominal domain. In general, minimally invasive surgery is suggested for small- and medium-sized hernias; laparoscopy can be challenging for large hernias and hernias with loss of domain [63]. One of the main reasons that minimally invasive surgery is challenging for large hernia defects is because of the growing interest on the benefits of primary fascial closure.

The role of primary fascial closure during minimally invasive hernia repair continues to be debated, as no high-quality, conclusive evidence currently exists that support this technique [64–67]. Proponents argue that fascial defect closure may be associated with fewer postoperative seromas and decreased long-term hernia recurrence as well as a lower risk of mesh eventration [66, 67]. A 2014 systematic review of 11 studies examining primary fascial closure with laparoscopic ventral hernia repair concluded that while only poor-quality data currently exists, primary fascial closure compared to non-closure resulted in lower recurrence rates (0–5.7 vs. 4.8–16.7%) and seroma formation (5.6–11.4 vs. 4.3–27.8%) rates over a follow-up period of 1–108 months [67]. In addition, patients reported improve patient centered outcomes including satisfaction with abdominal wall cosmesis and satisfaction. Currently, multiple randomized controlled trials are ongoing [68].

Defects between 6 and 10 cm in width may be challenging for surgeons to close with a minimally invasive technique [66, 67]. Compared to standard laparoscopic approach, the robotic platform may facilitate the intracorporeal suturing needed for fascial closure by allowing for ergonomic movements, seven degrees of motion, three-dimensional imaging, and dexterous wristed instrumentation [22, 59–61]. This theory is supported by the increased frequency of fascial closure in robotic intraperitoneal mesh placements and robotic retromuscular ventral hernia repairs [69, 70].

For large defects, myofascial release (component separation) may be needed to achieve fascial closure. While endoscopic component separation has been described and is feasible with laparoscopic surgery, the amount of release may be limited and associated with increased wound complications [71]. Among experts, endoscopic component separation is used sparingly due to the limited release and high seroma rates [6, 71]. The robotic platform has brought about an interest in performing minimally invasive retromuscular repairs and posterior component separation. Robotic posterior component separation has been shown to be feasible and efficacious when performed by experts. Short-term outcomes demonstrate similar outcomes compared to open with shorter hospital length of stay [72, 73]. However, existing studies are at high risk for bias and these conclusions can only be considered hypothesis generating. In addition, skeptics cite persistent concerns regarding value (cost/quality), missed enterotomy (which appears to be more common with robotic cases as compared to open procedures), and an overuse of component separation to achieve primary fascial closure. Both efficacy and effectiveness randomized controlled trials are needed.

Location

Lateral, suprapubic, subxiphoid, and subcostal ventral hernias typically are more challenging due to adjacent structures (e.g., bone, bladder, diaphragm, nerves) and the need for more complex dissection. Robotic ventral hernia repair may provide improved visualization for dissection and mesh fixation. Some authors have commented on being able to take precise bites of tissue to better anchor the mesh on or near lateral abdominal borders more easily with the robot. Mesh fixation with tacks, which is typically utilized during standard laparoscopic ventral hernia repair, can be challenging in these locations and risk injuring vital structures [7]. Alternatively, skeptics argue that surgeons may experience decreased haptic and tactile feedback with the robot that makes hernia repair in these locations more challenging [20–23]. Because these ventral hernias are uncommon, it is unlikely that any adequately powered, randomized controlled trials will be completed to compare robotic repair as opposed to open or laparoscopic repair of ventral hernias in these locations. Insight for these relatively uncommon hernias will likely need to be sought through examination of large databases or registries.

Contaminated Ventral Hernia Repairs

Contaminated cases include those falling within Wound Class II (clean contaminated; the respiratory, gastrointestinal, genital, or urinary tract is entered under controlled conditions), Wound

Class III (contaminated; the case involves gross spillage from the gastrointestinal tract or nonpurulent inflammation), or Wound Class IV (dirty or infected; infection is present in the initial operative field) [6, 7]. Higher wound classes are associated with increased surgical site infection rates, which in turn are associated with increased rates of hernia recurrence and reoperation [7, 74]. Much of the literature on contaminated cases has focused on mesh type and placement rather than surgical platform.

In contaminated ventral hernia repair, the desire to minimize recurrence through prosthetic mesh reinforcement must be balanced against potential infectious complications, reoperations, and possible need for mesh explanation. Choices include suture only repair, placement of mesh that is more resistant to bacterial contamination, staged repair, or leaving a planned ventral hernia and performing an elective repair in the future [6, 7]. Mesh reinforcement decreases hernia recurrence rates but the evidence supporting mesh use is derived from uncomplicated, elective ventral hernias with no contamination [5, 6]. In a study on of the National Surgical Quality Improvement Project, 33,832 cases of ventral hernia repair demonstrated that mesh reinforcement of contaminated ventral hernia repairs compared to suture repair substantially increases rates of surgical site infection and 30-day complications [75].

If mesh is utilized in a contaminated field, it may also be placed in one of several locations but there is also little data on the safety of each location [5]. It is widely believed that intraperitoneal mesh placement of synthetic mesh in the intraperitoneal (underlay) position is unsafe [76]. Alternatively, mesh placement in the retrorectus (sublay) or onlay position may be safer. The findings of a review of 1200 patients at seven academic centers involved with the Ventral Hernia Outcomes Collaborative undergoing Wound Class II-IV ventral hernia repair are summarized in Table 2.2 [7]. Most of these cases were open procedures as few laparoscopic procedures were performed in contaminated setting.

In standard laparoscopic ventral hernia repair where synthetic mesh is placed in the intraperito-

Table 2.2   Ventral hernia outcomes collaborative outcomes of mesh type and mesh location

		Wound class			Mesh location	
		II	III	IV	Sublay	Underlay
Suture (n = 136)	N	1	1	3		
	Width (cm)	2.3 ± 0.6	–	–		
	SSI (%)	1 (100%)	1 (100%)	0		
	Deep SSI (%)	0	0	0		
	Recurrence (%)	1 (100%)	0	0		
Synthetic[a] (n = 747)	N	107	5	1	131	578
	Width (cm)	3.9 ± 3.6	14.6 ± 9.0	8.0 ± 0	4.1 ± 4.8	5.1 ± 4.2
	SSI (%)	15 (14.0%)	2 (40.0%)	0	22 (16.8%)	89 (15.4%)
	Deep SSI (%)	7 (6.5%)	1 (20.0%)	0	6 (4.6%)	39 (6.7%)
	Recurrence (%)	15 (14.0%)	2 (40.0%)	0	10 (7.6%)	83 (14.4%)
Biologic (n = 336)	N	51	43	23	49	257
	Width (cm)	8.9 ± 5.4	10.0 ± 6.2	11.3 ± 5.8	12.3 ± 6.0	9.6 ± 5.6
	SSI (%)	7 (13.7%)	5 (11.6%)	4 (17.4%)	8 (16.3%)	33 (12.8%)
	Deep SSI (%)	5 (8.9%)	2 (4.7%)	2 (8.7%)	3 (6.1%)	12 (4.7%)
	Recurrence (%)	7 (13.7%)	10 (23.3%)	0	5 (10.2%)	46 (17.9%)

[a]Light- or mid-density (weight) mesh

neal (underlay) position, the risk of surgical site infection, in particular mesh infection, is high [76]. While small series have reported the efficacy laparoscopic repair clean-contaminated cases, these remain extremely small series in carefully selected patients with minimal contamination (e.g., tubal ligation or laparoscopic cholecystectomy for biliary colic with no spillage). The safety and effectiveness of routinely placing intraperitoneal synthetic mesh in patients with wound class II or higher is not supported by large nationwide database studies [76].

This leaves the minimally invasive surgeon a few options other than conversion to open: (1) laparoscopically suture the defect closed alone, (2) place a biologic mesh laparoscopically, or (3) place mesh in a location other than intraperitoneal/underlay (e.g., preperitoneal or retromuscular, sublay). While suture repair may be an acceptable therapy for primary ventral hernias in contaminated setting due to the lower absolute risk of hernia recurrence, it has an unacceptably high recurrence rate, even for small defects, for ventral incisional hernia repairs [2–5]. Alternatively, laparoscopic intraperitoneal mesh repair with a biologic mesh has been reported and is feasible. However, there are technical challenges associated with this practice and no high-quality data that exists to support the use of nonsynthetic mesh including biologic, biosynthetic, or bioabsorbable [77–79]. Technical challenges with nonsynthetic meshes include the risk of eventration with a bridged repair (i.e., need for primary fascial closure), challenges in fixation, and mesh selection given the wide variety and array of choices. Finally, placing a mesh in a sublay position (preperitoneal or retromuscular) may protect the mesh from intra-abdominal contamination. While this has been reported, it has substantial technical challenges, has unclear generalizability, and has not undergone the rigors of a randomized controlled trial [80–82].

Little literature has examined robotic hernia repair of contaminated cases. However, many of the technical challenges to performing a minimally invasive ventral hernia repair in the face of contamination may be simplified using the robotic platform. Primary fascial closure and mesh fixation of biologic mesh can be easier using the robotic platform [69, 70, 83]. In addition, sublay mesh repair seems to be more feasible with robotic platform as compared to laparoscopic approach [72, 73, 84]. However, these studies report on the results of high volume hernia experts with advanced minimally invasive skills. Safety, efficacy, and effectiveness of these approaches still require assessment through rigorously performed randomized controlled trials.

Primary Ventral Hernias

Primary ventral hernias are hernias that arise spontaneously on the abdominal wall and are not associated with any incision (e.g., umbilical hernia, epigastric hernia, Spigelian hernia, lumbar hernia) [1]. These hernias have substantially different outcomes, such as surgical site infection and hernia recurrence, when compared to ventral incisional hernias [5, 14]. While many treatments have similar reductions in relative risk, the differences in absolute risk reduction affect the nuances of treatment [2–5]. For example, mesh repair as opposed to suture repair has a similar relative risk reduction in hernia recurrence with primary ventral hernias and ventral incisional hernias (relative risk reduction of two- to threefold). However, the absolute risk reduction is substantially different (8% vs. 20% at 2–3 years postoperative). Because of this, while suture repair may be acceptable in certain settings with primary ventral hernias, suture repair of ventral incisional hernias should be avoided whenever possible. In a real-world example, while performing a laparoscopic cholecystectomy, a primary ventral hernia in a low-risk patient may be effectively treated with suture repair (11% recurrence at 2 years); however, a sutured ventral incisional hernia would not yield acceptable results (43% recurrence at 3 years) [2–5].

This similar risk/benefit consideration should be utilized when assessing minimally invasive surgery in primary ventral hernia. While laparoscopic surgery has a similar relative risk reduction of surgical site infection (two- to fourfold) the absolute risk reduction is highly variable [14]. Thus, a low-risk patient undergoing primary ventral hernia repair has a similar risk of surgical site infection with laparoscopic (<0.5%) vs. open (1%). This is quite different from the high-risk patient undergoing ventral incisional hernia repair that has a risk with laparoscopic of 1–5% but 20% with the open technique. In addition, many technical factors may affect the decision-making between minimally invasive repairs versus open repairs in patients with primary ventral hernias. Patients with multiple defects (umbilical and epigastric hernia), lateral defect (Spigelian or lumbar hernia), or concomitant diastasis recti may be easier to repair with a minimally invasive approach. We recommend minimally invasive ventral hernia repair in high-risk patients with a primary ventral hernia (overweight/obese, diabetes mellitus, smoker within the past year, chronic obstructive pulmonary disease, immunosuppression), multiple defects, lateral defects, and patients with diastasis recti [6, 7, 85].

The technical aspects of minimally invasive primary ventral hernia repair are also different from ventral incisional hernia repair. With primary ventral hernias, many predominantly contain preperitoneal fat and the hernia sac (peritoneum) which are easily separable from the other layers of the abdominal wall [85, 86]. If this tissue is not removed, patients often complain of a persistent bulge/mass and imaging will demonstrate tissue eventration (entrapment of preperitoneal fat and hernia sac). Because of this, we recommend that the hernia sac and preperitoneal fat be meticulously excised with all laparoscopic primary ventral hernia repairs. The role of primary fascial closure in primary ventral hernias may be substantially different as compared to ventral incisional hernias [87]. This effect is most likely due to hernia defect size rather than hernia type: the vast majority of primary ventral hernias are small (<2 cm fascial defect) as opposed to ventral incisional hernias which are commonly larger. Fascial closure may have a more substantial impact with a larger defect as opposed to smaller defects. The mesh is more likely to bulge or protrude (mesh eventration) through a large defect as opposed to a small defect [88]. We routinely close all fascial defects larger than 3 cm in width and bridge most defects smaller than 3 cm in width [7]. Most primary ventral hernias that we encounter have a fascial defect of less than 3 cm in width.

Existing Evidence Comparing Surgical Platforms

Open Versus Laparoscopic Incisional Hernia Repair

There is extensive, high-quality scientific literature evaluating open versus laparoscopic incisional hernia repair. Most meta-analyses and systematic reviews demonstrate that laparoscopic ventral hernia repair is associated with a decreased risk of surgical site infection but not wound complications (e.g., including seromas, hematomas) with no difference in risk of hernia recurrence [13–16]. A recent network meta-analysis of 19 randomized controlled trials demonstrated that laparoscopic repair had the lowest probability of being associated with a surgical site infection as compared to open mesh procedure, while no substantial difference existed in the risk of hernia recurrence comparing laparoscopic to open mesh repairs of ventral hernias [5]. Other meta-analyses have similar findings with decreased surgical site infection but no difference in hernia recurrence [13–16]. Some studies have demonstrated that although laparoscopic surgery is associated with a shorter hospital length of stay, the risk of bowel injury is higher compared to open ventral hernia repair (relative risk, 3.68; 95% CI, 1.56–8.67). Nationwide databases have validated the results of randomized controlled trials demonstrating that laparoscopy is associated with fewer early postoperative complications and shorter hospital length of stay [17, 89].

Open Versus Robotic Hernia Repair

Two published studies compare open and robotic ventral hernia repairs [72, 73]. Both studies are cohort studies at high risk for bias and the authors of both studies have significant financial conflicts of interest with industry. Robotic repair, in both studies, was associated with shorter hospital length of stay; however, the two articles differed in impact of surgical platform on the rate of surgical site occurrence and major complications.

These studies represent preliminary results of a limited number of highly specialized robotic hernia surgeons. Efficacy and effectiveness randomized controlled trials are needed to assess the true impact of robotic platform in the repair of complex ventral hernias. Currently, two randomized controlled trial are listed in clinicaltrials.gov to compare laparoscopic and robotic ventral hernia repair [90].

Laparoscopic Versus Robotic Incisional Hernia Repair

Four published studies compare laparoscopic and robotic ventral hernia repairs [69, 70, 83, 84]. All four studies are cohort studies at high risk for bias and the authors of all four of the studies have significant financial conflicts of interest with industry. Robotic repair was associated with clinical benefits in all four studies but differed in which outcomes were improved including ability to close the fascial defect, surgical site occurrence, and shorter length of stay. Three of the four studies demonstrated robotic ventral hernia repair was associated with increased hospital length of stay while the only study to assess cost demonstrates robotic repair was associated with higher costs.

These studies represent preliminary results of a limited number of highly specialized robotic hernia surgeons. Efficacy and effectiveness randomized controlled trials are needed to assess the true impact of robotic platform in the repair of complex ventral hernias. Currently, a single randomized controlled trial is listed in clinicaltrials. gov to compare open and robotic ventral hernia repair [91].

Conclusions

There is an intimate relationship between medical comorbidities such as obesity or diabetes and ventral incisional hernia. These diseases not only increase the risk of developing a ventral incisional hernia but also increase the risk of complications following repair of ventral incisional hernia. Minimally invasive surgical techniques have been demonstrated to decrease the risk of short-term surgical complications with similar long-term outcomes following ventral hernia repair with the greatest benefit in the comorbid patient. Despite this, adoption of laparoscopic ventral hernia repair remains limited. Barriers to adoption of minimally invasive techniques may be related to technical challenges of performing a complex procedure in a complex setting. The robotic platform may be able to overcome many of these challenges and "level" the playing field for even the most experienced surgeon when performing a minimally invasive hernia repair. High-quality studies (e.g., multi-surgeon/center randomized trials) comparing robotic ventral hernia repair to laparoscopic or open ventral hernia repair are needed to validate this assumption. The role of robotics in ventral hernia repair remains to be elucidated, but currently robotics may have the greatest role for surgeons who desire to perform minimally invasive retromuscular mesh repairs.

In addition, not all patients and hernias are suitable for ventral hernia repair, even a minimally invasive repair. Many patients can benefit from preoperative weight loss, glucose control, and smoking cessation prior to surgical intervention. Patient selection and preoperative optimization is key to a successful hernia practice in combination with evidence based surgical technique including minimally invasive surgery.

References

1. Muysoms FE, Miserez M, Berrevoet F, et al. Classification of primary and incisional abdominal wall hernias. Hernia. 2009;13(4):407–14.
2. Luijendijk RW, Hop WC, van den Tol MP, et al. A comparison of suture repair with mesh repair for incisional hernia. N Engl J Med. 2000;343(6):392–8.
3. Burger JW, Luijendijk RW, WCJ H, et al. Long-term follow-up of a randomized controlled trial of suture versus mesh repair of incisional hernia. Ann Surg. 2004;240(4):578–83; discussion 583–5
4. Mesh Versus Suture Repair for Umbilical Hernias (HUMP). Clinicaltrials.gov. NCT00789230. Accessed on July 29, 2017. Presented at the Americas Hernia Society Meeting, Washington, DC, 2016.
5. Holihan JL, Hannon C, Goodenough C, et al. Ventral hernia repair: a meta-analysis of randomized controlled trials. Surg Infect. 2017;18(6):647–58.
6. Liang MK, Holihan JL, Itani K, et al. Ventral hernia management: expert consensus guided by systematic review. Ann Surg. 2017;265(1):80–9.
7. Holihan JL, Alawadi ZM, Harris JW, et al. Ventral hernia: patient selection, treatment, and management. Curr Probl Surg. 2016;53(7):307–54.
8. Holihan JL, Flores-Gonzalez JR, Mo J, et al. A prospective assessment of clinical and patient-reported outcomes of initial non-operative management of ventral hernias. World J Surg. 2017;41(5):1267–73.
9. Kokotovic D, Sjølander H, Gögenur I, et al. Watchful waiting as a treatment strategy for patients with a ventral hernia appears to be safe. Hernia. 2016;20(2):281–7.
10. Verhelst J, Timmermans L, van de Velde M, et al. Watchful waiting in incisional hernia: is it safe? Surgery. 2015;157(2):297–303.
11. Bellows CF, Robinson C, Fitzgibbons RJ, et al. Watchful waiting for ventral hernias: a longitudinal study. Am Surg. 2014;80(3):245–52.
12. Holihan JL, Henchcliffe BE, Mo J, et al. Is non-operative management warranted in ventral hernia patients with comorbidities?: a case-matched, prospective, patient-centered study. Ann Surg. 2016;264(4):585–90.
13. Al Chalabi H, Larkin J, Mehigan B, McCormick P. A systematic review of laparoscopic versus open abdominal incisional hernia repair, with meta-analysis of randomized controlled trials. Int J Surg. 2015;20:65–74.
14. Arita NA, Nguyen MT, Nguyen DH, et al. Laparoscopic repair reduces incidence of surgical site infections for all ventral hernias. Surg Endosc. 2015;29(7):1769–80.
15. Zhang Y, Zhou H, Chai Y, al e. Laparoscopic versus open incisional and ventral hernia repair: a systematic review and meta-analysis. World J Surg. 2014;38(9):2233–40.
16. Sauerland S, Walgenbach M, Habermalz B, et al. Laparoscopic versus open surgical techniques for ventral or incisional hernia repair. Cochrane Database Syst Rev. 2011;3:CD007781.
17. Savitch SL, Shah PC. Closing the gap between the laparoscopic and open approaches to abdominal wall hernia repair: a trend and outcomes analysis of the ACS-NSQIP database. Surg Endosc. 2016;30(8):3267–78.
18. Aher CV, Kubasiak JC, Daly SC, et al. The utilization of laparoscopy in ventral hernia repair: an update of outcomes analysis using ACS-NSQIP data. Surg Endosc. 2015;29(5):1099–104.
19. Funk LM, Perry KA, Narula VK, et al. Current national practice patterns for inpatient management of ventral abdominal wall hernia in the United States. Surg Endosc. 2013;27(11):4104–12.
20. Stoikes N, Webb D, Voeller G. Robotic hernia repair. Surg Technol Int. 2016;XXIX:119–22.
21. Robotic Surgery. ECRI Institute. 2015. https://www.ecri.org. Accessed 29 July 2017.
22. Ahmad A, Ahmad ZF, Carleton JD, et al. Robotic surgery: current perceptions and the clinical evidence. Surg Endosc. 2017;31(1):255–63.
23. Boys JA, Alicuben ET, DeMeester MJ, et al. Public perceptions on robotic surgery, hospitals with robots, and surgeons that use them. Surg Endosc. 2016;30(4):1310–6.
24. National Institute of Diabetes and Digestive and Kidney Diseases. Overweight and obesity statistics. https://www.niddk.nih.gov/health-information/health-statistics/overweight-obesity. Accessed 29 July 2017.

25. Centers for Disease Control and Prevention. Obesity and overweight. https://www.cdc.gov/nchs/fastats/obesity-overweight.htm. Accessed 29 July 2017.

26. Regner JL, Mrdutt MM, Munoz-Maldonado Y. Tailoring surgical approach for elective ventral hernia repair based on obesity and National Surgical Quality Improvement Program outcomes. Am J Surg. 2015;210(6):1024–9; discussion 1029–30

27. Fekkes JF, Velanovich V. Amelioration of the effects of obesity on short-term postoperative complications of laparoscopic and open ventral hernia repair. Surg Laparosc Endosc Percutan Tech. 2015;25(2):151–7.

28. Fischer JP, Wink JD, Nelson JA, et al. Among 1,706 cases of abdominal wall reconstruction, what factors influence the occurrence of major operative complications? Surgery. 2014;155(2):311–9.

29. Lee J, Mabardy A, Kermani R, et al. Laparoscopic vs open ventral hernia repair in the era of obesity. JAMA Surg. 2013;148(8):723–6.

30. Novitsky YW, Orenstein SB. Effect of patient and hospital characteristics on outcomes of elective ventral hernia repair in the United States. Hernia. 2013;17(5):639–45.

31. Pernar LI, Pernar CH, Dieffenbach BV, Brooks DC, Smink DS, Tavakkoli A. What is the BMI threshold for open ventral hernia repair? Surg Endosc. 2017;31(3):1311–7.

32. Liang MK, Goodenough CJ, Martindale RG, et al. External validation of the ventral hernia risk score for prediction of surgical site infections. Surg Infect. 2015;16(1):36–40.

33. Berger RL, Li LT, Hicks SC, et al. Development and validation of a risk-stratification score for surgical site occurrence and surgical site infection after open ventral hernia repair. J Am Coll Surg. 2013;217(6):974–82.

34. Goodenough CJ, Liang MK, Nguyen MT, et al. Preoperative glycosylated hemoglobin and postoperative glucose together predict major complications after abdominal surgery. J Am Coll Surg. 2015;221(4):854–61.

35. Dronge AS, Perkal MF, Kancir S, et al. Long-term glycemic control and postoperative infectious complications. Arch Surg. 2006;141(4):375–80. discussion 380

36. van Rooijen SJ, Engelen MA, Scheede-Bergdahl C, et al. Systematic review of exercise training in colorectal cancer patients during treatment. Scand J Med Sci Sports. 2018;28(2):360–70.

37. Looijaard SM, Slee-Valentijn MS, Otten RH, et al. Physical and nutritional prehabilitation in older patients with colorectal carcinoma: a systematic review. J Geriatr Phys Ther. 2017. https://doi.org/10.1519/JPT.0000000000000125. [Epub ahead of print].

38. Moran J, Guinan E, McCormick P, et al. The ability of prehabilitation to influence postoperative outcome after intra-abdominal operation: a systematic review and meta-analysis. Surgery. 2016;160(5):1189–201.

39. Clinicaltrials.gov. Modifying Risk in Ventral Hernia Patients. Identifier NCT02365194. https://clinicaltrials.gov/ct2/show/NCT02365194. Accessed 29 July 2017.

40. Huntington C, Gamble J, Blair L, et al. Quantification of the effect of diabetes mellitus on ventral hernia repair: results from two national registries. Am Surg. 2016;82(8):661–71.

41. Danzig MR, Stey AM, Yin SS, et al. Patient profiles and outcomes following repair of irreducible and reducible ventral wall hernias. Hernia. 2016;20(2):239–47.

42. Kaoutzanis C, Leichtle SW, Mouawad NJ, et al. Risk factors for postoperative wound infections and prolonged hospitalization after ventral/incisional hernia repair. Hernia. 2015;19(1):113–23.

43. Fischer JP, Basta MN, Wink JD, et al. Optimizing patient selection in ventral hernia repair with concurrent panniculectomy: an analysis of 1974 patients from the ACS-NSQIP datasets. J Plast Reconstr Aesthet Surg. 2014;67(11):1532–40.

44. Lovecchio F, Farmer R, Souza J, et al. Risk factors for 30-day readmission in patients undergoing ventral hernia repair. Surgery. 2014;155(4):702–10.

45. Swenson BR, Camp TR, Mulloy DP, et al. Antimicrobial-impregnated surgical incise drapes in the prevention of mesh infection after ventral hernia repair. Surg Infect. 2008;9(1):23–32.

46. Finan KR, Vick CC, Kiefe CI, et al. Predictors of wound infection in ventral hernia repair. Am J Surg. 2005;190(5):676–81.

47. Thomsen T, Tønnesen H, Okholm M, Kroman N, Maibom A, Sauerberg ML, Møller AM. Brief smoking cessation intervention in relation to breast cancer surgery: a randomized controlled trial. Nicotine Tob Res. 2010;12(11):1118–24.

48. Lindström D, Sadr Azodi O, Wladis A, et al. Effects of a perioperative smoking cessation intervention on postoperative complications: a randomized trial. Ann Surg. 2008;248(5):739–45.

49. Sørensen LT, Hemmingsen U, Jørgensen T. Strategies of smoking cessation intervention before hernia surgery—effect on perioperative smoking behavior. Hernia. 2007;11(4):327–33.

50. Møller AM, Villebro N, Pedersen T, et al. Effect of preoperative smoking intervention on postoperative complications: a randomised clinical trial. Lancet. 2002;359(9301):114–7.

51. Kubasiak JC, Landin M, Schimpke S, et al. The effect of tobacco use on outcomes of laparoscopic and open ventral hernia repairs: a review of the NSQIP dataset. Surg Endosc. 2017;31(6):2661–6.

52. Ahonen-Siirtola M, Rautio T, Biancari F, et al. Laparoscopic versus hybrid approach for treatment of incisional ventral hernia. Dig Surg. 2017;34(6):502–6.

53. ten Broek RP, Schreinemacher MH, Jilesen AP, et al. Enterotomy risk in abdominal wall repair: a prospective study. Ann Surg. 2012;256(2):280–7.

54. Salameh JR, Sweeney JF, Graviss EA, et al. Laparoscopic ventral hernia repair during the learning curve. Hernia. 2002;6(4):182–7.

55. Sharma A, Khullar R, Soni V, et al. Iatrogenic enterotomy in laparoscopic ventral/incisional hernia

repair: a single center experience of 2,346 patients over 17 years. Hernia. 2013;17(5):581–7.

56. Tintinu AJ, Asonganyi W, Turner PL. Staged laparoscopic ventral and incisional hernia repair when faced with enterotomy or suspicion of an enterotomy. J Natl Med Assoc. 2012;104(3–4):202–10.

57. LeBlanc KA, Elieson MJ, Corder JM III. Enterotomy and mortality rates of laparoscopic incisional and ventral hernia repair: a review of the literature. JSLS. 2007;11(4):408–14.

58. LeBlanc KA. Laparoscopic incisional and ventral hernia repair: complications-how to avoid and handle. Hernia. 2004;8(4):323–31.

59. Allison N, Tieu K, Snyder B, et al. Technical feasibility of robot-assisted ventral hernia repair. World J Surg. 2012;36(2):447–52.

60. Ballantyne GH, Hourmont K, Wasielewski A. Telerobotic laparoscopic repair of incisional ventral hernias using intraperitoneal prosthetic mesh. JSLS. 2003;7(1):7–14.

61. Corcione F, Esposito C, Cuccurullo D, et al. Advantages and limits of robot-assisted laparoscopic surgery: preliminary experience. Surg Endosc. 2005;19(1):117–9.

62. Gonzalez A, Escobar E, Romero R, et al. Robotic-assisted ventral hernia repair: a multicenter evaluation of clinical outcomes. Surg Endosc. 2017;31(3):1342–9.

63. Earle D, Roth JS, Saber A, et al. SAGES Guidelines Committee. SAGES guidelines for laparoscopic ventral hernia repair. Surg Endosc. 2016;30(8):3163–83.

64. Papageorge CM, Funk LM, Poulose BK, et al. Primary fascial closure during laparoscopic ventral hernia repair does not reduce 30-day wound complications. Surg Endosc. 2017;31(11):4551–7.

65. Wennergren JE, Askenasy EP, Greenberg JA, et al. Laparoscopic ventral hernia repair with primary fascial closure versus bridged repair: a risk-adjusted comparative study. Surg Endosc. 2016;30(8):3231–8.

66. Tandon A, Pathak S, Lyons NJ, et al. Meta-analysis of closure of the fascial defect during laparoscopic incisional and ventral hernia repair. Br J Surg. 2016;103(12):1598–607.

67. Nguyen DH, Nguyen MT, Askenasy EP, et al. Primary fascial closure with laparoscopic ventral hernia repair: systematic review. World J Surg. 2014;38(12):3097–104.

68. Clinicaltrials.gov. Primary fascial closure with laparoscopic ventral hernia repair: a randomized controlled trial. NCT Number 02363790; The Influence of Closing the Gap on Postoperative Seroma and Recurrences in Laparoscopic Ventral Hernia Repair (CLOSURE). NCT Number 01719718; The Effect of Laparoscopically Closing the Hernia Defect in Laparoscopic Ventral Hernia Repair on Postoperative Pain (CLOSE-GAP). NCT Number 01962480.

69. Gonzalez AM, Romero RJ, Seetharamaiah R, et al. Laparoscopic ventral hernia repair with primary closure versus no primary closure of the defect: potential benefits of the robotic technology. Int J Med Robot. 2015;11(2):120–5.

70. Prabhu AS, Dickens EO, Copper CM, et al. Laparoscopic vs robotic intraperitoneal mesh repair for incisional hernia: an Americas Hernia Society Quality Collaborative Analysis. J Am Coll Surg. 2017;225(2):285–93.

71. Holihan JL, Askenasy EP, Greenberg JA, et al. Ventral Hernia Outcome Collaboration Writing Group. Component separation vs. bridged repair for large ventral hernias: a multi-institutional risk-adjusted comparison, systematic review, and meta-analysis. Surg Infect. 2016;17(1):17–26.

72. Bittner JG 4th, Alrefai S, Vy M, et al. Comparative analysis of open and robotic transversus abdominis release for ventral hernia repair. Surg Endosc. 2017;32(2):727–34.

73. Carbonell AM, Warren JA, Prabhu AS, et al. Reducing length of stay using a robotic-assisted approach for retromuscular ventral hernia repair: a comparative analysis from the Americas Hernia Society Quality Collaborative. Ann Surg. 2018;267(2):210–7.

74. Holihan JL, Alawadi Z, Martindale RG, et al. Adverse events after ventral hernia repair: the vicious cycle of complications. J Am Coll Surg. 2015;221(2):478–85.

75. Choi JJ, Palaniappa NC, Dallas KB, et al. Use of mesh during ventral hernia repair in clean-contaminated and contaminated cases: outcomes of 33,832 cases. Ann Surg. 2012;255(1):176–80.

76. Orr NT, Davenport DL, Roth JS. Outcomes of simultaneous laparoscopic cholecystectomy and ventral hernia repair compared to that of laparoscopic cholecystectomy alone. Surg Endosc. 2013;27(1):67–73.

77. Atema JJ, de Vries FE, Boermeester MA. Systematic review and meta-analysis of the repair of potentially contaminated and contaminated abdominal wall defects. Am J Surg. 2016;212(5):982–95.

78. Kissane NA, Itani KM. A decade of ventral incisional hernia repairs with biologic acellular dermal matrix: what have we learned? Plast Reconstr Surg. 2012;130(5 Suppl 2):194S–202S.

79. Primus FE, Harris HW. A critical review of biologic mesh use in ventral hernia repairs under contaminated conditions. Hernia. 2013;17(1):21–30.

80. Luque JA, Luque AB, Menchero JG, et al. Safety and effectiveness of self-adhesive mesh in laparoscopic ventral hernia repair using transabdominal preperitoneal route. Surg Endosc. 2017;31(3):1213–8.

81. Prasad P, Tantia O, Patle NM, et al. Laparoscopic transabdominal preperitoneal repair of ventral hernia: a step towards physiological repair. Indian J Surg. 2011;73(6):403–8.

82. Prasad P, Tantia O, Patle NM, et al. Laparoscopic ventral hernia repair: a comparative study of transabdominal preperitoneal versus intraperitoneal onlay mesh repair. J Laparoendosc Adv Surg Tech A. 2011;21(6):477–83.

83. Walker PA, May AC, Mo J, et al. Multicenter review of robotic versus laparoscopic ventral hernia repair: is there a role for robotics? Surg Endosc. 2018;32(4):1901–5.

84. Warren JA, Cobb WS, Ewing JA, et al. Standard laparoscopic versus robotic retromuscular ventral hernia repair. Surg Endosc. 2017;31(1):324–32.

85. Holihan JL, Liang MK. Umbilical hernias. In: Hope WW, Cobb WS, Adrales GL, editors. Textbook of hernias. 2017;1(1):305–15.
86. Liang MK, Berger RL, Li LT, Davila JA, Hicks SC, Kao LS. Outcomes of laparoscopic vs open repair of primary ventral hernias. JAMA Surg. 2013;148(11):1043–8.
87. Lambrecht JR, Vaktskjold A, Trondsen E, et al. Laparoscopic ventral hernia repair: outcomes in primary versus incisional hernias: no effect of defect closure. Hernia. 2015;19(3):479–86.
88. Carter SA, Hicks SC, Brahmbhatt R, et al. Recurrence and pseudorecurrence after laparoscopic ventral hernia repair: predictors and patient-focused outcomes. Am Surg. 2014;80(2):138–48.
89. Colavita PD, Tsirline VB, Walters AL, et al. Laparoscopic versus open hernia repair: outcomes and sociodemographic utilization results from the nationwide inpatient sample. Surg Endosc. 2013;27(1):109–17.
90. Clinicaltrials.gov. Laparoscopic "DA VINCI" Robot Assisted Abdominal Wall Hernia Repair (ARTE). NCT 0297414, 00908193. https://clinicaltrials.gov/ct2/show/NCT00908193?term=00908193&rank=1. Accessed 29 July 2017.
91. Clinicaltrials.gov. Open Versus Robotic Retromuscular Ventral Hernia Repair (ORREO). NCT 03007758. https://clinicaltrials.gov/ct2/show/NCT03007758. Accessed 29 July 2017.

Preoperative Optimization and Enhanced Recovery After Surgery Protocols in Ventral Hernia Repair

Sean B. Orenstein and Robert G. Martindale

Introduction

Many factors go into achieving success following ventral hernia repair. Besides technical factors that affect outcomes such as which repair technique, tissue plane dissected and the mesh prosthetic being implanted, there are multiple aspects of pre- and postoperative care that greatly affect outcomes. What is highly beneficial is that many of the patient-specific factors are modifiable. Therefore, with the assistance of their surgeons, patients have an opportunity to positively affect the outcomes of their own repair.

Hernia recurrence is a major indicator of the quality of the hernia repair. While extremely important, hernia recurrence may not be apparent for months, years, or even decades. In the short term, wound morbidity has a greater influence on the quality of life of the patient, as significant wound morbidity (e.g., surgical site infection [SSI]) can lead to increased visits to the emergency department, readmission to the hospital, greater time and effort within the clinic setting, or possible reoperation(s) to manage complex postoperative wound complications. Additionally, perioperative surgical site occurrences (SSOs), including SSI, seroma, wound ischemia, and

dehiscence, can greatly increase the risk of recurrent hernia [1]. Therefore, it is in the best interest of the patient and surgeon to optimize all measures that promote optimal wound healing, reduce infection, and enhance early postoperative recovery. In the ventral hernia population, the most common complication in the immediate perioperative period is surgical site infection (SSI) [2].

Minimally invasive surgical (MIS) techniques have been developed over the last few decades and encompass a wide breadth of surgical disciplines. While robotic-assisted procedures have been present for some time, a recent surge of hernia repairs are being performed robotically. Additionally, robotic-assisted techniques are being used for more complex hernia repairs, including component separation techniques for ventral hernias. Of the many benefits of MIS procedures, reduced wound morbidity and length of hospitalization are two of the principal advantages. With the rising popularity and use of robotic-assisted herniorrhaphy, there should be a reduction in wound complications, just as we have seen a reduction in wound complications with the utilization of laparoscopic hernia repair techniques. That said, it is still of utmost importance that we optimize our patients to ensure the highest quality hernia repair and prevent or reduce complications. This chapter will briefly review several pre- and perioperative measures that have been reported to decrease SSOs (surgical site

S. B. Orenstein (✉) · R. G. Martindale
Oregon Health and Science University,
Portland, OR, USA
e-mail: orenstei@ohsu.edu

© Springer International Publishing AG, part of Springer Nature 2018
K. A. LeBlanc (ed.), *Laparoscopic and Robotic Incisional Hernia Repair*,
https://doi.org/10.1007/978-3-319-90737-6_3

occurrences) and shorten length of hospital stay. Limited robotic-specific data exist regarding enhanced recovery after surgery (ERAS) for various surgeries [3], with the bulk of ERAS literature pertaining to open as well as laparoscopic surgery optimization and complication reduction. However, much of the information is still relevant in a population requiring complex (and simple) hernia repairs performed in a minimally invasive approach such as robotics.

Preoperative Optimization

There are multiple patient factors that contribute to wound healing and should be optimized prior to surgery. Factors such as obesity, smoking, diabetes, malnutrition, and surgical site contamination are all detrimental to wound healing and can lead to infection or hernia recurrence, among other complications. Obesity and smoking have been shown to be independent risk factors for increased rate of hernia recurrence as well as SSO. Poor glycemic control in the remote preoperative period, perioperative and postoperative periods has repeatedly demonstrated increased risk for superficial and deep tissue infections. Similarly, patients with malnutrition have significant alterations in wound healing and immune function, and will consequently have an increased incidence of postoperative SSOs as well as hernia recurrence. Unfortunately, many of our patients had multiple detrimental factors at the time of hernia repair. While all these factors influence surgical outcomes and work congruently on morbidity, many can be evaluated and treated as separate entities.

Obesity

Obesity represents one of the most significant threats for the development of incisional hernias as well as recurrence following ventral hernia repair. Hernia recurrence rate increases linearly as BMI increases regardless of the technique of repair [4–6]. In our practice we have found that in patients with BMI $\geq$ 50, the recurrence and

wound morbidity rate is prohibitively high. Therefore, we no longer perform elective herniorrhaphies in this group of high-risk patients unless they have stigmata of acutely worsening symptomology (e.g., recurrent obstruction, evolving ischemia, strangulation).

A lifetime of poor eating habits and insufficient physical activity are the likely culprits for many patients, making management of obesity quite challenging. Much time is spent during clinic visits, counseling patients on methods to improve dietary habits and increase physical activity. Following weight loss strategy discussions and objective rationale for the necessity of weight loss, we will set an attainable weight loss goal (e.g. 15–30 lbs) and have the patient return to the clinic in 3–6 months for reevaluation. Having a dietary consult with a nutritionist well versed in perioperative optimization can also provide valuable information and assist with motivated patients in reaching obtainable weight loss goals. If the patient fails to lose sufficient weight, or gains weight in the interim, elective surgery is postponed and other more aggressive methods of weight loss are discussed. If attempts at medical weight loss fail, it is our practice to refer patients to our bariatric surgery colleagues for discussion for surgical weight loss. Alternatively, newer endoscopic and other minimally invasive devices have been developed to assist with weight loss. The long-term efficacy of such devices is still under investigation, but early results are encouraging.

Ideally, if an MIS bariatric procedure is being performed in a patient with an incisional hernia, we will wait to definitively repair the hernia until adequate weight loss has been achieved. The simplest hernia repair is performed at this time (e.g., primary fascial closure) of the bariatric procedure, saving more complex hernia repairs (e.g., component separation) until after sufficient weight loss from their bariatric procedure. Some have advocated concomitant hernia repair at the time of sleeve gastrectomy, as sleeve gastrectomy does not put the patient at the extreme nutritional risk for poor wound healing and perioperative morbidity compared to bypass procedures [7]. However, the patient is still not optimized until adequate weight loss has been achieved.

Smoking

The multiple detrimental effects of smoking are well known, with reduction of both blood and tissue oxygen tension, as well as the negative effects on collagen deposition of at the site of healing wounds [8–10]. These effects adversely influence healing of surgical wounds. Numerous animal and human models have studied the detrimental physiological effects of smoking and have compared wound complications in smokers versus nonsmokers. Several authors have examined the effect of smoking on postoperative wound infection and have found wound infection following repair of ventral hernias to be increased in smokers [11–13]. Smoking is also a risk factor for developing an incisional hernia along with other postoperative complications following gastrointestinal or other abdominal surgery [14]. Because complex ventral hernia repair frequently requiring a combination of prosthetics, tissue flaps, and possibly some form of concomitant gastrointestinal procedure, these studies reinforce the need for smoking cessation prior to complex hernia repair and abdominal wall reconstruction (AWR). One study looking at smoking versus cessation with nicotine patches in patient undergoing primary hernia repair, hip or knee prosthesis, or laparoscopic cholecystectomy demonstrated almost a 50% reduction in total complications in the cessation + patch group [15]. This study confirms another landmark study by this group in which volunteers were divided into four groups: smokers, nonsmokers, those who quit smoking for 30 days preoperatively, and those who quit smoking and had a nicotine patch placed. This study indicated that smoking cessation for 30 days allows for the deleterious effects smoking to be alleviated, and the nicotine patch did not alter the beneficial influence of cessation [16]. Thus, 4 weeks may be an effective time of abstinence to reverse the complications associated with smoking. The other interesting and unexpected phenomenon is that nicotine patches did not have a deleterious effect on complications, suggesting that it is not nicotine but something else in the cigarette smoke that is deleterious.

Because of the substantial high-quality literature demonstrating a clear correlation between active tobacco use and impaired wound healing and its sequelae, we require patients to cease all smoking activity for a minimum of 30 days preoperatively for those undergoing elective complex VHR by any method, be it open, laparoscopically or robotic [11]. While robotic-assisted and other minimally invasive techniques benefit patients with reduced wound complications, active tobacco use still adds substantial impairments to adequate wound healing. We do allow the use of nicotine patches, as the data is reasonably good indicating that nicotine is not a factor in cigarette smoke that causes problems with wound healing.

Diabetes

While glucose management is important for all stages of patient care related to hernia repair, preoperative glycemic control is essential for optimal outcomes. This is routinely measured using glycosylated hemoglobin (Hgb A1c). Studies have demonstrated reduced wound healing and increased postoperative complications in diabetic patients undergoing a variety of surgical procedures [17–19]. In elective cases, it has been shown that glucose control in the 30–60 days prior to surgery is beneficial in decreasing perioperative complications [20]. At our institution, we postpone elective hernia repair in patients with elevated Hgb A1c levels (>7.5%), with attempts at achieving a Hgb A1c goal closer to 6.5%. The patient is referred to a diabetic nurse educator or endocrinologist, and the VHR repair is rescheduled when glycemic levels are sufficiently controlled. Postoperative glycemic management is discussed later in this chapter in the Postoperative Optimization section.

Nutrition and Metabolic Control

Multiple large observational studies, over 40 randomized controlled trials (RCTs), as well as numerous meta-analyses and systematic reviews demonstrate the role that nutritional therapy plays in the ability of patients to heal and recover following surgery. Despite substantial evidence supporting the role that nutrition plays on perioperative outcomes and healing, insufficient emphasis is placed on optimizing the patient's nutritional status in the preoperative setting [21].

The concept of preoperative preparation of the patient with specific metabolic and immune active nutrients gained popularity after several landmark studies by Gianotti and colleagues [22–24]. These well-done RCT investigations demonstrated benefit in lowering perioperative complications by adding the amino acid arginine along with the omega-3 fatty acids, docosahexaenoic acid (DHA) and eicosapentaenoic acid (EPA), for 5 days preoperatively. They reported major morbidity could be reduced by approximately 50% in patients undergoing major foregut surgery, including esophageal, stomach, or pancreas procedures. Similar benefit was noted in both the well-nourished and malnourished patient populations [24, 25].

Interestingly, even well-nourished patients have demonstrated benefits from nutritional metabolic and immune modulation [22, 24]. In these studies, the patients consumed 750 mL to 1 L per day of the metabolic-modulating formula in addition to their regular diet. The formula used by Gianotti and Braga and most of the other major studies contained additional arginine, [omega]-3 fatty acids, and nucleic acids, and resulted in significant decreases in infectious morbidity, length of hospital stay, and hospital-related expenses [22–24]. The exact mechanisms of all of the active ingredients are yet to be completely elucidated. However, it has been shown that fish oils have multiple mechanisms, including attenuating the metabolic response to stress, altering gene expression to minimize the proinflammatory cytokine production, beneficially modifying the Th1 to Th2 lymphocyte population to lower the inflammatory response, increasing production of EPA and DHA derived pro-resolving lipid compounds "Specialized Proresolving Molecules" (SPMs), and regulating bowel motility via vagal efferents [26–31]. Arginine has been reported to have a multitude of potential benefits in the surgical populations. These include improved wound healing, optimizing lymphocyte proliferation and function, and enhancing blood flow via the nitric oxide vasodilation effects [32, 33].

Another area of metabolic manipulation of growing interest is preoperative carbohydrate-loading [34]. This metabolic strategy utilizes an isotonic carbohydrate solution given 3 h preoperatively to alter stress metabolism and decrease insulin resistance [35]. In most Western surgical settings, the "routine" is for the patient to fast after dinner the night before surgery and remain nothing by mouth (*nil* per os, NPO) after midnight prior to surgery in the am. Essentially following this "routine," glycogen stores are nearly depleted at the time of surgery. Soop et al. [36], Fearon et al. [37], and more recently Awad [38, 39] have demonstrated the beneficial effects of carbo-loading in several animal and clinical studies reporting primarily benefits in insulin resistance. Caution with direct cause and effect conclusions here is needed as most large human studies dealing with carbo-loading were done as part of several preoperative interventions with the experimental groups receiving multimodality treatment, including avoidance of drains, controlled perioperative sodium and fluid administration, epidural anesthesia, and early mobilization in addition to the carbo-loading [34]. These carbohydrate-loading studies have consistently reported several metabolic benefits including significantly reduced insulin resistance, decreased postoperative nitrogen loss, and better retention of muscle function [36, 37].

Peri- and Postoperative Care

Surgical Site Infection

Attention to SSIs plays an important role with far-reaching ramifications for hernia repairs. SSI rates are noted to be higher for hernia repairs compared to other clean non-hernia surgeries [40]. Traditionally, if a permanent synthetic mesh was implanted at the time of hernia repair and it becomes infected, the ability to sterilize the mesh and completely eradicate the infection without removing the mesh was essentially zero. Synthetic mesh salvage rates following mesh related wound infections are reported between 10 and 70% and depend on the type of mesh involved. The bacterial clearance rates are dependent on the type of mesh used, location of mesh placement and the extent of contamination, as well as the viability of the tissue and host defenses [1, 41]. PTFE-based meshes remain the most difficult and virtually impossible to clear of infection, followed by multi-filament polyester, while macroporous polypropylene yields the best chance of salvage [41, 42]. In addition, infected mesh is associated with costly and serious morbidity including prolonged wound management, enterocutaneous fistulae as well as recurrent hernia. These complications can be quite severe and expose the patient to significant morbidity, mortality, and significant additional cost of care [42].

Skin Preparation and Decolonization Protocols

Proper disinfection of the surgical site with the use of skin preparations has been well elucidated. Multiple major trials have been published which essentially show equality with either an iodine or chlorhexidine skin prep as long as alcohol is included [43–45].

Hair trimming at the time of surgery has been the standard of care for several years, with the notion that clippers rather than razor be used to clear the surgical site hair [46]. Surgical site barriers and skin sealants have not been studied well in ventral hernia repair. The data on these products are widely variable with reports from beneficial to detrimental. The data on skin sealants and surgical site barriers are far too inconsistent to make any recommendation to use these in ventral hernia repair or AWR. That said, the use of iodine-impregnated sealant drapes can be beneficial from a draping standpoint, allowing wide draping and sealing at various edges of the sterile field. Also, the use of preoperative showers with antiseptic soaps to decrease SSIs has been inconsistent [47–49]. Showering with anti-septic agents such as chlorhexidine or Betadine, when compared to showering with soap, has not shown significant benefit in lowering SSI, and may alter the normal protective skin flora (microbiome) [50].

The nares are the most common site for colonization of *Staphylococcus aureus*. As such, nasal clearance of *S. aureus* in the preoperative setting has gained significant popularity in the last several years following a landmark paper published by Bode et al. in the *New England Journal of Medicine* in 2010. They reported a 42% decrease in *S. aureus* postoperative infections in the treated group [51]. Other studies have been carried out in orthopedic joint replacement or spine surgery, as hardware infection has devastating and costly consequences. In our practice we favor treating high-risk patient populations instead of random methicillin-resistant *S. aureus* (MRSA) nasal screening. High-risk patients include previous MRSA infection, co-habitant with MRSA, recently hospitalized within 6 months, living in a nursing facility or prison, currently on broad-spectrum antibiotics, etc. These patients are treated with a protocol combining mupirocin ointment applied in each nostril twice daily along with chlorhexidine showers once daily for 5 days prior to the date of surgery. A povidone-iodine based preparation has recently been released and may offer a single treatment option [52].

Perioperative Antibiotics

According to Guidelines that were developed jointly by the American Society of Health-System Pharmacists (ASHP), the Infectious Diseases Society of America (IDSA), the Surgical Infection Society (SIS), and the Society for Healthcare Epidemiology of America (SHEA), patients undergoing routine ventral hernias repair should be given prophylactic antibiotics using a first generation cephalosporin [53]. The antibiotics should be given with adequate time to allow for levels in the tissue to reach a level above the minimum inhibitory concentration (MIC) for the bacteria for which one is trying to inhibit, usually this is within 30 min prior to incision [54]. Antibiotics should be redosed, if necessary, during the operation as indicated based on duration of surgery, half-life of antibiotic being used, blood loss, and use of cell saver. Regarding the use of postoperative antibiotics, several well-done randomized trials have shown no benefit of dosing prophylactic antibiotics after the skin has been closed [53, 55–58]. These outcomes have been similar across several surgical disciplines. One challenge with regard to antibiotic dosing is in the obese population. In a recent large survey, only 66% of patients received prophylactic dosing to reach adequate serum levels when BMI was over 30 [59]. According to ASHP guidelines it is recommended that all patients under 120 kg receive 2 g cefazolin, while those at or above 120 kg be given 3 g cefazolin, then redosed every 4 h for extended surgeries. Interestingly, because of shorter half-lives antibiotics such as ampicillin-sulbactam, cefoxitin, and piperacillin-tazobactam are redosed every 2 h when used for intraoperative prophylaxis, according to ASHP recommendations [53]. Additionally, because of increased risk of methicillin-*sensitive S. aureus* (MSSA) wound infection when vancomycin is used [60], we routinely use both cefazolin in addition to vancomycin for prophylaxis in patients with high risk for MRSA infection. This ensures adequate coverage of both MSSA and MRSA, especially in the setting of a mesh prosthetic implant; this is also discussed in the ASHP therapeutic guidelines [53].

For patients with active wound infections, chronic draining sinuses, infected mesh, enterocutaneous or enteroatmospheric fistulae, and so on, our primary goal is removal of all foreign bodies and niduses of infection. Prior to definitive hernia repair the goal is removal of all infected meshes and other foreign bodies (e.g., suture material), debridement all infected and poor integrity tissue, and perform any necessary gastrointestinal resections with anastomoses, as indicated. For many cases where the bioburden of bacteria is high we will stage the repair with a negative pressure dressing and close the abdomen with native tissue or absorbable mesh and

perform a subsequent hernia repair, likely with a biologic or biosynthetic resorbable mesh, at some point in the future depending on the patient's condition, nutritional status, and degree of contamination [61].

Postoperative Blood Glucose Management

The immediate postoperative period is a critical period with regard to glucose management. Hyperglycemia has been shown to alter chemotaxis, phagocytosis, and oxidative burst which can prevent the early optimal killing of bacteria which entered the wound during surgery [62]. Therefore, meticulous glycemic control is vital within the first 24 h of the postoperative period to maximize neutrophil activity. Multiple large randomized clinical trials have confirmed the target blood glucose level in the immediate perioperative period appears optimal in the 120–160 mg/dL range [63–66].

Multimodal Pain Control

Adequate pain control remains a challenging entity following hernia repair. This holds true for minimally invasive approaches including laparoscopy and robotic-assisted repairs, along with their open repair counterpart. Because of the innervation of the abdominal wall, defect closure and trans-fascial suturing all play roles in postoperative pain. That said, because robotic-assisted surgery allows for improved intracorporeal suturing, with less transabdominal suturing, there is potential for reduced pain compared to standard laparoscopy. While narcotics represent a common component of multimodal approaches, their use is lessened when combined with an array of non-opiates in an effort to reduce the deleterious effects of opiates such as constipation, sedation, and respiratory depression. The principal components of our postoperative multimodal pain regimen include an immediate-acting narcotic such as hydromorphone or oxycodone, acetaminophen, along with gabapentin. Other agents, including antispasmodics may be added but are less routine. The multimodal approach should be tailored to the degree of hernia repair, as more complex repairs (e.g., robotic TAR or flank hernia repairs) will likely require greater breadth of analgesics. Conversely, simpler umbilical hernia repairs may only require one or two analgesic agents.

Commonly, patients are given an opiate-based analgesic for immediate pain relief. Patients undergoing same-day surgery can be discharged with oral oxycodone, hydromorphone, or hydrocodone. However, patients that are admitted are routinely given a hydromorphone patient-controlled analgesia (PCA) pump for narcotic-assisted analgesia. Once a patient is tolerating a diet, we transition to oral oxycodone or hydromorphone as needed for breakthrough pain. Acetaminophen is routinely given as well to aid in analgesia, as there is lack of side effects seen with opiates such as sedation, respiratory depression, and ileus, and no concern of bleeding or impaired renal function seen with nonsteroidal anti-inflammatory drugs (NSAIDs) [13]. However, because acetaminophen is primarily metabolized in the liver, its use should be cautioned in patients with hepatic dysfunction. These benefits result in decreased postoperative pain while significantly reducing opioid consumption. While the precise mechanism of acetaminophen remains unknown, it appears to have a central analgesic effect on multiple target pathways [67]. For those that are unable to receive oral medications, IV acetaminophen can be very helpful. However, IV acetaminophen is expensive, and many hospital pharmacies will require documentation stating a patient's inability to accept oral or rectal acetaminophen before allowing IV infusion. Principal benefits of IV acetaminophen include rapid onset and high peak concentration compared to equivalent oral and rectal doses, along with its ability to be used in patients without adequate bowel function. Because of its safety profile when dosed appropriately, patients will routinely be discharged with acetaminophen as a primary analgesic.

Another useful analgesic for patients admitted following hernia repair is gabapentin, which serves as an adjunct for postoperative pain control at the neuronal level, with mechanisms of action on calcium channels and GABA receptors [68–70]. Multiple randomized controlled trials (RCTs) have demonstrated the benefits of pain control as well as reduced opioid use without the side effect profile of opiates [70–74]. While some patients experience sedative effects from gabapentin, this effect is less frequent than opiates, though monitoring for sedation with the use of multiple analgesics is necessary. For our pain pathway, we routinely provide oral gabapentin (300 mg TID) immediately postoperatively until the day of discharge. Rarely, patients are prescribed gabapentin upon discharge, and this is typically reserved for patients with known chronic pain syndromes or if significant lateral wall dissection was performed.

Another medication of usefulness following abdominal wall hernia repair is diazepam. While typically thought as an anxiolytic, we administer diazepam as a postoperative muscle relaxant. There is limited literature regarding the use of diazepam for postoperative pain control in hernia repair, though studies do support the use in a multimodal fashion with narcotics [75, 76]. Because significant abdominal wall dissection can result in muscle spasm, diazepam's antispasmodic properties can be a useful component, especially if trans-fascial fixation or numerous tacks are utilized. Diazepam is initiated on postoperative day 1 or 2, allowing for evaluation of sedation with other multimodal medications. 2–5 mg of diazepam is scheduled every 6 h around the clock for the first 48 postoperative hours, excluding elderly patients over 65 years old and all patients with a history of obstructive sleep apnea. Caution must be used with diazepam, as an added sedative effect can be seen with patients sensitive to sedatives, prompting strict holding parameters for any signs of somnolence or lethargy. Because of the sedative effects and greater addictive profile of benzodiazepines, we routinely exclude diazepam as a discharge medication.

While oral and intravenous analgesics represent the mainstay of a multimodal pain regimen, local-regional blockade is a useful adjunct for ventral hernia repair. Transversus abdominis plane (TAP) blocks have gained greater popularity given its blockade of intercostal, subcostal, ilioinguinal, and iliohypogastric nerves (T6-L1) [77, 78]. TAP blocks employ local anesthetic infusion between the internal oblique and transversus abdominis muscles and are performed either via ultrasound-guidance, indirect visualization laparoscopically/robotically, or direct visualization of the planes if performing a transversus abdominis release (TAR). TAP blocks have shown to reduce postoperative pain, overall narcotic usage, length of stay, as well as reduction of opioid-specific side effects [79–83]. If available, long-acting liposomal bupivacaine can provide up to 72 h of local anesthetic blockade, though many hospital pharmacies restrict their use due to high cost compared to standard bupivacaine.

Other analgesics are being utilized by surgical and anesthesia teams to help alleviate peri- and postoperative pain following ventral hernia repair. NSAIDS are a useful adjunct, but should be used in caution with elderly patients given the risk of postoperative kidney injury. Therefore, NSAIDS are reserved for non-elderly patients, with only a short duration in the postoperative setting. Given the opiate crisis that is more publicly apparent, a reduction in narcotic use is favored. Therefore, multimodal pain regimens will no doubt change in the upcoming years, and patients should be tailored for their own personal analgesic needs in the postoperative setting.

Early Enteral Feeding

No longer do we keep our patients *nil* per os (NPO) for extended periods of time awaiting return of bowel function. Multiple studies have demonstrated success with tolerance to early enteral feeding, in addition to multiple metabolic benefits, all while reducing postoperative ileus and decreasing length of hospitalization [84–87]. For our early recovery pathway, patients receive unlimited clear liquids with the addition of a clear liquid protein supplement on postoperative day #1, then are advanced to a regular diet on postoperative day #2. Antiemetics are provided for patients on an as needed basis. However, most patients tolerate this rapid progression without deleterious sequelae. The exceptions are for patients that required significant adhesiolysis and/or bowel resection; such patients are at higher risk for ileus development. Therefore, any significant nausea and emesis prompt nasogastric tube decompression and holding enteral feeds.

Conclusion

As discussed above, many factors influence the outcomes following ventral hernia repair. Optimizing the patient in the preoperative setting, including smoking cessation, appropriate weight loss, and diabetes control, among others, can greatly impact success after ventral hernia repair. While most preoperative optimization studies pertain to open repairs, it is still of great benefit to maximize outcomes for patients undergoing minimally invasive approaches such as robotic-assisted ventral hernia repair. As we accrue more data from robotic-assisted surgeries, there will no doubt be advancements in patient outcomes as we combine the positive returns of preoperative optimization with the benefits of minimally invasive surgeries.

References

1. Sanchez VM, Abi-Haidar YE, Itani KMF. Mesh infection in ventral incisional hernia repair: incidence, contributing factors, and treatment. Surg Infect. 2011;12(3):205–10. https://doi.org/10.1089/sur.2011.033.
2. Hawn MT, Gray SH, Snyder CW, Graham LA, Finan KR, Vick CC. Predictors of mesh explantation after incisional hernia repair. Am J Surg. 2011;202(1):28–33. https://doi.org/10.1016/j.amjsurg.2010.10.011.
3. Collins JW, Patel H, Adding C, Annerstedt M, Dasgupta P, Khan SM, Artibani W, Gaston R, Piechaud T, Catto JW, Koupparis A, Rowe E, Perry M, Issa R, McGrath J, Kelly J, Schumacher M, Wijburg C, Canda AE, Balbay MD, Decaestecker K, Schwentner C, Stenzl A, Edeling S, Pokupic S, Stockle M, Siemer S, Sanchez-Salas R, Cathelineau X, Weston R, Johnson M, D'Hondt F, Mottrie A, Hosseini A, Wiklund PN. Enhanced recovery after robot-assisted radical cystectomy: EAU robotic urology section scientific working group consensus

view. Eur Urol. 2016;70(4):649–60. https://doi.org/10.1016/j.eururo.2016.05.020.

4. Sauerland S, Korenkov M, Kleinen T, Arndt M, Paul A. Obesity is a risk factor for recurrence after incisional hernia repair. Hernia. 2004;8(1):42–6. https://doi.org/10.1007/s10029-003-0161-x.

5. Lin HJ, Spoerke N, Deveney C, Martindale R. Reconstruction of complex abdominal wall hernias using acellular human dermal matrix: a single institution experience. Am J Surg. 2009;197(5):599–603. https://doi.org/10.1016/j.amjsurg.2008.12.022.

6. Desai KA, Razavi SA, Hart AM, Thompson PW, Losken A. The effect of BMI on outcomes following complex abdominal wall reconstructions. Ann Plast Surg. 2016;76(Suppl 4):S295–7. https://doi.org/10.1097/SAP.0000000000000673.

7. Spaniolas K, Kasten KR, Mozer AB, Sippey ME, Chapman WH, Pories WJ, JRt P. Synchronous ventral hernia repair in patients undergoing bariatric surgery. Obes Surg. 2015;25(10):1864–8. https://doi.org/10.1007/s11695-015-1625-7.

8. Jensen JA, Goodson WH, Hopf HW, Hunt TK. Cigarette smoking decreases tissue oxygen. Arch Surg. 1991;126(9):1131–4.

9. Knuutinen A, Kokkonen N, Risteli J, Vahakangas K, Kallioinen M, Salo T, Sorsa T, Oikarinen A. Smoking affects collagen synthesis and extracellular matrix turnover in human skin. Br J Dermatol. 2002;146(4):588–94. https://doi.org/10.1046/j.1365-2133.2002.04694.x.

10. Sørensen LT, Toft BG, Rygaard J, Ladelund S, Paddon M, James T, Taylor R, Gottrup F. Effect of smoking, smoking cessation, and nicotine patch on wound dimension, vitamin C, and systemic markers of collagen metabolism. Surgery. 2010;148(5):982–90. https://doi.org/10.1016/j.surg.2010.02.005.

11. Sorensen LT, Hemmingsen UB, Kirkeby LT, Kallehave F, Jorgensen LN. Smoking is a risk factor for incisional hernia. Arch Surg. 2005;140(2):119–23. https://doi.org/10.1001/archsurg.140.2.119.

12. Finan KR, Vick CC, Kiefe CI, Neumayer L, Hawn MT. Predictors of wound infection in ventral hernia repair. Am J Surg. 2005;190(5):676–81. https://doi.org/10.1016/j.amjsurg.2005.06.041.

13. Yang GP, Longaker MT. Abstinence from smoking reduces incisional wound infection. Ann Surg. 2003;238(1):6–8. https://doi.org/10.1097/01.sla.0000074966.51219.eb.

14. Sorensen LT, Hemmingsen U, Kallehave F, Wille-Jorgensen P, Kjaergaard J, Moller LN, Jorgensen T. Risk factors for tissue and wound complications in gastrointestinal surgery. Ann Surg. 2005;241(4):654–8.

15. Lindström D, Azodi OS, Wladis A, Tønnesen H, Linder S, Nåsell H, Ponzer S, Adami J. Effects of a perioperative smoking cessation intervention on postoperative complications. Ann Surg. 2008;248(5):739–45. https://doi.org/10.1097/sla.0b013e3181889d0d.

16. Sorensen LT, Karlsmark T, Gottrup F. Abstinence from smoking reduces incisional wound infection. Ann Surg. 2003;238(1):1–5. https://doi.org/10.1097/01.sla.0000074980.39700.31.

17. Christman AL, Selvin E, Margolis DJ, Lazarus GS, Garza LA. Hemoglobin A1c predicts healing rate in diabetic wounds. J Invest Dermatol. 2011;131(10):2121–7. https://doi.org/10.1038/jid.2011.176.

18. Humphers J, Shibuya N, Fluhman BL, Jupiter D. The impact of glycosylated hemoglobin and diabetes mellitus on postoperative wound healing complications and infection following foot and ankle surgery. J Am Podiatr Med Assoc. 2014:140626130507002. https://doi.org/10.7547/13-026.1.

19. Armaghani SJ, Archer KR, Rolfe R, Demaio DN, Devin CJ. Diabetes is related to worse patient-reported outcomes at two years following spine surgery. J Bone Joint Surg Am. 2016;98(1):15–22. https://doi.org/10.2106/JBJS.O.00297.

20. Dronge AS, Perkal MF, Kancir S, Concato J, Aslan M, Rosenthal RA. Long-term glycemic control and postoperative infectious complications. Arch Surg. 2006;141(4):375–80.; discussion 380. https://doi.org/10.1001/archsurg.141.4.375.

21. Martindale RG, McClave SA, Vanek VW, McCarthy M, Roberts P, Taylor B, Ochoa JB, Napolitano L, Cresci G. Guidelines for the provision and assessment of nutrition support therapy in the adult critically ill patient: Society of Critical Care Medicine and American Society for Parenteral and Enteral Nutrition: Executive Summary*. Crit Care Med. 2009;37(5):1757–61. https://doi.org/10.1097/ccm.0b013e3181a40116.

22. Braga M, Gianotti L, Nespoli L, Radaelli G, Di Carlo V. Nutritional approach in malnourished surgical patients. Arch Surg. 2002;137(2). https://doi.org/10.1001/archsurg.137.2.174.

23. Braga M, Gianotti L, Vignali A, Schmid A, Nespoli L, Di Carlo V. Hospital resources consumed for surgical morbidity: effects of preoperative arginine and ω-3 fatty acid supplementation on costs. Nutrition. 2005;21(11–12):1078–86. https://doi.org/10.1016/j.nut.2005.05.003.

24. Gianotti L, Braga M, Nespoli L, Radaelli G, Beneduce A, Di Carlo V. A randomized controlled trial of preoperative oral supplementation with a specialized diet in patients with gastrointestinal cancer. Gastroenterology. 2002;122(7):1763–70. https://doi.org/10.1053/gast.2002.33587.

25. Drover JW, Dhaliwal R, Weitzel L, Wischmeyer PE, Ochoa JB, Heyland DK. Perioperative use of arginine-supplemented diets: a systematic review of the evidence. J Am Coll Surg. 2011;212(3):385–399.e381. https://doi.org/10.1016/j.jamcollsurg.2010.10.016.

26. Calder PC. Fatty acids and inflammation: the cutting edge between food and pharma. Eur J Pharmacol. 2011;668:S50–8. https://doi.org/10.1016/j.ejphar.2011.05.085.

27. Calder PC. Omega-3 polyunsaturated fatty acids and inflammatory processes: nutrition or pharmacology? Br J Clin Pharmacol. 2013;75(3):645–62. https://doi.org/10.1111/j.1365-2125.2012.04374.x.

28. Calder PC. Mechanisms of action of (n-3) fatty acids. J Nutr. 2012;142(3):592S–9S. https://doi.org/10.3945/jn.111.155259.

29. Lee H-N, Surh Y-J. Therapeutic potential of resolvins in the prevention and treatment of inflammatory disorders. Biochem Pharmacol. 2012;84(10):1340–50. https://doi.org/10.1016/j.bcp.2012.08.004.

30. Pluess T-T, Hayoz D, Berger MM, Tappy L, Revelly J-P, Michaeli B, Carpentier YA, Chioléro RL. Intravenous fish oil blunts the physiological response to endotoxin in healthy subjects. Intensive Care Med. 2007;33(5):789–97. https://doi.org/10.1007/s00134-007-0591-5.

31. Spite M, Norling LV, Summers L, Yang R, Cooper D, Petasis NA, Flower RJ, Perretti M, Serhan CN. Resolvin D2 is a potent regulator of leukocytes and controls microbial sepsis. Nature. 2009;461(7268):1287–91. https://doi.org/10.1038/nature08541.

32. Marik PE, Flemmer M. The immune response to surgery and trauma. J Trauma Acute Care Surg. 2012;73(4):801–8. https://doi.org/10.1097/ta.0b013e318265cf87.

33. Rudolph FB, Van Buren CT. The metabolic effects of enterally administered ribonucleic acids. Curr Opin Clin Nutr Metab Care. 1998;1(6):527–30. https://doi.org/10.1097/00075197-199811000-00009.

34. Burden S, Todd C, Hill J, Lal S. Pre-operative nutrition support in patients undergoing gastrointestinal surgery. Cochrane Database Syst Rev. 2012;11:CD008879. https://doi.org/10.1002/14651858.cd008879.pub2.

35. Svanfeldt M, Thorell A, Hausel J, Soop M, Nygren J, Ljungqvist O. Effect of "preoperative" oral carbohydrate treatment on insulin action—a randomised cross-over unblinded study in healthy subjects. Clin Nutr. 2005;24(5):815–21. https://doi.org/10.1016/j.clnu.2005.05.002.

36. Soop M, Nygren J, Myrenfors P, Thorell A, Ljungqvist O. Preoperative oral carbohydrate treatment attenuates immediate postoperative insulin resistance. Am J Physiol Endocrinol Metab. 2001;280(4):E576–83.

37. Fearon KCH, Ljungqvist O, Von Meyenfeldt M, Revhaug A, Dejong CHC, Lassen K, Nygren J, Hausel J, Soop M, Andersen J, Kehlet H. Enhanced recovery after surgery: a consensus review of clinical care for patients undergoing colonic resection. Clin Nutr. 2005;24(3):466–77. https://doi.org/10.1016/j.clnu.2005.02.002.

38. Awad S, Constantin-Teodosiu D, Constantin D, Rowlands BJ, Fearon KCH, Macdonald IA, Lobo DN. Cellular mechanisms underlying the protective effects of preoperative feeding. Ann Surg. 2010;252(2):247–53. https://doi.org/10.1097/sla.0b013e3181e8fbe6.

39. Awad S, Fearon KCH, Macdonald IA, Lobo DN. A randomized cross-over study of the metabolic and hormonal responses following two preoperative conditioning drinks. Nutrition. 2011;27(9):938–42. https://doi.org/10.1016/j.nut.2010.08.025.

40. Houck JP, Rypins EB, Sarfeh IJ, Juler GL, Shimoda KJ. Repair of incisional hernia. Surg Gynecol Obstet. 1989;169(5):397–9.

41. Cevasco M, Itani KMF. Ventral hernia repair with synthetic, composite, and biologic mesh: characteristics, indications, and infection profile. Surg Infect. 2012;13(4):209–15. https://doi.org/10.1089/sur.2012.123.

42. Le D, Deveney CW, Reaven NL, Funk SE, McGaughey KJ, Martindale RG. Mesh choice in ventral hernia repair: so many choices, so little time. Am J Surg. 2013;205(5):602–7. https://doi.org/10.1016/j.amjsurg.2013.01.026.

43. Swenson Brian R, Hedrick Traci L, Metzger R, Bonatti H, Pruett Timothy L, Sawyer Robert G. Effects of preoperative skin preparation on postoperative wound infection rates: a prospective study of 3 skin preparation protocols. Infect Control Hosp Epidemiol. 2009;30(10):964–71. https://doi.org/10.1086/605926.

44. Darouiche RO, Wall MJ Jr, Itani KM, Otterson MF, Webb AL, Carrick MM, Miller HJ, Awad SS, Crosby CT, Mosier MC, Alsharif A, Berger DH. Chlorhexidine-alcohol versus povidone-iodine for surgical-site antisepsis. N Engl J Med. 2010;362(1):18–26. https://doi.org/10.1056/NEJMoa0810988.

45. Swenson BR, Sawyer RG. Importance of alcohol in skin preparation protocols. Infect Control Hosp Epidemiol. 2010;31(9):977. https://doi.org/10.1086/655843.

46. Tanner J, Norrie P, Melen K. Preoperative hair removal to reduce surgical site infection. Cochrane Database of Syst Rev. 2011. https://doi.org/10.1002/14651858.cd004122.pub4.

47. Dumville JC, McFarlane E, Edwards P, Lipp A, Holmes A. Preoperative skin antiseptics for preventing surgical wound infections after clean surgery. Cochrane Database Syst Rev. 2013. https://doi.org/10.1002/14651858.cd003949.pub3.

48. Edmiston CE, Okoli O, Graham MB, Sinski S, Seabrook GR. Evidence for using chlorhexidine gluconate preoperative cleansing to reduce the risk of surgical site infection. AORN J. 2010;92(5):509–18. https://doi.org/10.1016/j.aorn.2010.01.020.

49. Chlebicki MP, Safdar N, O'Horo JC, Maki DG. Preoperative chlorhexidine shower or bath for prevention of surgical site infection: a meta-analysis. Am J Infect Control. 2013;41(2):167–73. https://doi.org/10.1016/j.ajic.2012.02.014.

50. Prabhu AS, Krpata DM, Phillips S, Huang LC, Haskins IN, Rosenblatt S, Poulose BK, Rosen MJ. Preoperative chlorhexidine gluconate use can increase risk for surgical site infections after ventral hernia repair. J Am Coll Surg. 2017;224(3):334–40. https://doi.org/10.1016/j.jamcollsurg.2016.12.013.

51. Bode LGM, Kluytmans JAJW, Wertheim HFL, Bogaers D, Vandenbroucke-Grauls CMJE, Roosendaal R, Troelstra A, Box ATA, Voss A, van der Tweel I, van Belkum A, Verbrugh HA, Vos MC. Preventing surgical-site infections in nasal carriers of Staphylococcus aureus. N Engl J Med. 2010;362(1):9–17. https://doi.org/10.1056/nejmoa0808939.

52. Anderson MJ, David ML, Scholz M, Bull SJ, Morse D, Hulse-Stevens M, Peterson ML. Efficacy of skin and nasal povidone-iodine preparation against mupirocin-resistant methicillin-resistant Staphylococcus aureus and S. aureus within the anterior nares. Antimicrob Agents Chemother. 2015;59(5):2765–73. https://doi.org/10.1128/AAC.04624-14.

53. Bratzler DW, Dellinger EP, Olsen KM, Perl TM, Auwaerter PG, Bolon MK, Fish DN, Napolitano LM, Sawyer RG, Slain D, Steinberg JP, Weinstein RA, American Society of Health-System Pharmacists, Infectious Disease Society of America, Surgical Infection Society, Society for Healthcare Epidemiology of America. Clinical practice guidelines for antimicrobial prophylaxis in surgery. Am J Health Syst Pharm. 2013;70(3):195–283. https://doi.org/10.2146/ajhp120568.

54. Junker T, Mujagic E, Hoffmann H, Rosenthal R, Misteli H, Zwahlen M, Oertli D, Tschudin-Sutter S, Widmer AF, Marti WR, Weber WP. Prevention and control of surgical site infections: review of the Basel Cohort Study. Swiss Med Wkly. 2012. https://doi.org/10.4414/smw.2012.13616.

55. Berbari EF, Osmon DR, Lahr B, Eckel-Passow JE, Tsaras G, Hanssen AD, Mabry T, Steckelberg J, Thompson R. The Mayo prosthetic joint infection risk score: implication for surgical site infection reporting and risk stratification. Infect Control Hosp Epidemiol. 2012;33(08):774–81. https://doi.org/10.1086/666641.

56. Enzler MJ, Berbari E, Osmon DR. Antimicrobial prophylaxis in adults. Mayo Clin Proc. 2011;86(7):686–701. https://doi.org/10.4065/mcp.2011.0012.

57. Fonseca SNS. Implementing 1-dose antibiotic prophylaxis for prevention of surgical site infection. Arch Surg. 2006;141(11):1109. https://doi.org/10.1001/archsurg.141.11.1109.

58. Suehiro T, Hirashita T, Araki S, Matsumata T, Tsutsumi S, Mochiki E, Kato H, Asao T, Kuwano H. Prolonged antibiotic prophylaxis longer than 24 hours does not decrease surgical site infection after elective gastric and colorectal surgery. Hepato-Gastroenterology. 2008;55(86–87):1636–9.

59. Hanley MJ, Abernethy DR, Greenblatt DJ. Effect of obesity on the pharmacokinetics of drugs in humans. Clin Pharmacokinet. 2010;49(2):71–87. https://doi.org/10.2165/11318100-000000000-00000.

60. Bull AL, Worth LJ, Richards MJ. Impact of vancomycin surgical antibiotic prophylaxis on the development of methicillin-sensitive Staphylococcus aureus surgical site infections. Ann Surg. 2012;256(6):1089–92. https://doi.org/10.1097/sla.0b013e31825fa398.

61. Diaz JJ Jr, Conquest AM, Ferzoco SJ, Vargo D, Miller P, Wu YC, Donahue R. Multi-institutional experience using human acellular dermal matrix for ventral hernia repair in a compromised surgical field. Arch Surg. 2009;144(3):209–15. https://doi.org/10.1001/archsurg.2009.12.

62. Turina M, Fry DE, Polk HC. Acute hyperglycemia and the innate immune system: clinical, cellular, and molecular aspects. Crit Care Med. 2005;33(7):1624–33. https://doi.org/10.1097/01.ccm.0000170106.61978.d8.

63. Van den Berghe G, Wouters P, Weekers F, Verwaest C, Bruyninckx F, Schetz M, Vlasselaers D, Ferdinande P, Lauwers P, Bouillon R. Intensive insulin therapy in critically ill patients. N Engl J Med. 2001;345(19):1359–67. https://doi.org/10.1056/nejmoa011300.

64. Investigators N-SS, Finfer S, Liu B, Chittock DR, Norton R, Myburgh JA, McArthur C, Mitchell I, Foster D, Dhingra V, Henderson WR, Ronco JJ, Bellomo R, Cook D, McDonald E, Dodek P, Hebert PC, Heyland DK, Robinson BG, The NICE-SUGAR Study Investigators. Hypoglycemia and risk of death in critically ill patients. N Engl J Med. 2012;367(12):1108–18. https://doi.org/10.1056/NEJMoa1204942.

65. Ramos M, Khalpey Z, Lipsitz S, Steinberg J, Panizales MT, Zinner M, Rogers SO. Relationship of perioperative hyperglycemia and postoperative infections in patients who undergo general and vascular surgery. Ann Surg. 2008;126:228–34. https://doi.org/10.1097/sla.0b013e31818990d1.

66. Ata A, Lee J, Bestle SL, Desemone J, Stain SC. Postoperative hyperglycemia and surgical site infection in general surgery patients. Arch Surg. 2010;145(9):858–64. https://doi.org/10.1001/archsurg.2010.179.

67. Svensson LG, Adams DH, Bonow RO, Kouchoukos NT, Miller DC, O'Gara PT, Shahian DM, Schaff HV, Akins CW, Bavaria J, Blackstone EH, David TE, Desai ND, Dewey TM, D'Agostino RS, Gleason TG, Harrington KB, Kodali S, Kapadia S, Leon MB, Lima B, Lytle BW, Mack MJ, Reece TB, Reiss GR, Roselli E, Smith CR, Thourani VH, Tuzcu EM, Webb J, Williams MR. Aortic valve and ascending aorta guidelines for management and quality measures: executive summary. Ann Thorac Surg. 2013;95(4):1491–505. https://doi.org/10.1016/j.athoracsur.2012.12.027.

68. Abdi A, Farshidi H, Rahimi S, Amini A, Tasnim Eftekhari SF. Electrocardiologic and echocardiographic findings in patients with scorpion sting. Iran Red Crescent Med J. 2013;15(5):446–7. https://doi.org/10.5812/ircmj.2853.

69. Sills GJ. Not another gabapentin mechanism! Epilepsy Curr. 2005;5(2):75–7. https://doi.org/10.1111/j.1535-7597.2005.05210.x.

70. Hurley RW, Cohen SP, Williams KA, Rowlingson AJ, Wu CL. The analgesic effects of perioperative gabapentin on postoperative pain: a meta-analysis. Reg Anesth Pain Med. 2006;31(3):237–47. https://doi.org/10.1016/j.rapm.2006.01.005.

71. Ho KY, Gan TJ, Habib AS. Gabapentin and postoperative pain—a systematic review of randomized controlled trials. Pain. 2006;126(1–3):91–101. https://doi.org/10.1016/j.pain.2006.06.018.

72. Tiippana EM, Hamunen K, Kontinen VK, Kalso E. Do surgical patients benefit from perioperative gabapentin/pregabalin? A systematic review of efficacy and safety. Anesth Analg. 2007;104(6):1545–56, table of contents. https://doi.org/10.1213/01.ane.0000261517.27532.80.

73. Dauri M, Faria S, Gatti A, Celidonio L, Carpenedo R, Sabato AF. Gabapentin and pregabalin for the acute post-operative pain management. A systematic-narrative review of the recent clinical evidences. Curr Drug Targets. 2009;10(8):716–33.

74. Peng PW, Wijeysundera DN, Li CC. Use of gabapentin for perioperative pain control—a meta-analysis. Pain Res Manage. 2007;12(2):85–92.

75. Paulson DM, Kennedy DT, Donovick RA, Carpenter RL, Cherubini M, Techner L, Du W, Ma Y, Schmidt WK, Wallin B, Jackson D. Alvimopan: an oral, peripherally acting, mu-opioid receptor antagonist for the treatment of opioid-induced bowel dysfunction—a 21-day treatment-randomized clinical trial. J Pain. 2005;6(3):184–92. https://doi.org/10.1016/j.jpain.2004.12.001.

76. Caumo W, Hidalgo MP, Schmidt AP, Iwamoto CW, Adamatti LC, Bergmann J, Ferreira MB. Effect of preoperative anxiolysis on postoperative pain response in patients undergoing total abdominal hysterectomy. Anaesthesia. 2002;57(8):740–6.

77. Petersen PL, Hilsted KL, Dahl JB, Mathiesen O. Bilateral transversus abdominis plane (TAP) block with 24 hours ropivacaine infusion via TAP catheters: a randomized trial in healthy volunteers. BMC Anesthesiol. 2013;13(1):30. https://doi.org/10.1186/1471-2253-13-30.

78. Cohen SM. Extended pain relief trial utilizing infiltration of Exparel((R)), a long-acting multivesicular liposome formulation of bupivacaine: a phase IV health economic trial in adult patients undergoing open colectomy. J Pain Res. 2012;5:567–72. https://doi.org/10.2147/JPR.S38621.

79. Petersen PL, Mathiesen O, Torup H, Dahl JB. The transversus abdominis plane block: a valuable option for postoperative analgesia? A topical review. Acta Anaesthesiol Scand. 2010;54(5):529–35. https://doi.org/10.1111/j.1399-6576.2010.02215.x.

80. McDonnell JG, O'Donnell B, Curley G, Heffernan A, Power C, Laffey JG. The analgesic efficacy of transversus abdominis plane block after abdominal surgery: a prospective randomized controlled trial. Anesth Analg. 2007;104(1):193–7. https://doi.org/10.1213/01.ane.0000250223.49963.0f.

81. McDonnell JG, Curley G, Carney J, Benton A, Costello J, Maharaj CH, Laffey JG. The analgesic efficacy of transversus abdominis plane block after cesarean delivery: a randomized controlled trial. Anesth Analg. 2008;106(1):186–91, table of contents. https://doi.org/10.1213/01.ane.0000290294.64090.f3.

82. Carney J, McDonnell JG, Ochana A, Bhinder R, Laffey JG. The transversus abdominis plane block provides effective postoperative analgesia in patients undergoing total abdominal hysterectomy. Anesth Analg. 2008;107(6):2056–60. https://doi.org/10.1213/ane.0b013e3181871313.

83. Aveline C, Le Hetet H, Le Roux A, Vautier P, Cognet F, Vinet E, Tison C, Bonnet F. Comparison between ultrasound-guided transversus abdominis plane and conventional ilioinguinal/iliohypogastric nerve blocks for day-case open inguinal hernia repair. Br J Anaesth. 2011;106(3):380–6. https://doi.org/10.1093/bja/aeq363.

84. Stewart BT, Woods RJ, Collopy BT, Fink RJ, Mackay JR, Keck JO. Early feeding after elective open colorectal resections: a prospective randomized trial. Aust N Z J Surg. 1998;68(2):125–8.

85. Lewis SJ, Egger M, Sylvester PA, Thomas S. Early enteral feeding versus "nil by mouth" after gastrointestinal surgery: systematic review and meta-analysis of controlled trials. BMJ. 2001;323(7316):773–6.

86. Barlow R, Price P, Reid TD, Hunt S, Clark GW, Havard TJ, Puntis MC, Lewis WG. Prospective multicentre randomised controlled trial of early enteral nutrition for patients undergoing major upper gastrointestinal surgical resection. Clin Nutr. 2011;30(5):560–6. https://doi.org/10.1016/j.clnu.2011.02.006.

87. McClave SA, Codner P, Patel J, Hurt RT, Allen K, Martindale RG. Should we aim for full enteral feeding in the first week of critical illness? Nutr Clin Pract. 2016;31(4):425–31. https://doi.org/10.1177/0884533616653809.

Philip E. George, Benjamin Tran,
and Brian P. Jacob

Introduction and Brief History

Incisional hernias are unfortunately very common despite modern advances in surgical technique. With around two million laparotomies being performed annually and an incidence rate ranging from 3 to 20% [1, 2], incisional ventral hernias are one of the biggest problems that a surgeon addresses. About 100,000–200,000 incisional hernia repairs are performed in the United States annually with a recurrence rate of up to 25% [3]. Knowing how to handle incisional hernias is therefore very important to the surgeons training, and limiting their recurrence is critical.

Incisional hernias are defined as a fascial defect in which any amount of intra-abdominal content can protrude through the opening. These hernias can cause pain, intolerance to oral intake, and can possibly lead to bowel obstruction or perforation. The types of incisional hernias can range from asymptomatic trocar site defects to massive midline defects which cause extreme lateralization of fascia and loss of abdominal wall domain. Because of the wide variety of incisional hernias, there exists no one classification system or accepted method of repair. Currently, there are numerous surgical techniques a surgeon may employ to repair ventral hernias. These include multiple open approaches and the minimally invasive approaches consisting of laparoscopy and robotic-assisted procedures.

The idea of minimally invasive surgery was first described by Hippocrates in the fourth century for the application of visualizing anatomy and pathology through natural orifices [4]. This method was improved upon throughout the centuries using various illumination technology, with major advances following the invention of the electric light bulb by Edison in 1879. By the second half of the nineteenth century, rigid endoscopic instruments with built-in light sources were widely used. The first true laparoscopic procedure was performed in 1901, in which an instrument was inserted through a posterior wall vaginal incision to visualize the pelvic and abdominal viscera. A Swedish surgeon, Hans Christian Jacobaeus, published the first clinical series in laparoscopic surgery and in doing so coined the term laparoscopy to define this revolutionary technique [5].

The first laparoscopic ventral hernia repair was described by LeBlanc in 1992 in a published case series demonstrating its feasibility [6]. After the widespread adoption of laparoscopy in the late twentieth century, many surgeons began employing this technique in the hopes of reducing patient's postoperative pain, length of stay and rates of hernia recurrence or de novo ventral hernias. However, the laparoscopic ventral hernia repair was not

P. E. George (✉) · B. Tran · B. P. Jacob
Department of Surgery, Mount Sinai Hospital of
New York, Icahn School of Medicine,
New York, NY, USA
e-mail: Philip.george@mountsinai.org

© Springer International Publishing AG, part of Springer Nature 2018
K. A. LeBlanc (ed.), *Laparoscopic and Robotic Incisional Hernia Repair*,
https://doi.org/10.1007/978-3-319-90737-6_4

regarded as a standard practice in many hospitals until the 2000s. Currently, the laparoscopic approach accounts for approximately 20–27% of all incisional hernia repairs [7, 8]. However, laparoscopy has inherent limitations including the limited degrees of motion of rigid laparoscopic instruments, a two-dimensional image through an unstable camera platform, and unfavorable ergonomics for the surgeon. These shortcomings have pushed the field of robot-assisted procedures and their application to hernia repair.

The use of robotic technology for surgical application was developed by the military in the 1970s. The incorporation of such technology in the operating room occurred in 1985, and was followed by the introduction and popularization of the da Vinci Surgical System (Intuitive Surgical, Sunnyvale, CA, USA) in the early 2000s. While the utilization of this technology has been well established in the fields of gynecology and urology, the operative applications of robotic surgery in hernia surgery remains a growing field. Benefits of robotic technology for surgery include three-dimensional imaging, improved ergonomics for the surgeon, and six degrees of motion to each instrument. Specific to ventral hernia repairs, the use of robotic technology when compared to the laparoscopic approach facilitates the surgeon's ability to suture mesh to the anterior abdominal wall [9]. However, there are limitations to the use of robotic technology as a tool for the general surgeon. The cost-effectiveness of robotic surgery has yet to be fully established, and studies have demonstrated an increase in the operative times of robotic-assisted versus laparoscopic procedures [10]. Given the current benefits and drawbacks of robotic-assisted surgery, it is our stance that such robotic-assisted surgery has an integral role in operations where the current minimally invasive approach of laparoscopy is not feasible. In such cases, robotic-assisted surgery can play a future role in replacing the historically standard open approach.

Primary Suture Repair

In the twentieth century, incisional hernia repairs were primarily completed using suture alone. This operation involves an open approach. An incision is made at the site of the prior scar, after which a careful dissection is completed down to the defect to locate the hernia sac. The hernia sac is excised, with any protruding abdominal viscera manually reduced into the peritoneum. Healthy fascial edges are then identified and approximated in a standard fascial closure fashion using nonabsorbable or slowly absorbable sutures. Many surgeons consider this technique to be suitable for defects less than 2 cm. While there is no data to support this indication, the argument is that the long-term risk of recurrence as compared to a repair with mesh is negligible. Another use for a primary suture repair is in grossly contaminated cases in which the use of nonabsorbable mesh is contraindicated. Overall, it is thought that over half of all primary incisional hernia repairs with this method will lead to recurrence, and its use has decreased in popularity with the advent of laparoscopy and utilization of mesh for such repairs.

Laparoscopic Repair

Following technological advancements such as the video camera and computer, minimally invasive surgery quickly gained a foothold in incisional hernia repair surgery. This technique involves achieving pneumoperitoneum, inserting trocars, and visualizing the fascial defect from the inside of the abdominal cavity. After careful examination, any adhesions to surrounding omentum and intestine are lysed. Following this, a primary suture repair can be achieved, but in most instances, laparoscopic incisional hernia repair involves mesh. The mesh is inserted through a trocar, limiting contact with skin flora, and fixed to the peritoneum with tacks and/or suture. There is debate over the optimal technique for fixing mesh during laparoscopic repair. Sole use of suture is associated with less postoperative pain, but also results in an increase in operative time, while observational studies have shown no difference in recurrence rate based on the use of suture or tacks [11, 12].

In a randomized controlled study by Itani et al. comparing laparoscopic and open ventral hernia repair, the laparoscopic group was found to have significantly lower postoperative pain, accelerated return to work, and fewer rates of seroma formation and wound infection postoperatively. Inherent to all laparoscopic procedures is the risk of injury to abdominal viscera and vasculature. This same study noted serious operative complications such as bowel injury and anesthesia-related complications as solely arising in the laparoscopic arm of the trial [13].

Mesh-Based Repair: Materials

The invention and adoption of prosthetic mesh redefined the field of incisional hernia repair. In the late nineteenth century, Theodor Billroth conceptualized the application of mesh in hernia repair, believing an artificial material with the density and strength of fascia would provide a cure to hernias. The ideal prosthetic mesh must be cost-effective, inert, sterile, cause a limited immune response, noncarcinogenic, and be resistant to significant force. Initially, prosthetic mesh was made of various materials including silver and stainless steel. These materials had a propensity to cause patient discomfort due to their rigidity and stiffness.

In the mid-twentieth century the first plastic-based mesh, made of the monofilament nylon, was developed. Reports of its use for inguinal repair showed distinct advantages over earlier materials, including fever, foreign body reactions, sepsis, and sinus tract infection [14]. However, future generations of plastic-based mesh replaced nylon, as nylon had a propensity to lose tensile strength over time and required removal in cases of infection. This ushered the use of polypropylene, a material that gained popularity for ventral hernia repair as it proved to be relatively inexpensive and flexible. Studies by its original investigator, Francis Usher, found that this plastic prosthesis could be incorporated into contaminated abdominal wall defects in animal models and still result in wound strengthening [15]. Other advantages of this material included the ability to cut the mesh to the desired specifications without fraying the edges, and the inflammatory response and fibrosis of the mesh around the surrounding tissues further increasing the strength of the repair.

A recent development in the field of hernia repair is biologic mesh. Biologic mesh utilizes acellular animal or human sources, free of cells and immunogenic material, as a scaffold of extracellular matrix for the host cells to propagate. Theoretical benefits of this technology include its use in cases at high infectious risk as the incorporation of native cells leads to revascularization around the mesh. Additionally, it is thought that these materials lead to a diminished inflammatory response compared to synthetic mesh and form fewer adhesions [16]. While these materials are being used by surgeons performing incisional hernia repairs today, data from randomized control trials is limited to its usefulness as prophylaxis for incisional hernia occurrence following elevated risk open surgery cases including organ transplant and open bariatric surgery [17–19]. Biologic mesh, currently more expensive than its synthetic counterpart, deserves further evaluation and study to determine its application in the diverse field of incisional hernia repair.

Mesh-Based Repair: Technique

Usher pioneered the field of mesh in hernia repair with his description of mesh placement "to bridge the defect" rather than reinforce tissues approximated under stress [20]. Incisional hernia repairs with mesh apply Laplace's Law by redistributing intra-abdominal pressure across the mesh. One randomized clinical trial comparing incisional hernia repair with mesh versus primary suture found the use of mesh significantly superior regarding lowering recurrence of hernia irrespective of hernia size. At 3 years, the rates of recurrence among patients with mesh was 24%, as compared to 43% in patient who underwent an operation with the primary suture technique [21]. For optimal distribution of such forces, it is necessary for the prosthesis to overlap the defect by at least 2 cm, with some surgeons opting for a more conservative 5 cm in each direction. The mesh is traditionally sutured and/or tacked to surrounding tissues. Some surgeons also use transfascial sutures which allow there to be less of a need for overlap of mesh in some spaces such as the pre-vesicular space or near the subcostal margins. However, the use of these sutures is thought to contribute to postoperative pain, with the sutures having the potential to strangulate muscle and entrap nerves.

Mesh can be placed anterior to the fascia, in the retro-rectus plane, in the preperitoneal or intraperitoneal space. The intraperitoneal space can be opened through an open repair but only with a large vertical wound and with extensive dissection, leading to higher incidences of morbidity including surgical site infections, postoperative pain, and recurrence. Laparoscopy with placement of an intraperitoneal mesh mitigates the incidence of these morbidities since it avoids a large incision but still includes placement of a covering mesh [22].

Tacking devices have been a large part of hernia surgeons' arsenal for some time, but the correct type and amount and use of tacks have never been fully researched. A study by Schoenmaeckers et al. determined that decreasing the number of tacks used per case from 40 to 20 significantly reduced pain as determined by the visual analog scale at 3 months, but there were several faults in the study such as not controlling for type of mesh [23]. Also, the results might not have any clinical significance. Multiple comparisons have been done comparing suture-only repairs versus tack-only repairs, but most studies have found to show no difference in recurrence or other complications with either techniques.

Component Separation

During the advancements of incisional hernia repairs in the twentieth century, surgeons became keenly aware of the necessity to reduce abdominal wall tension to obtain lasting repairs. An early technique utilized by surgeons involved incisions in the aponeurosis to relax the abdominal wall musculature. In 1990, Ramirez described the component separation technique adopted by the modern-day hernia surgeon [24]. The surgeon has the option between an anterior or posterior component separation. In the anterior approach, an extensive dissection of the skin and subcutaneous tissues is completed to isolate the anterior rectus sheath and external oblique muscle. The external oblique aponeurosis is then incised 2 cm lateral to the rectus sheath. The incision is extended superiorly and inferiorly to release tension on the abdominal wall. The posterior approach involves isolating the transverse abdominis muscle and releasing the muscle fibers off the posterior rectus sheath approximately 1 cm from the rectus muscle. Both techniques are essential to repairing select large, complex abdominal wall hernias, although a retrospective study has noted the incidence of wound infection to be higher with the anterior approach due to the extensive exposure of the subcutaneous tissue with this technique [25]. Further development of this technique has seen the implementation of laparoscopy and robotic surgery for posterior component separation to further limit wound infection, although this approach is technically challenging and limits the exposure necessary to perform an optimal abdominal wall release. These techniques have been shown to be feasible, but lacking evidence showing superiority towards previous repairs.

Access to the Reoperative Abdomen

In comparison to open technique, entry into the abdomen using a laparoscopic approach can be dangerous. As a rule of thumb, the safest point of entry is usually the patient's left upper quadrant, which is away from most midline defects and the effects of adhesions. Two or three finger breadths below the left subcostal margin at the mid-clavicular line is generally regarded as a good access point, also known as Palmer's point [26]. Using either Veress needle or "Optiview technique" is preferred. Using a Veress needle, the abdomen is entered by tactile sense and feedback until the layers of fascia are traversed and no resistance is encountered, at which point the abdomen is insufflated. The "Optiview technique" is where a laparoscope is inserted into a trocar, and the layers of the abdominal wall are visualized upon introduction of the trocar and allows the abdomen to be insufflated in the correct layer.

These techniques are not without their flaws and complications. Injury to bowel, bladder, vascular and other intra- or retroperitoneal organs can occur. Up to 50% of bowel and vascular injuries are undiagnosed at the time of surgery, with mortality rates ranging from 2 to 15%. Reducing the incidence of, and increasing the recognition of bowel or vascular injury is paramount to sound laparoscopy. A study of 10,837 patients undergoing laparoscopic hernia repair found that there were 76 (2.5%) cases of minor vascular injury, mostly to the epigastric vessels. Minimizing these injuries can be helped with direct visualization of primary or secondary trocars along with transillumination of the abdominal wall.

Open visualization of the abdominal cavity or Hassons technique might be useful in primary surgeries, but in repair of incisional hernias, open entry into the lateral abdominal wall might not be as fast or effective as other techniques. Some investigators believe that the incisions for direct entry might be too large and be subject to increased wound infections, as well as leakage of gas. There is also a decrease in visualization in obese patients that might be more suited to optical trocar insertion.

Once pneumoperitoneum is established, ideally two additional ports should be placed so that two instruments can work in tandem. Performing adhesiolysis in reoperative cases can be dangerous and time consuming. It is generally accepted to try to avoid electrocautery as much as possible in cases of adhesiolysis, as electrocurrent or heat can be transmitted to nearby bowel very easily. A laparoscopic scissor device can be used to sharply lyse adhesions, and generous use of clips should be used for visibly bleeding vessels (Figs. 4.1 and 4.2).

When undergoing an open repair of an incisional hernia on the other hand, the surgeon uses the old incision itself as the entry point which allows direct visualization of the bowel and abdominal wall. This approach however, identified by numerous prospective and randomized studies has a higher incidence of overall complications.

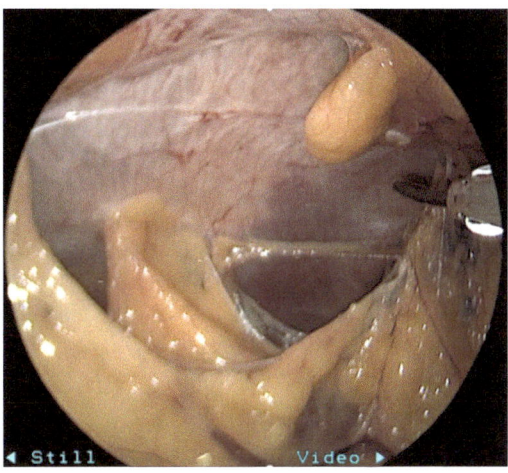

Fig. 4.1 Intra-abdominal adhesions in a patient with prior laparotomies

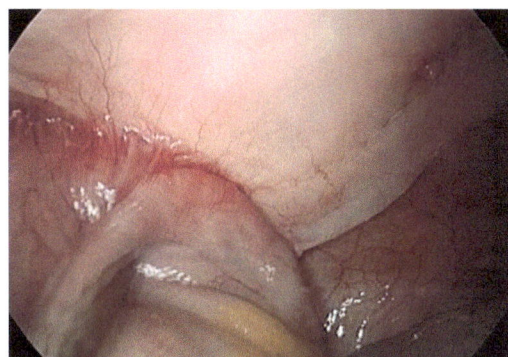

Fig. 4.2 Adhesions can also cause bowel to be adherent directly against the abdominal wall. This is a patient with small bowel adhesed to a prior trocar site

Comparison of Techniques

After measuring the defect in preparation for closure, some surgeons choose to close the primary defect before laying a mesh over the closure. There are multiple reasons for this, such as greater surface area of interface of the mesh with the abdominal wall, as well as prevention of possible bulging of the mesh back into the defect during the healing process. There are multiple ways of closing the defects which include intracorporeal suturing, extracorporeal suturing using a laparoscopic suture passer, or a hybrid open approach prior to a laparoscopic mesh placement. Clapp et al. studied the difference in outcomes with patients who underwent primary closure vs. those without and found that those who underwent primary closure prior to mesh placement had significantly lower recurrence rates, seroma rates, and higher patient satisfaction scores [27].

It is widely known that placing a mesh reduces recurrence rates, but when placing a mesh, where does one decide to place it? There are several different layers of the abdominal wall where a mesh can be placed but no consensus on how to describe the layers. Recently, a large Facebook-based hernia collaboration, The International Hernia Collaboration was polled on how to describe the placements of the certain layers of mesh, to simplify discussion [28]. A mesh that overlies the rectus muscles should be referred to as an "onlay," a mesh that is between the rectus muscles to bridge the gap should be referred to as an "inlay," mesh that lies behind the rectus muscles should be referred to as "retro-muscular," a mesh that is below the muscle but above the peritoneum should be referred to as "preperitoneal," and a mesh that is below the peritoneum should be called "intraperitoneal."

The intraperitoneal onlay mesh (IPOM) procedure is the most commonly practiced ventral hernia repair, and is generally regarded as a better repair than open repair for simpler cases without loss of abdominal wall domain with faster return to work, decreased blood loss and decreased postoperative pain. Some studies show that there is a decrease in hernia recurrence rate as well. A possible reasoning behind this is that the intraperitoneal pressure is distributed along the entire surface of the mesh as opposed to just the suture line like in conventional repair [29]. The technique involves placement of a mesh intraperitoneally with suture or tack fixation along the perimeter as well as the inside, with or without primary suture repair of the hernia. There has never been shown to be any difference in recurrence rates between cases in which the primary hernia defect was repaired or not. The difficulty of the repair lies in the lysis of adhesions that sometimes must be performed as well as obtaining the angle for placement of the tacks if they are used, or even more so the placement of intraperitoneal sutures.

Preperitoneal placement of the mesh involves careful dissection of the peritoneum from all areas of the projected mesh placement in one solid piece, to reattach it over top of the mesh. In theory, this reduces the risk of complications involving mesh contact to bowel such as erosion or adhesions, but has never panned out in actual studies. Many studies have evaluated laparoscopic preperitoneal mesh placement and intraperitoneal mesh placement with almost no differences in patient outcomes but showing that the cost of preperitoneal placement of the mesh is less than intraperitoneal, factoring in tacking devices.

Single Incision/Port Surgery

Single port surgery has been in use for appendectomy and cholecystectomy with widespread use. Its use for ventral incisional hernia repair has been limited. Limiting port sites and potential future hernias is always of great interest to the hernia surgeon, but few studies have been published on the matter. A recent case series show the use of the S-PORT platform (Storz, Tuttlingen, Germany) and its feasibility of use with similar costs to standard laparoscopic repair, with similar incision size to the largest incision in the standard repair. However, larger studies with randomization must be undergone before recommendations for its use can be made. A recent 2017 meta-analysis showed that in comparison to conventional laparoscopy, single site incision surgery through the umbilicus was shown to have a higher rate of trocar site hernias [30].

Robotic Incisional Hernia Repair

Robotic use with ventral hernia repair has been contemplated since its inception, but the first reported use of suture only intracorporeal mesh fixation which was published in 2007. This was one of the first studies to document both feasibility of using robotics in ventral hernia care, but also that there was no need for tacking devices or extracorporeal suturing (Fig. 4.3).

Some surgeons started using robotic-assistance during cases to more easily suture the primary defect close prior to mesh placement. In a study comparing defect closure with robotic assistance versus no closure and laparoscopic mesh placement, there was found to be no difference in wound complications or recurrence with an additional operative time for robotic cases [31] (Fig. 4.4).

Because of the ease of use of the robot, several groups are using it routinely to try to make more difficult open hernia repair operations simpler. The Rives-Stoppa retro-muscular mesh placement is sometimes difficult with increased complication rates because of the large open incision but can be performed robotically by certain groups. A study by Warren et al. showed, with a small group, that robotic Rives-Stoppa repair had a decrease in surgical site infection rate, shorter length of stay and less blood loss with no difference in cost or operating time [32]. The study did remark on the learning curve

of the procedure, with the initial procedure taking about 6 h to perform, with their latest taking only 2.5 h.

Conclusion

Laparoscopic and robotic incisional hernia repairs have evolved greatly since the course of their inception. Reducing the size of the incisions, using mesh as adjunct coverage, and reducing postoperative pain have all been sequelae from the minimally invasive techniques. If laparoscopy is not available or the surgeon is not comfortable with laparoscopy, the use of robotic technology might offer an advantage still over the open approach for some surgeries. As technology improves and different strategies are formed, the reduction in patient morbidity will follow.

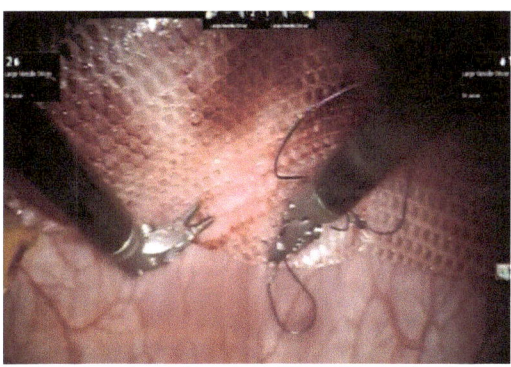

Fig. 4.3 Example of robotic intracorporeal suturing

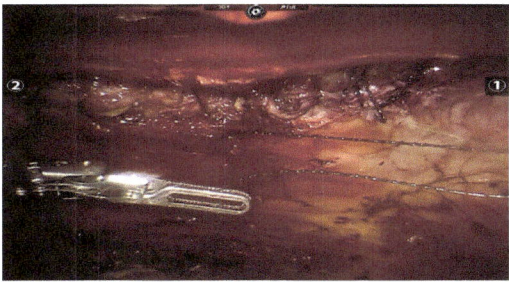

Fig. 4.4 Example of the robotic assistance of primary defect closure

References

1. Bucknall TE, Cox PJ, Ellis H. Burst abdomen and incisional hernia: a prospective study of 1129 major laparotomies. Br Med J. 1982;284(6320):931.
2. Sanders DL, Kingsnorth AN. The modern management of incisional hernias. Br Med J. 2012;344:e2843.
3. Flum DR, Horvath K, Koepsell T. Have outcomes of incisional hernia repair improved with time? A population-based analysis. Ann Surg. 2003;237(1):129–35.
4. Kaiser AM. Evolution and future of laparoscopic colorectal surgery. World J Gastroenterol. 2014;20:15119–24.
5. Jacobaeus HC. Ueber die Möglichkeit die Zystoskopie bei Untersuchungen seröser Höhlungen anzuwenden. Munch Med Wochenschr. 1910;57:2090–19.
6. LeBlanc KA, Booth WV. Laparoscopic repair of incisional abdominal hernias using expanded polytetrafluoroethylene: preliminary findings. Surg Laparosc Endosc. 1993;3:39–41.
7. Alexander AM, Scott DJ. Laparoscopic ventral hernia repair. Surg Clin North Am. 2013;93:1091–110.
8. Funk LM, Perry KA, Narula VK, Mikami DJ, Melvin WS. Current national practice patterns for inpatient management of ventral abdominal wall hernia in the United States. Surg Endosc. 2013;27:4104–12.
9. Vorst AL, Kaoutzanis C, Carbonell A, Franz M. Evolution and advances in laparoscopic ventral and incisional hernia repair. World J Gastrointest Surg. 2015;7(11):293–305.
10. Chen JY, Huynh D, Nguyen S, Chin E, Divino C, Zhang L. Outcomes of robot assisted versus laparoscopic repair of small-sized ventral hernias. Surg Endosc. 2017;31:1275–9.

11. Bansal VK, Misra MC, Kumar S, Rao YK, Singhal P, Goswami A, Guleria S, Arora MK, Chabra A. A prospective randomized study comparing suture mesh fixation versus tacker mesh fixation for laparoscopic repair of incisional and ventral hernias. Surg Endosc. 2011;25(5):1431–8.

12. Greenstein AJ, Nguyen SQ, Buch KE, Chin EH, Weber KJ, Divino CM. Recurrence after laparoscopic ventral hernia repair: a prospective pilot study of suture versus tack fixation. Am Surg. 2008;74(3):227–31.

13. Itani KMF, Hur K, Kim LT, Anthony T, Berger DH, Reda D, Neumayer L. for the Veterans Affairs Ventral Incisional Hernia Investigators. Comparison of laparoscopic and open repair with mesh for the treatment of ventral incisional hernia: a randomized trial. Arch Surg. 2010;145(4):322–8.

14. Read RC. Milestones in the history of hernia surgery: prosthetic repair. Hernia. 2004;8:8–14.

15. Handley WS. A method for the radical cure of inguinal hernia (darn and stay-lace method). Practitioner. 1918;100:466–71.

16. Ibrahim AM, Vargas CR, Colakoglu S, Nguyen JT, Lin SJ, Lee BT. Properties of meshes used in hernia repair: a comprehensive review of synthetic and biologic meshes. J Reconstr Microsurg. 2015;31:83–94.

17. Sarr MG, Hutcher NE, Snyder S, Hodde J, Carmody B. A prospective, randomized, multicenter trial of Surgisis Gold, a biologic prosthetic, as a sublay reinforcement of the fascial closure after open bariatric surgery. Surgery. 2014;156:902–8.

18. Llaguna OH, Avgerinos DV, Nagda P, Elfant D, Leitman IM, Goodman E. Does prophylactic biological mesh placement protect against the development of incisional hernia in high-risk patients? World J Surg. 2011;35:1651–5.

19. Brewer MB, Rada EM, Milburn ML, Goldberg NH, Singh DP, Cooper M, Silverman RP. Human acellular dermal matrix for ventral hernia repair reduces morbidity in transplant patients. Hernia. 2011;15:141–5.

20. Read RC, Usher FC. Herniologist of the twentieth century. Hernia. 1999;3:167–71.

21. Luijendijk RW, Hop WC, van den Tol MP, de Lange DC, Braaksma MM, IJzermans JN, Boelhouwer RU, de Vries BC, Salu MK, Wereldsma JC, Bruijninckx CM, Jeekel J. A comparison of suture repair with mesh repair for incisional hernia. N Engl J Med. 2000;343:392–8.

22. Cobb WS, Kercher KW, Heniford BT. Laparoscopic repair of incisional hernias. Surg Clin North Am. 2005;85:91–103.

23. Schoenmaeckers EJ, de Haas RJ, Stirler V, Raymakers JT, Rakic S. Impact of the number of tacks on postoperative pain in laparoscopic repair of ventral hernias: do more tacks cause more pain? Surg Endosc. 2012;26:357–60.

24. Ramirez OM, Ruas E, Dellon AL. "Components separation" method for closure of abdominal-wall defects: an anatomic and clinical study. Plast Reconstr Surg. 1990;86(3):519–26.

25. Krpata DM, Blatnik JA, Novitsky YW, Rosen MJ. Posterior and open anterior components separations: a comparative analysis. Am J Surg. 2012;203:318–22.

26. Krishnakumar S, Tambe P. Entry complications in laparoscopic surgery. J Gynecol Endosc Surg. 2009;1(1):4–11.

27. Clapp ML, Hicks SC, Awad SS, Liang MK. Transcutaneous Closure of Central Defects (TCCD) in laparoscopic ventral hernia repairs (LVHR). World J Surg. 2013;37:42–51.

28. Muysoms F, Jacob B. International hernia collaboration consensus on nomenclature of abdominal wall hernia repair. World J Surg. 2018;42(1):302–4.

29. Prasad P, Tantia OM, Patle NM, Khanna S, Sen B. Laparoscopic ventral hernia repair: a comparative study of transabdominal preperitoneal versus intraperitoneal onlay mesh repair. J Laparoendosc Adv Surg Tech. 2011;21(6):477–83.

30. Antoniou SA, Garcia-Alamino JM, Hajibandeh S, Hajibandeh S, Weitzendorfer M, Muysoms FE, Granderath FA, Chalkiadakis GE, Emmanuel K, Antoniou GA, Gioumidou M, Iliopoulou-Kosmadaki S, Mathioudaki M, Souliotis K. Single-incision surgery trocar-site hernia: an updated systematic review meta-analysis with trial sequential analysis by the Minimally Invasive Surgery Synthesis of Interventions Outcomes Network (MISSION). Surg Endosc. 2018;32(1):14–23.

31. Gonzalez AM, Romero RJ, Seetharamaiah R, Gallas M, Lamoureux J, Rabaza JR. Laparoscopic ventral hernia repair with primary closure versus no primary closure of the defect: potential benefits of the robotic technology. Int J Med Robot. 2015;11:120–5.

32. Warren JA, Cobb WS, Ewing JA, Carbonell AM. Standard laparoscopic versus robotic retromuscular ventral hernia repair. Surg Endosc. 2017;31(1):324–32.

Karl A. LeBlanc

Introduction

The use of prosthetic biomaterials in the repair of hernias of the abdominal wall is now very commonplace throughout the world. In the USA over 95% of all inguinal and ventral hernias are repaired with a prosthetic material or device and some countries are also beginning to approach this figure. In other parts of the world, this is not the case. Limitations on the use of these products include a natural reluctance to place a biomaterial into a primary hernia or the cost of these products. Increasing usage of these products is due to the fact that recurrence rates are markedly decreased with their use (this is described in other chapters in this text).

Incisional hernias will develop in at least 13% and perhaps as many as 20% of laparotomy incisions. The risk of herniation is increased by fivefold if a postoperative wound infection occurs. Other factors that predispose to the development of a fascial defect include smoking, obesity, poor nutritional status, steroid usage, etc. While some of these may be avoided, those patients that are found to have such a hernia can present difficult

management problems due to the high potential for recurrence. It has been known for many years that without the use of a prosthetic material, the recurrence rate for ventral hernia repair is as high as 51% [1]. The use of a synthetic material will reduce this rate to 10–24% [2]. While these publications are older, they are still relevant in today's management of hernia repair. Recent data still reveals a recurrence rate of 17.1% without the use of mesh, 12.3% with open mesh repair, and 10.6% with laparoscopic mesh repair [3]. There are numerous other papers that reinforce this fact.

The laparoscopic repair of incisional and ventral hernias was first performed in 1991 using the Soft Tissue Patch made by W.L. Gore and Associates (Elkhart, DE, USA) [4]. The recurrence rate that has been reported in other recent literature varies from 0 to 11% but averages approximately 5.5%. There are a variety of factors that influence recurrence rates that are discussed in other chapters of this text. The "ideal" prosthetic product has yet to be found. The hernia that is being repaired and the status of the patient into which this material will be placed should dictate the type of material that will be chosen. This chapter will identify these goals and the properties of the various biomaterials that are on the market today.

There are many different products that can be used in the repair of hernias of the abdominal wall. In many of the products listed below there is a paucity of published literature that verifies the claims that are made by the manufacturers. It is

K. A. LeBlanc
Surgeons Group of Baton Rouge, Our Lady of the Lake Physician Group, Clinical Professor, Surgery, Louisiana State University Health Sciences Center, Baton Rouge, LA, USA

© Springer International Publishing AG, part of Springer Nature 2018
K. A. LeBlanc (ed.), *Laparoscopic and Robotic Incisional Hernia Repair*,
https://doi.org/10.1007/978-3-319-90737-6_5

very difficult to find Level 1 studies that evaluate the success or failure of the respective materials. While this is the situation at the time of the production of this textbook, the reader is advised to reference the available journals to identify the uses and results of these materials. Much of the information discussed was obtained from the respective manufacturer directly but not in all cases. Therefore, the reader should reference the particular manufacturer for in-depth information and current product availability that cannot be provided in this text.

Indications for Use of Prosthetic Materials

Surgeons recognize that the main purpose in the use of these materials will be the repair of a fascial defect in the abdominal wall. The main indications of use of the materials are listed in Table 5.1.

Musculofascial tissue strength can be lost in a variety of ways. The most common, of course, would be due to the external etiology of the weakness that develops after a laparotomy or other abdominal incision that is larger than that of the 5 mm laparoscopic trocar (although even this small incision can rarely develop a hernia). Another example would be the loss of tissue with trauma such as gunshot wounds and/or treatment with an open abdomen. The increase of intra-abdominal pressure that results from significant weight gain will result in an internal source of weakening of the abdominal wall musculature. Poor nutrition and/or protein malnutrition are also sources of such problems. Other predisposing factors such as emphysema

or the chronic bronchitis of individuals that smoke tobacco products results in a constant increase in intra-abdominal pressure because of a frequent cough. Life-threatening infections such as fasciitis and gangrene will produce large areas of necrosis and resultant tissue loss. More frequently, the development of a postoperative wound infection will increase the risk of herniation by as much a five times. In fact, almost 30% of patients that develop a postoperative incisional wound infection will eventually develop an incisional hernia [5]. Modern needs of patients have resulted in the development of products that are not permanent such as biologic meshes or synthetic products that resorb over varying lengths of time.

The effects of aging and the declining ability of the elderly patients to repair the native tissues will lead to the loss of fascial integrity. This is commonly seen with the direct inguinal hernia. It also occurs with the enlargement of the linea alba that is referred to as diastasis recti. These latter defects can enlarge and occasionally become symptomatic, requiring repair. The disruption of collagen that is seen by the effects of smoking will have a similar effect (i.e., metastatic emphysema).

The most common defect that results from a denervation phenomenon follows the flank incision that is utilized in a nephrectomy, lumbar sympathectomy or an anterior approach to the lumbar interbody fusion for degenerative disc disease or traumatic events. In these entities, there is no defined fascial edge that is seen with the more common anterior abdominal wall defects. This is due to the broad surface of the denervated musculature that has intact fascia but lacks the reinforcement of healthy muscle tissue. These are very challenging to repair and such methods are described elsewhere in this text. Mesh materials are necessary for these problems to assure as durable a repair as feasible.

All of these biomaterials were attempting to address the "ideal characteristics" that were promulgated by Cumberland and Scales [6, 7]. While it is widely felt that the ideal material has yet to be found, these criteria are the goals that are sought by the manufacturers (Table 5.2).

Table 5.1 Indications for prostheses

Replacement of lost musculofascial tissue caused by:
Trauma
External
Internal
Infection
Reinforcement of native tissue weakness
Aging (laxity of tissues)
Neurological deficit (denervation)

Table 5.2 Ideal characteristics of synthetic products

No physical modification by tissue fluids	Chemically inert
Does not incite inflammatory or foreign body reaction	Does not produce allergy or hypersensitivity
Noncarcinogenic	Resistant to mechanical strains
Can be fabricated to the form required	Sterilizable

Table 5.3 Ideal surgical clinical characteristics of synthetic products

Permanent repair of the abdominal wall (i.e., no recurrences)
Ingrowth characteristics that result in a normal pattern of tissue repair and healing
No alteration of the compliance of the abdominal wall musculature
Lack of adhesion predisposition
Cuts easily and without fraying
Inexpensive
Lack of long-term complications such as pain or fistualization

While the clinical uses of these prosthetic materials share these considerations, the operating surgeon does, in fact, desire slightly different priorities in the use of the prosthesis within his or her individual patient. Disregarding the obvious need to be noncarcinogenic, the clinical characteristics of the "ideal surgical" material are listed in Table 5.3.

Biologic prostheses are based upon the use of porcine, bovine, or cadaveric tissues to produce a collagen matrix. These materials are not truly absorbable as they are intended to provide a scaffold for the native fibroblasts to incorporate natural collagen to repair a fascial defect. It is the goal of these devices to repair the hernia defect with the tissues of the patient as these will be degraded and replaced over time.

The synthetic prosthetic materials can be divided into the absorbable and nonabsorbable products. The synthetic nonabsorbable materials are of many types, sizes, and shapes. The use of these products is commonplace in the repair of virtually all hernias. There has been an increase in the number of synthetic absorbable products over the last several years. More recently there are hybrid products that include both absorbable and nonabsorbable layers. These attempt to capitalize on the attributes of both of these technologies.

The materials that are presented below are given in an arbitrary arrangement and with an accurate information that could be obtained. An effort was made, however, to stratify these products in a classification that grouped similar products together. I have attempted to identify all of the currently available products that are used in most parts of the world at the time of publication. Some of these materials have either no published clinical data or scant information as to the clinical performance characteristics. Therefore, it is certain, that some products and/or details have been overlooked despite my efforts to present all that I could identify. Due to the very large variation in the sizes of the products, little comment regarding the sizes of these products will be given. Additionally, due to the recent surge in techniques that allow the placement of mesh in different layers of the abdominal wall, the reader should be certain that the products described here can be used in the location that is selected during the operation in which it is used.

The reader is referred to the respective manufacturer for these details. It should also be noted that not all of these products are available in all countries. Manufacturers have limited the release of many of them to only selected areas of the world or have not obtained the necessary governmental approvals for clinical distribution at the time of this writing. Finally, it is certain that all of the available products are not included in this compilation or that some of those listed are no longer available due to the lag in this research and actual publication. Many companies are quite small and/or have limited distribution. Therefore, if any of these are not included it was not because of an intended omission but rather a lack of obtainable information.

Absorbable Prosthetic Biomaterials

The general purpose of these products is the temporary replacement of absent tissue (Table 5.4).

Table 5.4 Absorbable products

Bio-A, W. L. Gore & Associates, Elkhart, DE, USA
Dexon, Medtronic, Minneapolis, MN, USA
Safil Mesh, B. Braun Surgical, Germany
TIGR mesh, Novus Scientific Pte Ltd., Singapore
Phasix mesh, CR Bard, Providence, RI, USA
Phasix ST mesh, CR Bard, Providence, RI, USA
Vicryl (knitted) mesh, Ethicon, Inc., Somerville, NJ, USA
Vicryl (woven) mesh, Ethicon, Inc., Somerville, NJ, USA

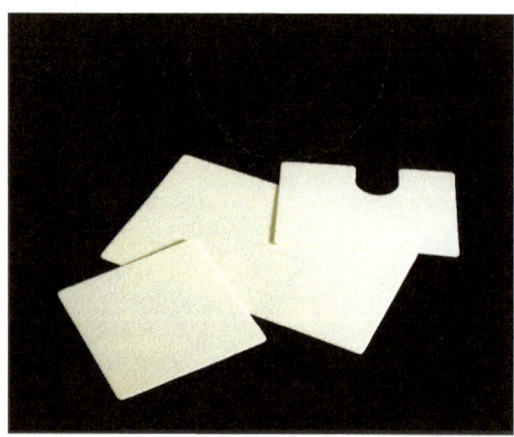

Fig. 5.1 Bio-A

The strength of these materials and the lack of permanency make some of them unsuitable for the permanent repair of any hernia (although research is being conducted on this question). Newer research has suggested that they might be preferred in some circumstances rather than a true biologic. This may be due to the fact that biologics require degradation then rebuilding of the collagen of the patient's fascia. These materials do not require the extent of cellular degradation that true biological materials require and seem to progress to reconstructive metabolism more rapidly. This is an area of ongoing research. Clinical usage will be dependent upon the longevity of the material that is sought by the surgeon.

Bio-A, *Phasix*, and *TIGR* meshes represent a somewhat newer concept in synthetic materials. This field of materials perhaps represents part of the next phase of mesh development. As will be seen below, combination products have now been developed with a permanent backbone and the absorbable materials listed here. The *Bio-A* product is supplied in flat sheet (Fig. 5.1). It is made of trimethylene carbonate and polyglycolic acid. It will maintain approximately 70% of its tensile strength for 21 days. It serves as a scaffold to allow for fibroblastic infiltration and replacement by the patient's native collagen. Recent studies have shown efficacy for complex situations [8].

Safil Mesh is a warp-knitted polyglycolic acid material that will retain 50% of its strength at 20 days and is totally resorbed in 60–90 days (Fig. 5.2). It is used to strengthen the closure of the abdominal and chest walls. The above photo

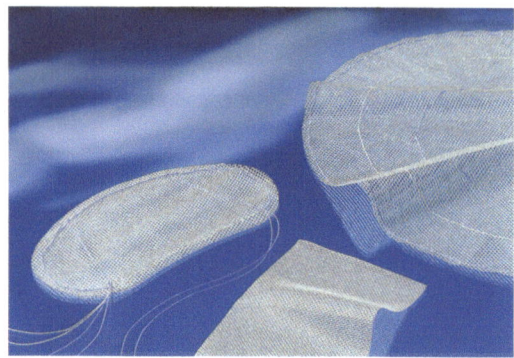

Fig. 5.2 Safil mesh

also shows the bags into which this material is also shaped for use in splenic preservation.

Phasix is composed of poly-4-hydroxybutyrate (P4HB). This is produced from byproducts of *E. coli* metabolism (Fig. 5.3). It is degraded by hydrolysis and hydrolytic enzymatic processes. The absorption of the material is minimal until about 26 weeks postimplantation and is essentially complete in about 52 weeks. The material is also available with a barrier coating of carboxymethylcellulose and hyaluronic acid as *Phasix ST* (Fig. 5.4). This product is placed in the intraperitoneal position against the intestine. There are many investigations that are ongoing to learn the unique properties of this product.

TIGR Matrix Surgical Mesh is knitted from two different synthetic resorbable fibers, polyglycolic acid and polylactic acid (Fig. 5.5). The Matrix is warp-knitted in a proprietary way, allowing it to

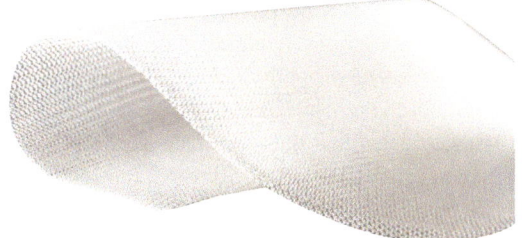

Fig. 5.3 Phasix mesh

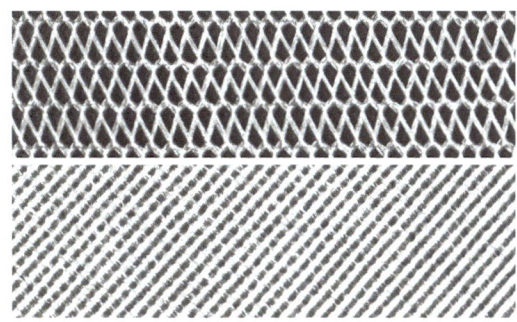

Fig. 5.6 Vicryl (knitted) and woven (lower). (Images courtesy of Ethicon, Inc.)

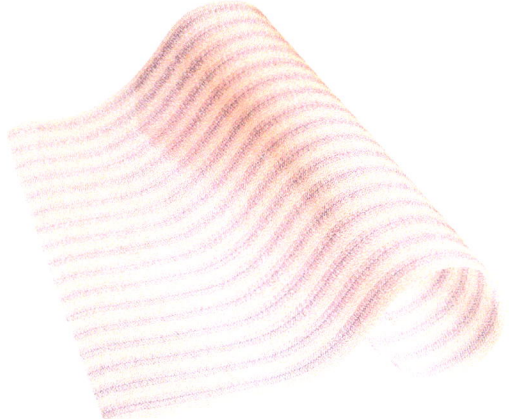

Fig. 5.4 Phasix ST

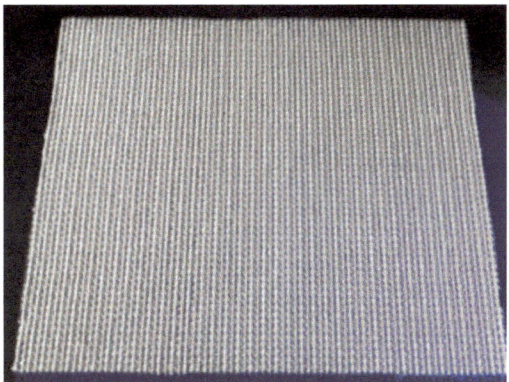

Fig. 5.7 Dexon mesh

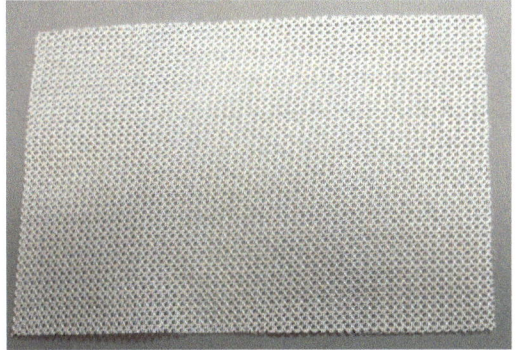

Fig. 5.5 TIGR mesh

gradually degrade over time. The strength of the Matrix is comparable to conventional mesh implants for the initial 6–9 months following implantation. The first fiber (polyglycolic acid) appears to lose its functional capabilities in 2 weeks while the second fiber (polylactic acid) maintains its strength for approximately 9 months.

The *Vicryl* and *Dexon* meshes are primarily polylactic acid (Figs. 5.6 and 5.7). The Vicryl is available in a knitted or woven configuration as noted in the figure. These products can be affixed onto the fascia directly with sutures but are not of sufficient durability to formally repair a defect. Most frequently these are used to provide a buttress of support for the temporary closure of an infected incisional wound of the abdomen or in the patient with intra-abdominal sepsis or abdominal compartment syndrome. They have also been used in the treatment of complex or very large hernias that will be repaired in a staged fashion. In that instance, this product will be placed as a bridge and the patient will be returned to the operating room within a few days to perform the definitive procedure. These represent a less costly alternative to biologic materials for this application.

Biologic Products

These products do not represent a new concept in hernia repair and were used in the early 1900's. They are a marked improvement over the materials developed earlier in the last century. They are based upon a harvested collagen matrix that is manufactured into sheets of tissue-engineered materials that can be used to repair defects in the abdominal wall. The concept of these materials is that the biologic material will allow the migration of the patient's own fibroblasts onto them so that collagen will be deposited to form a "neo-fascia." For the most part, these are used in open techniques but there has been some usage in laparoscopic methods especially in the repair of hiatal hernias.

There are similarities of all of the biologic products. They are the most expensive of all prosthetic materials that repair or replace the abdominal wall fascia. They are all harvested from an organism that was once alive. The source will dictate the size of the material and, in most cases, the thickness of the product. The thickness will be variable in nearly all of them. Some manufacturers have found creative techniques to increase the size of the materials available. All of the products are processed to eliminate all cellular and nuclear material as well as any prions. Following this, another process can be applied to crosslink the collagen at the molecular level. There is only one product that is currently cross-linked as discussed below. The final stage is the sterilization of the prosthesis. It is beyond the scope of this chapter to cover all of these in detail. However, it should be considered, when using any of these materials, that the processing plays a large part into the characteristics and the clinical behavior of them postimplantation.

In general, the biologic products were introduced for use in contaminated fields such as a synthetic mesh infection. While they can be used in this manner, it is recommended that the wound should not possess gross pus as the collagenases of some bacteria and inflammatory cells can degrade these products. These products are sometimes used in the repair of very complex noninfected hernias as well. One concern will be that if the patient possesses an undiagnosed collagen deficiency disorder, the remodeling of these products will not occur properly, leading to a predictable failure of the repair. It has also be learned over the last few years that these products perform best if they have direct contact with some type of vascularized tissue. Intuitively, if the expectation of these biologic scaffolds to become infiltrated by fibroblasts and subsequent collagen deposition, blood supply will deliver these cells more rapidly. Consequently, a higher failure rate will be noted if a biologic prosthesis is used as a "bridge" between fascial edges. It is recommended that if a bridge is unavoidable, then use of the peritoneum of the hernia sac can provide a source of vascular supply.

Bovine Products

The bovine products are from dermis or pericardium (Table 5.5). Only the *SurgiMend* is fetal (dermal) tissue (Fig. 5.8). As shown in the figure, it is available in four different sizes. The associated numbers are the thickness of the four different products in millimeters. *SurgiMend-e* is specifically designed for ventral hernia repair

Table 5.5 Bovine biologic prostheses

SurgiMend 1.0,2.0,3.0,4.0, Integra LifeSciences, USA
SurgiMend-e, Integra LifeSciences, USA
SurgiMend MP, Integra LifeSciences, USA
Tutomesh, RTI Biologics, Alachua, FL, USA
Tutopatch, RTI Biologics, Alachua, FL, USA
Veritas, Baxter Healthcare Corporation, Deerfield, IL, USA

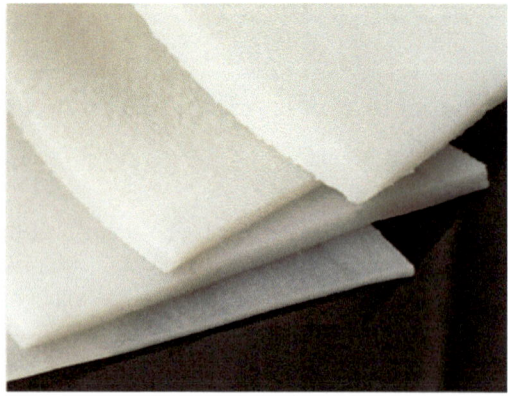

Fig. 5.8 SurgiMend 1-2-3-4

(Fig. 5.9). It is elliptical in shape, perforated, and available in 3 mm or 4 mm thicknesses. *Surgimend MP* is similar to the former product in that it is available in four different thicknesses but is also perforated over its entirety (Fig. 5.10).

Tutomesh and *Tutopatch* are of the same source (pericardium) and are processed in the same manner (Figs. 5.11 and 5.12). The only difference in

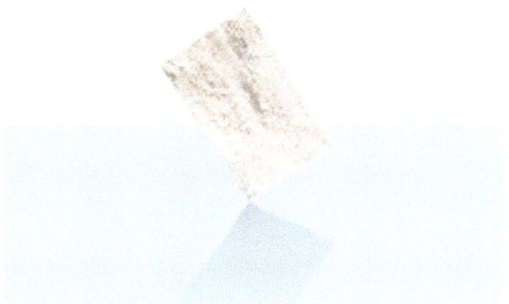

Fig. 5.12 Tutopatch

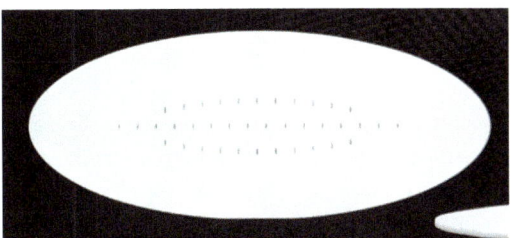

Fig. 5.9 SurgiMend-e

Fig. 5.10 Surgimend MP

Fig. 5.13 Veritas

these two is that the Tutomesh is perforated while Tutopatch is not. *Veritas* is also pericardium and does not require rehydration (Fig. 5.13). The use of all of these bovine products has generally been limited to the incisional hernia repair.

Cadaveric Products

The human cadaveric products have a long history (Table 5.6). There is significant variability in the amount of stretch that each of these will undergo either at the time of implantation and subsequent to the procedure. This stretch varies from product to product and should be accounted for at the time of implantation. These products are not cross-linked and require rehydration. These are also used in the repair of hiatal hernias. *AlloMax* Surgical Graft is 0.8–1.8 mm thick (Fig. 5.14). *Cortiva* and *Cortiva 1 mm* are similar materials that are in two different thicknesses. *Cortiva* is thicker at 1.3 mm (0.8–1.8 mm) and *Cortiva 1 mm* is 1 mm (0.8–1.2 mm) (Fig. 5.15). *DermaMatrix* is used for hernia repair but is additionally used for purposes other than hernia

Fig. 5.11 Tutomesh

Table 5.6 Cadaveric biologic prostheses

AlloMax, Davol, Inc., Warwick, RI, USA
Cortiva, RTI Surgical, Alachua, FL, USA
Cortiva 1 mm, RTI Surgical, Alachua, FL, USA
DermaMatrix, Synthes CMF, West Chester, PA, USA
FlexHD STRUCTURAL, Ethicon, Inc., Somerville, NJ, USA

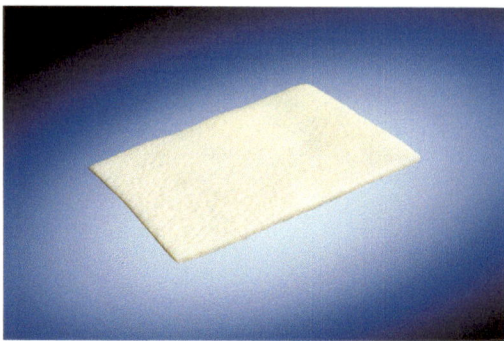

Fig. 5.14 Allomax

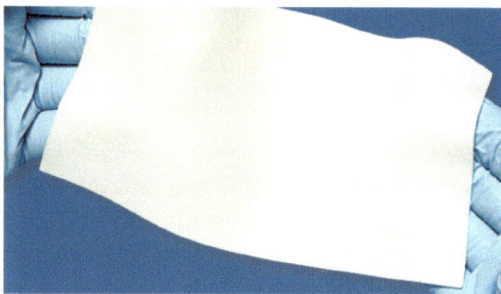

Fig. 5.15 Cortiva

Fig. 5.16 DermaMatrix

repair (Fig. 5.16). It is available in thicknesses of 0.2–0.4 mm, 0.4–0.8 mm, 0.8–1.7 mm, and ≥1.8 mm. It is notched so that if the notch is in the upper left the epidermal side (basement membrane) is facing up. It is recommended that the dermal side be placed against vascularized tissue. *Flex HD Structural* is available in a thick version (0.8–1.7 mm) or an Ultra Thick version (1.8–4 mm). The Musculoskeletal Transplant Foundation produces the latter two products.

Porcine Products

There are a number of these materials that are available (Table 5.7). Depending on the manufacturer, they are in different sizes and shapes and construction. Some are laminated, some are cross-linked, some are perforated, some require rehydration, and others do not. These are specific to the product and it is recommended that the user follow the instructions for use (IFU) that is provided with each product.

BioDesign Hernia Grafts are three products that are designed for the repair of specific hernias, ventral, inguinal, and hiatal (Figs. 5.17, 5.18, and 5.19). They are all developed from por-

Table 5.7 Porcine biologic prostheses

Biodesign, Cook Surgical, Inc., Bloomington, IN, USA
Cellis, Meccellis Biotech, La Rochelle, France
Fortiva, RTI Biologics, Alachua, FL, USA
Gentrix Surgical Matrix, ACell, Columbia, MD, USA
Permacol, Medtronic, Minneapolis, MN, USA
Strattice RTM, Acelity, San Antonio, TX, USA
XenMatrix, Davol, Inc., Warwick, RI, USA
XenMatrix AB, Davol, Inc., Warwick, RI, USA
XCM Biologic Tissue Matrix, Ethicon, Somerville, NJ, USA

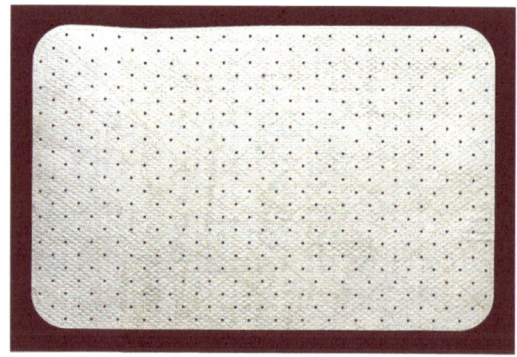

Fig. 5.17 Biodesign hernia graft

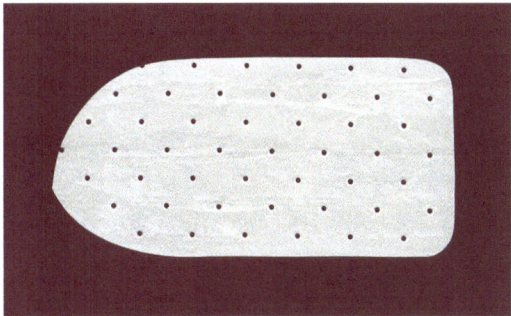

Fig. 5.18 Biodesign inguinal hernia graft

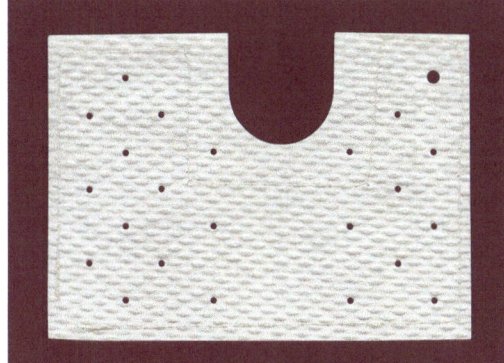

Fig. 5.19 Biodesign hiatal hernia graft

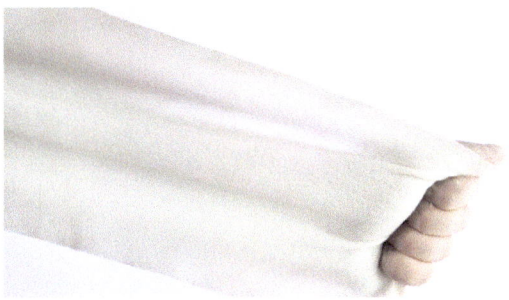

Fig. 5.20 Cellis

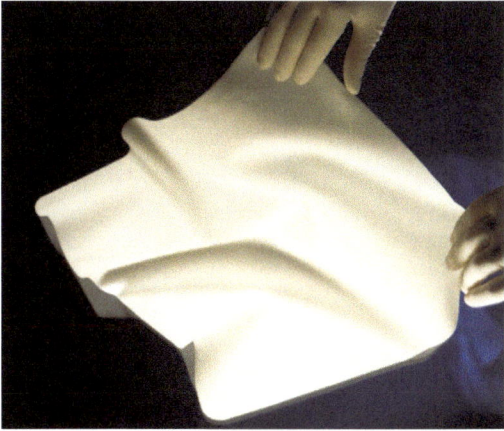

Fig. 5.21 Fortiva

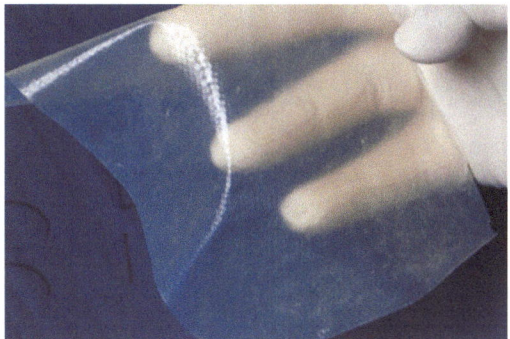

Fig. 5.22 Gentrix RS

cine small intestinal submucosa and are the only products with such a source. These are laminated, sewn together, and fenestrated. These must be rehydrated. *Cellis* is porcine dermal collagen and is available in many sizes and different thicknesses (Fig. 5.20). It also requires rehydration. *Fortiva* originates from dermis but does not require hydration (Fig. 5.21). *Gentrix Surgical Matrix* is also a laminated product. It is unique in

this biologic category as it is the only one that is made from the urinary bladder of the pig. All of these products have a notch to identify the correct positioning of the material. If the notch is placed in the upper top outside corner, then the basement membrane is facing up. The membrane should be placed away from the defect according to the product literature. *Gentrix* is available as *RS* (three ply), *PSM* (six ply), or *PSMX* (eight ply) and *Plus* (eight ply). The only real difference in the latter is the size of the product itself, the latter being the larger available material (Figs. 5.22, 5.23, 5.24, and 5.25). *Permacol* is a dermal collagen-based product that is the only material listed that is cross-linked and does not require rehydration (Fig. 5.26). It is known to be present for a prolonged period of time due to the cross-linkage of the collagen fibers. It is available in thicknesses of 0.5, 1.0, and 1.5 mm.

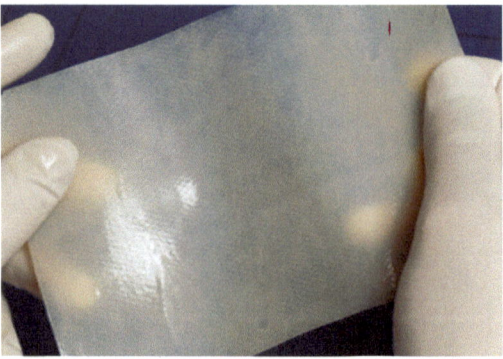

Fig. 5.23 Gentrix PSM

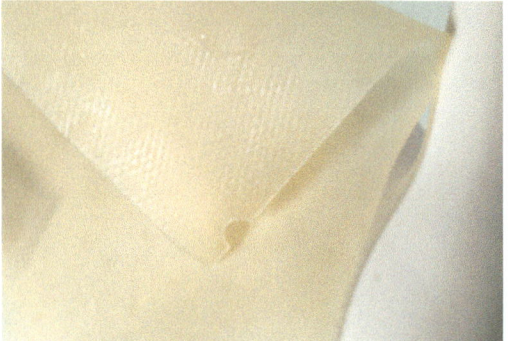

Fig. 5.24 Gentrix PSMX

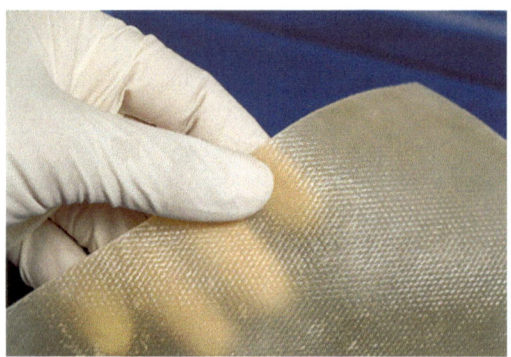

Fig. 5.25 Gentrix Plus

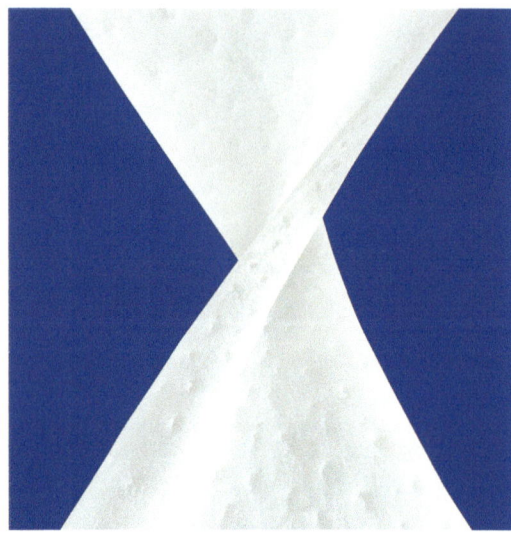

Fig. 5.26 Permacol (All rights reserved. Used with permission of Medtronic)

Fig. 5.27 Strattice firm

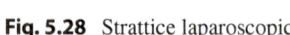

Fig. 5.28 Strattice laparoscopic

Strattice Reconstructive Tissue Matrix (RTM) is available in two thicknesses, firm and pliable. It is made from dermis and does require rehydration. It is available in many sizes, which depend upon which version is selected. These versions include a pliable and preshaped pliable, a firm (Fig. 5.27), a laparoscopic (Fig. 5.28), and a per-

forated version (Fig. 5.29). The Strattice Firm has a thickness 1.76 ± 0.012. The selection will

Fig. 5.29 Strattice perforated

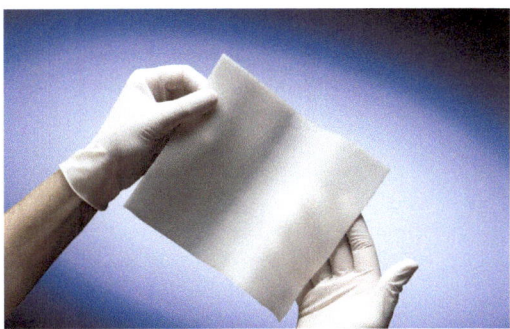

Fig. 5.30 XenMatrix

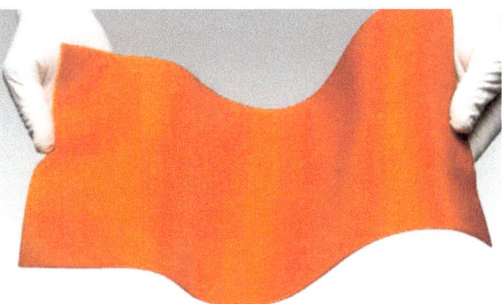

Fig. 5.31 XenMatrix AB

Fig. 5.32 XCM

depend on type of hernia to be repaired and the area to be covered. This is the only biologic product that has a specific version that is designed for use laparoscopically. *XenMatrix* is also dermal based and is not cross-linked (Fig. 5.30). It does require rehydration but not refrigeration. It is one of the thickest porcine biologics due to its 1.95 ± 0.012 measurement. It has recently been modified to contain the antimicrobials, rifampin and minocycline, which are present for over 7 days. *XenMatrix AB* has a distinct orange color due to the presence of the rifampin (Fig. 5.31). It

is unique in all of the biologic materials in that it contains antimicrobial agents. *XCM Biologic Tissue Matrix* is also a non-cross-linked porcine dermal product and does not require rehydration (Fig. 5.32). It is approximately 1.5 mm thick (±0.3 mm).

Hybrid Products

This is a relatively new concept in mesh development. There are clear reasons to use a permanent material in the repair of fascial defects. There are real reasons to consider the use of products that are not permanent but seek to increases the levels

Table 5.8 Hybrid products

OviTex, OviTex 1S, Ovitex 2S, Permanent, TelaBio, Malvern, PA, USA
OviTex, OviTex 1S, Ovitex 2S, Resorbable, TelaBio, Malvern, PA, USA
Synecor, W. L. Gore & Associates, Elkhart, DE, USA
Synecor Pre, W. L. Gore & Associates, Elkhart, DE, USA
Zenapro, Cook Medical, Bloomington, IL, USA

of collagen deposition to enhance the healing process. These materials seek to capitalize on the benefits of both of these concepts (Table 5.8). There is relatively little data on the actual results of the use of these materials but these data will undoubtedly be researched in the future.

OviTex, OviTex 1S and 2S is the most recent additions to these class of meshes. They are a combination of ovine gastric submucosal extracellular matrix and embedded polypropylene or polyglycolic acid. There is a four-layer core of this matrix in the *OviTex* version (Fig. 5.33). *OviTex 1S* has an additional two layers of matrix on one side and the *OviTex 2S* has the core plus two layers on both sides of the product (Fig. 5.33, middle and lower). Because of these differing designs, the thickness varies from 0.9 to 1.1 to 1.6 mm. The absorbable component option makes it the only biologic hybrid option with such a concept. The non-biologic portion is constructed with 6 mm pores. These figures are of the permanent component option. The resorbable polymer option is clear and will not be seen. Both *OviTex 1S* and *OviTex 2S* can be placed with visceral contact.

Synecor IP has combined some older materials together (Fig. 5.34). The internal permanent material is polytetrafluoroethylene. This is woven into a structure that is similar to other macroporous materials and is not the same as ePTFE. This is sandwiched between two types of polyglycolic acid/trimethylene carbonate (PGA/TMC). The parietal surface is similar to the Bio-A that is described above (Fig. 5.34, left). The visceral (tissue-separating) side is PGA/TMC and is a different structural weave which is quite tight to prevent ingrowth (Fig. 5.34, right). This material can be used either dry or wet. *Synecor Pre* is has the

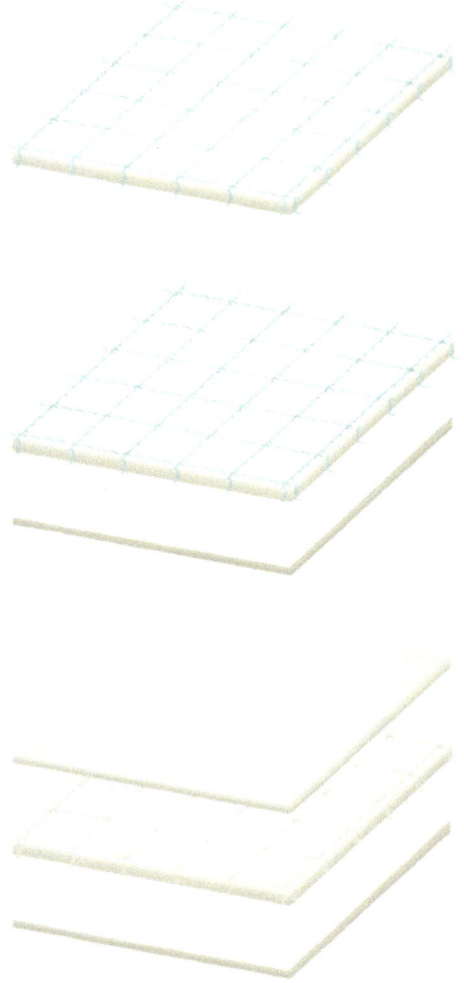

Fig. 5.33 Ovitex 1S, 2S

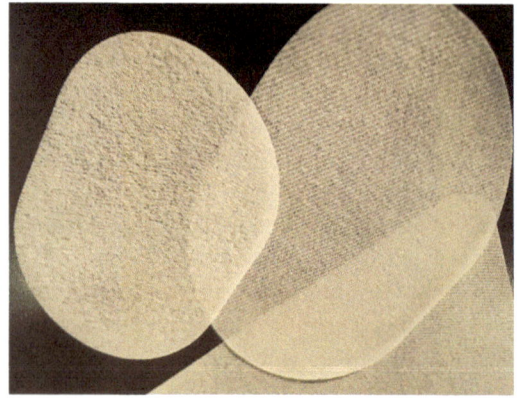

Fig. 5.34 Synecor IP

Bio-A coating on both sides of the PTFE and is designed to be placed in the extraperitoneal plane and should not be used against the viscera (Fig. 5.35).

Zenapro is the oldest of these three products (Fig. 5.36). It is a combination of the small intestinal submucosa that is found in the BioDesign materials described above. It has two layers of the submucosa on one side and four on the other and is perforated, unlike the other two hybrid products. Between these two layers is a large pore (5 mm) polypropylene mesh. It is not indicated in contaminated fields and requires rehydration. There is a rough and a smooth side with the rough side going against the abdominal wall in the repair of a hernia. The Instructions for Use state "The liberal use of transfascial sutures is recommended. Tacking devices alone may not provide adequate fixation to prevent recurrence." It is no longer available.

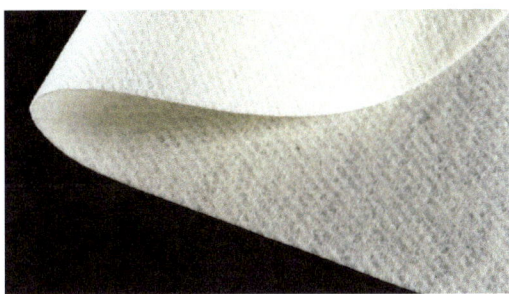

Fig. 5.35 Synecor Pre

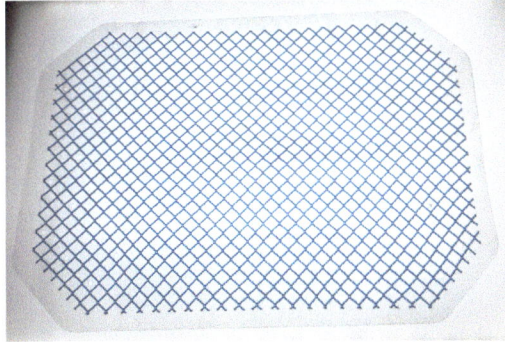

Fig. 5.36 Zenapro

Flat Prosthetic Products

The currently available products in use today are polypropylene (PP), polyester (POL), polytetrafluoroethylene (PTFE), expanded PTFE (ePTFE), or condensed PTFE (cPTFE). All are available in a variety of sizes and can be cut to conform to the dimensions that are necessary. There are currently so many products on the market today that it is quite difficult to become well versed in all of these materials. In fact, the similarities of these materials may result in many of them to be considered a "commodity" type of a product, whereupon only the pricing of the material will influence the use of it. The most prominent and commonly used are PP materials (Table 5.9). These should be used either in laparoscopic

Table 5.9 Flat polypropylene products

2D PPT Std, Microval, Saint-Just-Malmont, France
2D PPT LW, Microval, Saint-Just-Malmont, France
2D PPNT, Microval, Saint-Just-Malmont, France
Basic mesh, Di.pro Medical Devices, Torino, Italy
Basic Evolution mesh, Di.pro Medical Devices, Torino, Italy
Bard mesh, Davol, Inc., Warwick, RI, USA
Bard Soft mesh, Davol, Inc., Warwick, RI, USA
Biomesh P1, Cousin Biotech, Wervicq-Sud, France
Bulev UL, Di.pro Medical Devices, Torino, Italy
Bulev B5050, Di.pro Medical Devices, Torino, Italy
DynaMesh PP-Standard, FEG Textiltechnik mbH, Aachen, Germany
DynaMesh PP- Light, FEG Textiltechnik mbH, Aachen, Germany
EasyProthes, TransEasy Medical Tech.Co.Ltd., Beijing, China
Hertra 0, HerniaMesh, S.R.L., Torino, Italy
Hermesh 3,4,5,6,7,8, HerniaMesh, S.R.L., Torino, Italy
Lapartex, Di.pro Medical Devices, Torino, Italy
Optilene, B. Braun Melsungen AG, Melsungen, Germany
Optilene LP, B. Braun Melsungen AG, Melsungen, Germany
Optilene Mesh Elastic, B. Braun Melsungen AG, Melsungen, Germany
Parietene Flat Sheet, Medtronic, Minneapolis, MN, USA
Parietene Lightweight, Medtronic, Minneapolis, MN, USA

(continued)

Table 5.9 (continued)

Premilene, B. Braun Melsungen AG, Melsungen, Germany
Premium, Cousin Biotech, Wervicq-Sud, France
Prolene, Ethicon Inc., Somerville, NJ, USA
Prolene Soft Mesh, Ethicon Inc., Somerville, NJ, USA
Prolite, Atrium Medical Corporation, Hudson, NH, USA
Repol Angimesh 0,1,8,9, Angiologica, S. Martino Sicc., Italy
SMX, THT Bio-Science, Montpelier, France
SMH2, THT Bio-Science, Montpelier, France
SMH, THT Bio-Science, Montpelier, France
Surgimesh WN, Aspide Medical, St. Etienne, France
Surgipro Monofilamented, Covidien plc, Dublin, Ireland
Surgipro Multifilamented, Covidien plc, Dublin, Ireland
Surgipro Open Weave, Covidien plc, Dublin, Ireland
TiMESH, GfE Medizintechnik, Nuremburg, Germany
TiLENE, GfE Medizintechnik, Nuremburg, Germany
TiLENE Blue, GfE Medizintechnik, Nuremburg, Germany
VitaMesh—Getinge Group, Wayne, NJ, USA
VitaMesh Blue—Getinge Group, Wayne, NJ, USA

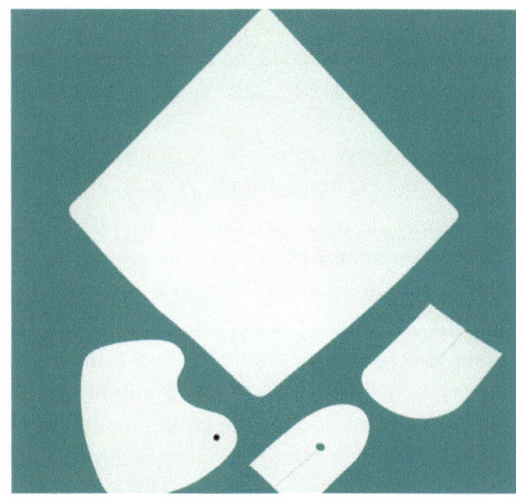

Fig. 5.37 2D PPNT

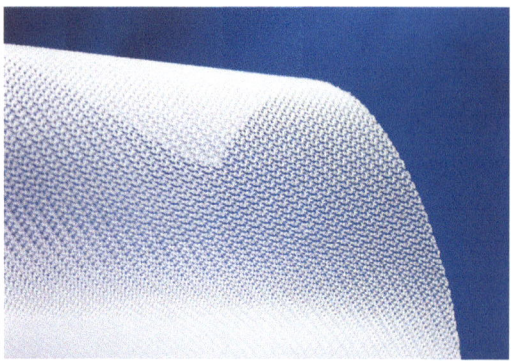

Fig. 5.38 Basic mesh

applications if not exposed to the viscera. Because of the complexities of pore sizes and the multitude of differing weights and shapes of the PPM within each of these materials, this chapter could not expound upon all of them. The reader is referred to the manufacturer for further information in the exact densities, weights, and pore sizes of these products. Many of the figures below include the configurations of the inguinal applications due to the fact that most are available for this use.

The *2D* products are available in a variety of products and weights. The *2D PPT Std* and the *2D PPT LW* are both knitted and differ in the weight and pore size. The former is heavy weight while the latter is medium weight and more macroporous. The 2D PPNT is a nonwoven PP material that is available in three different weights and thicknesses (Fig. 5.37). These meshes are configured in a variety of shapes and sizes as shown.

Basic mesh is a lightweight mesh (Fig. 5.38). Di.pro has developed an ultra lightweight version that is called *Basic Evolution* mesh (Fig. 5.39). *Bard Mesh* is probably the oldest flat sheet of

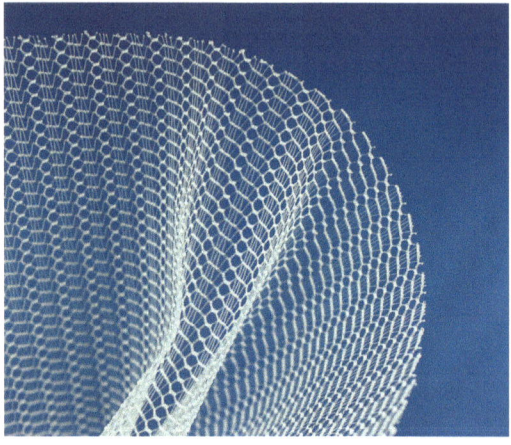

Fig. 5.39 Basic evolution

heavy weight polypropylene in existence, having been brought to market in the early 1960s (Fig. 5.40). It is still in use today and like many of these prostheses, a lightweight and more macroporous version has been developed, the *Bard Soft Mesh* (Fig. 5.41). *Biomesh P1* is the standard weight material compared to the *Premium* (Figs. 5.42 and 5.43). It is available for extraperitoneal placement in various shapes and sizes to accommodate open or laparoscopic inguinal and ventral hernias. *Bulev B* and *Bulev UL* are somewhat similar to the Basic and Basic Evolution meshes discussed above (Figs. 5.44 and 5.45). The weights of the Bulev products are 48 g/m² and 39 g/m², respectively. They are different in that they possess blue lines to differentiate them from the other meshes and aid in positioning of the product.

DynaMesh comes in two weights; the standard is twice the weight of the lightweight product

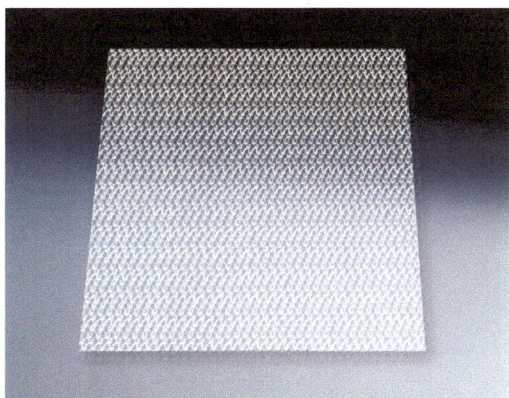

Fig. 5.42 Biomesh P1

Fig. 5.43 Premium mesh

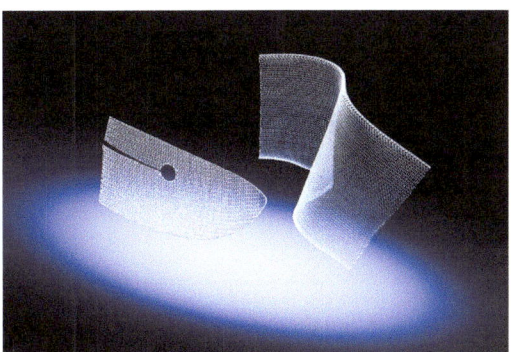

Fig. 5.40 Bard mesh flat and preshape

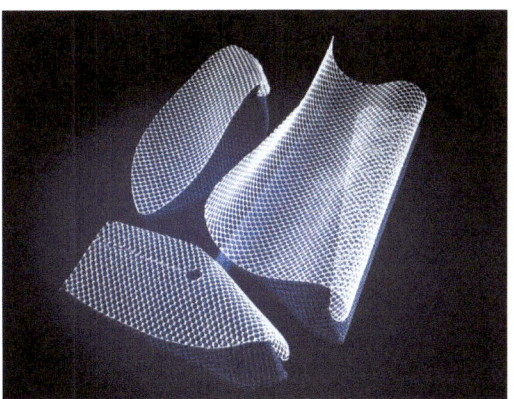

Fig. 5.41 Bard soft mesh

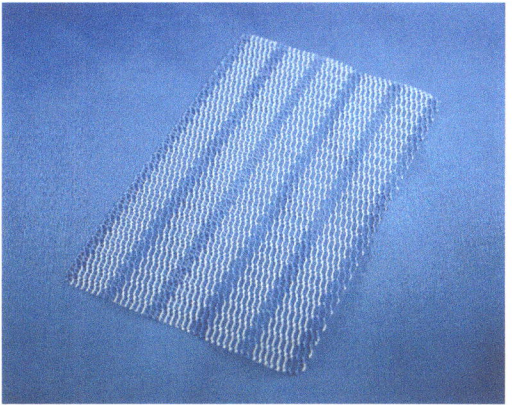

Fig. 5.44 Bulev B

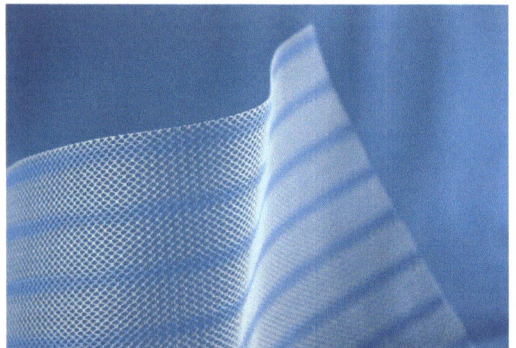

Fig. 5.45 Bulev UL

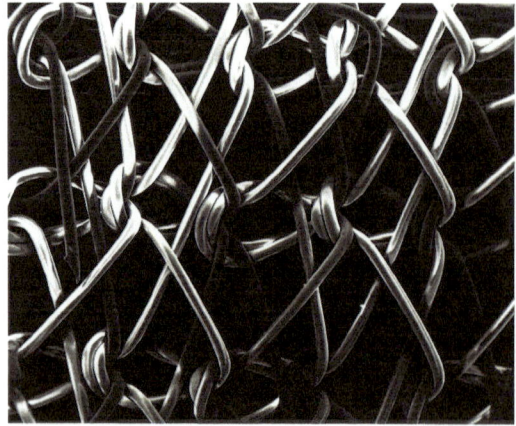

Fig. 5.48 Easy Prothes 70

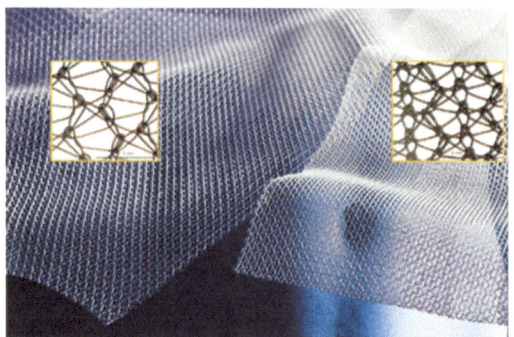

Fig. 5.46 DynaMesh light and standard

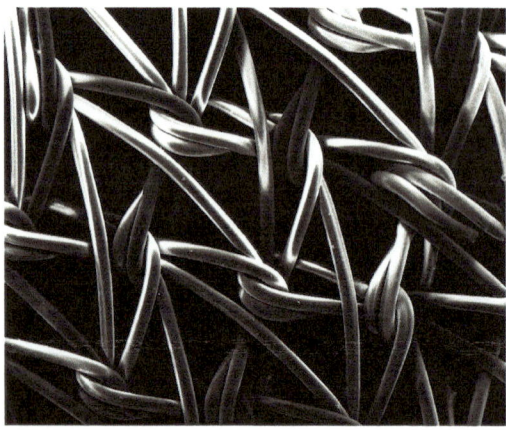

Fig. 5.47 Easy Prothes heavy weight PP.

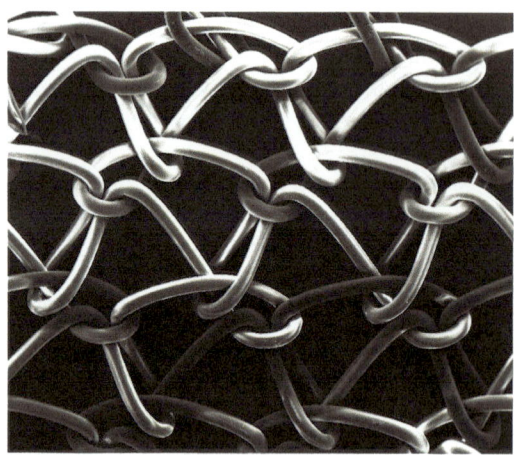

Fig. 5.49 Easy Prothes 60

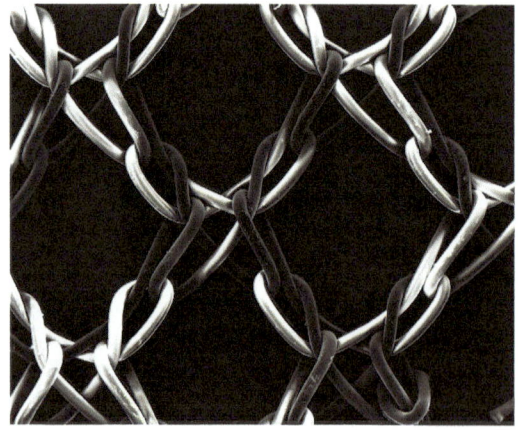

Fig. 5.50 Easy Prothes lightweight

(Fig. 5.46). *Easy Prothes* is available as a heavy weight material (90 g/m^2), two medium products (70 and 60 g/m^2), and a lightweight version (40 g/m^2). Figures 5.47, 5.48, 5.49, and 5.50 detail the differences in the weaves of the products. Figures 5.51 and 5.52 compare the medium and

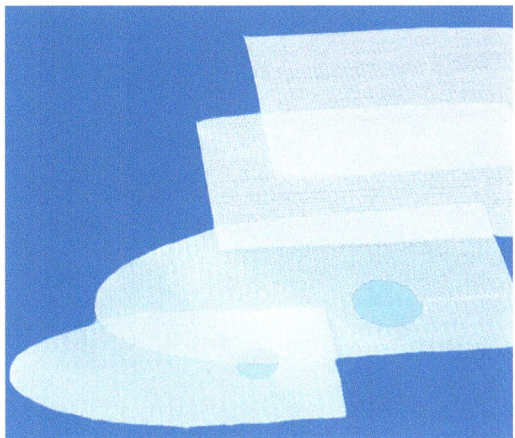

Fig. 5.51 Easy Prothes 60

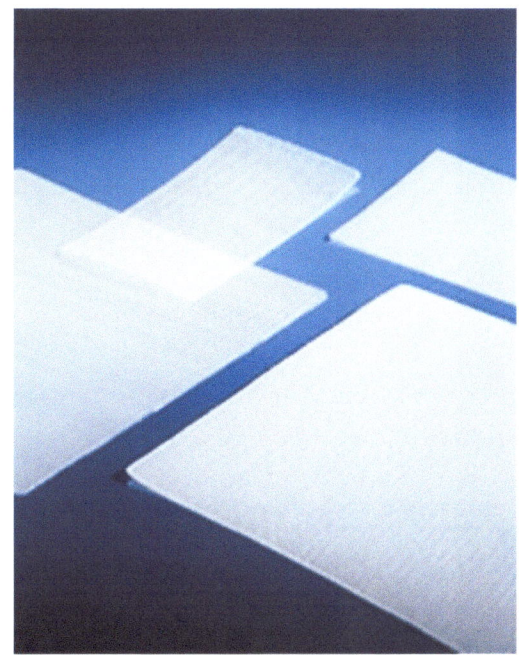

Fig. 5.53 Hermesh variety

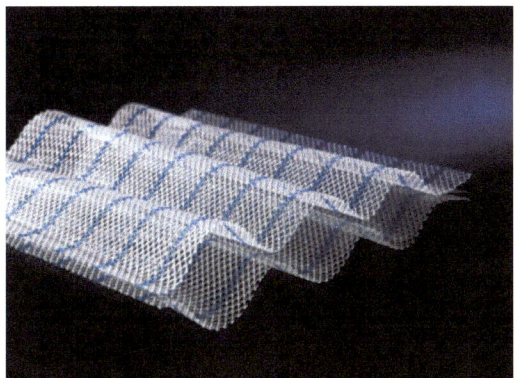

Fig. 5.52 Easy Prothes lightweight

Fig. 5.54 Lapartex (It is no longer available)

lightweight versions. The *Hermesh 3–8* have a huge variety of weights and sizes and can be used in either open or laparoscopic repairs (Fig. 5.53). The graduated weights of these vary from the heaviest (3) to the lightest (8). *Lapartex* is a heavier product than some of the other materials (Fig. 5.54). The production of this product was stopped prior to the publication of this textbook).

Optilene products are all lightweight materials that vary from the heaviest by that name (60 g/m^2) to the *Elastic* (48 g/m^2) and the lighter *LP* (36 g/m^2). The Elastic version has unequal pore sizes (3.6 × 2.8 mm) to allow for multidirectional elasticity (Figs. 5.55, 5.56, and 5.57). Unlike some of the other prostheses, the blue lines in the Optilene do not signify an absorbable component. *Parietene Flat Sheet and Parietene*

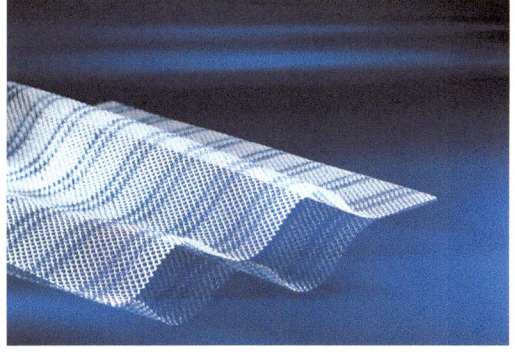

Fig. 5.55 Optilene

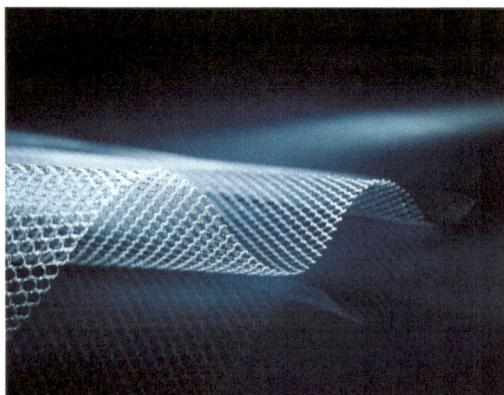

Fig. 5.56 Optilene mesh Elastic

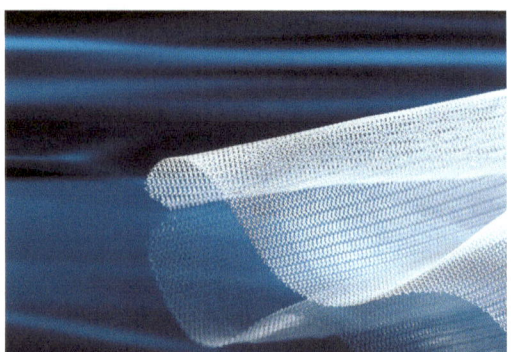

Fig. 5.57 Optilene mesh LP

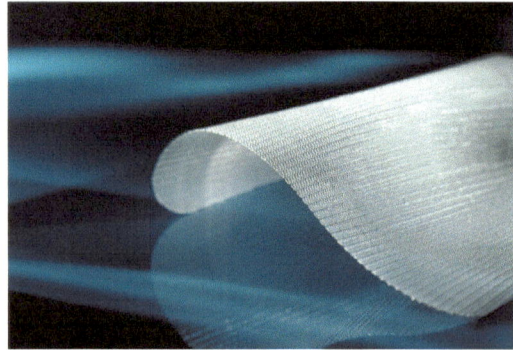

Fig. 5.59 Premilene mesh

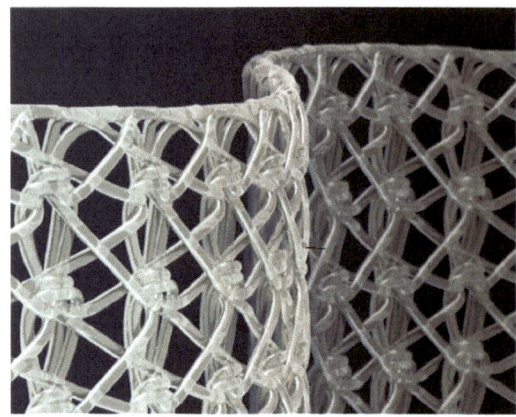

Fig. 5.60 Prolene (Image courtesy of Ethicon, Inc.)

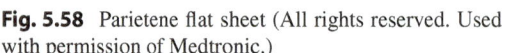

Fig. 5.58 Parietene flat sheet (All rights reserved. Used with permission of Medtronic.)

Lightweight products are monofilament flat sheet products (Fig. 5.58). *Premilene* is the heaviest weight (82 g/m^2) product in the Braun flat mesh product line (Fig. 5.59). *Prolene* is also a heavier weight mesh material and it is one of the older products available (Fig. 5.60). *Prolene Soft Mesh*

is the lighter weight version that has larger pores than the original mesh and blue lines to help differentiate it (Fig. 5.61). *ProLite* was one of the earliest meshes that were introduced as a lighter weight material (Fig. 5.62). Today, it is considered a mid-weight mesh. *ProLite Ultra* possesses even less weight of mesh than ProLite (Fig. 5.63).

Repol Angimesh 0, 1, 8, 9 are all similar and differentiated in the weights and weaves from each other. The 0 is the lightest and 9 is the heaviest. *SurgiMesh WN* is a nonwoven microfiber PP product that is extremely lightweight and has a differing microstructure than the other materials listed in this section (Fig. 5.64). It is available in several configurations for open or laparoscopic procedures but cannot be placed against the viscera. *Surgipro* was originally introduced as a multifilament mesh (Fig. 5.65). Because of the demand for a monofilament product, the second-generation

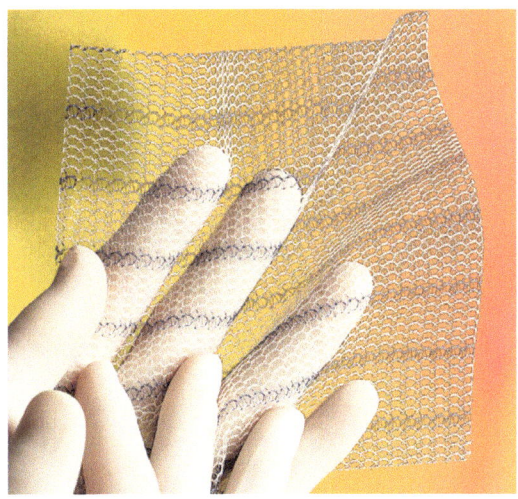

Fig. 5.61 Prolene soft mesh (Image courtesy of Ethicon, Inc.)

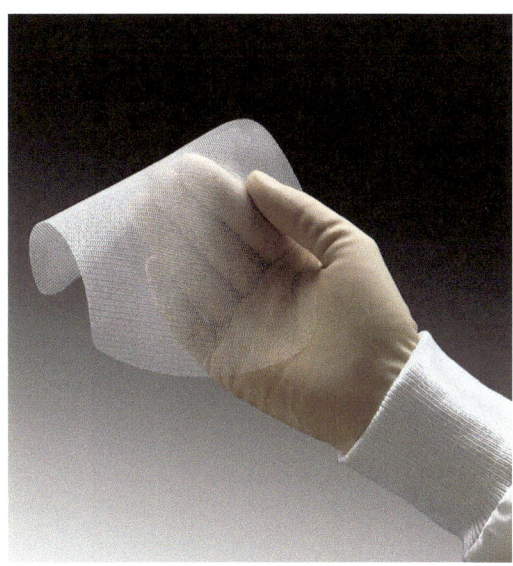

Fig. 5.63 ProLite Ultra

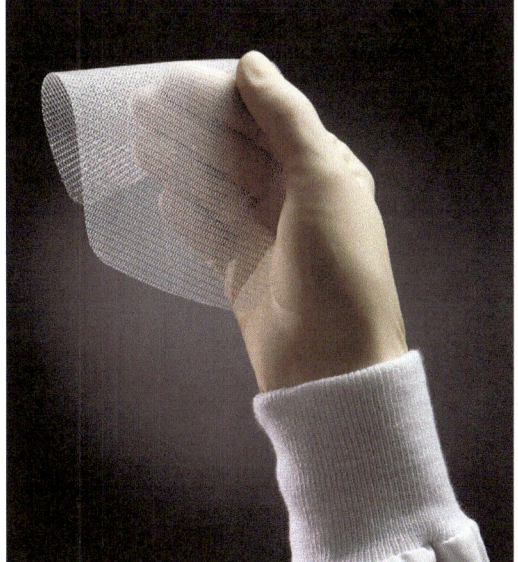

Fig. 5.62 ProLite

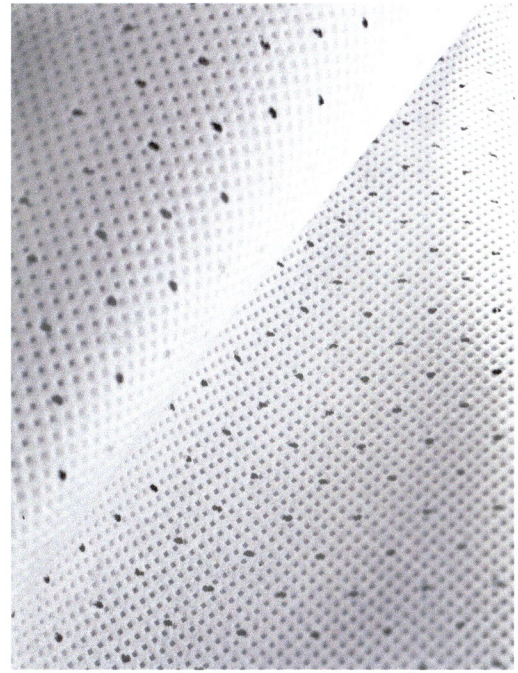

Fig. 5.64 SurgiMeshWN

product was released (Fig. 5.66). The multifilament material is noticeably softer than the monofilament one. There is now an open weave product called the *Surgipro Open Weave* (Fig. 5.67). *SMX* is a heavy product designed for all hernia repairs (Fig. 5.68). It is part of the "Swing-mesh" product line. It is available in a lightweight and ultra light material as *SMH2* and *SMH,* respectively (Fig. 5.69).

TiMESH is similar to the lightweight materials but has a bonded layer of titanium on the fibers of the PP using nanotechnology (Figs. 5.70 and 5.71). This is supposed to allow ingrowth in a flexible manner while inhibiting the development of a scar plate. It can be used in either

Fig. 5.65 Surgipro multifilamented (All rights reserved. Used with permission of Medtronic.)

Fig. 5.67 Surgipro open weave (All rights reserved. Used with permission of Medtronic.)

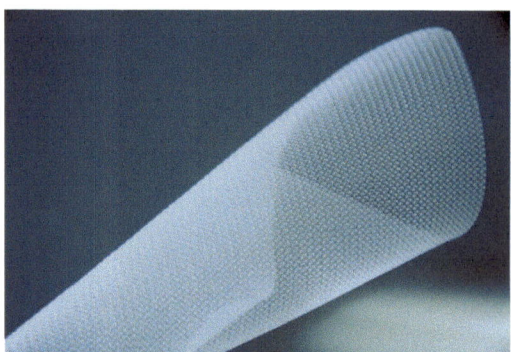

Fig. 5.68 SMX

Fig. 5.66 Surgipro monofilamented (All rights reserved. Used with permission of Medtronic.)

the intraperitoneal or extraperitoneal positions. TiLENE Blue has blue lines incorporated into the material to aid in positioning and can also be used in the intra- or extraperitoneal planes (Fig. 5.72). It is also available without the blue lines as *TiLENE*. *VitaMesh* is of a single macroporous material (50 g/m²) available for open and

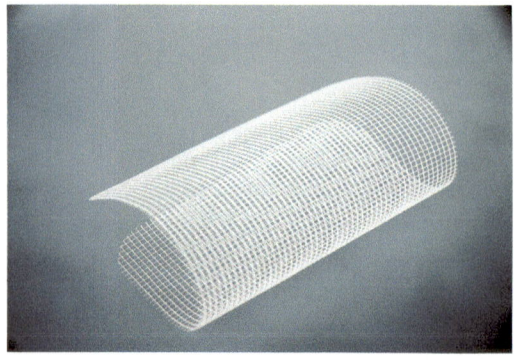

Fig. 5.69 SMH2

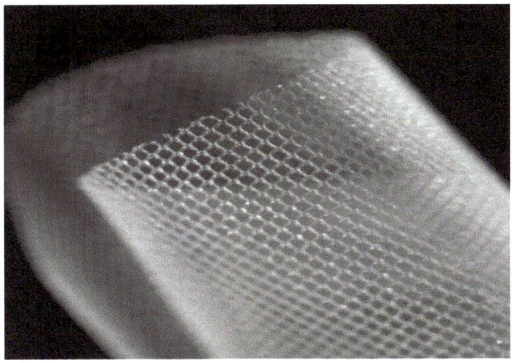

Fig. 5.70 TiMESH

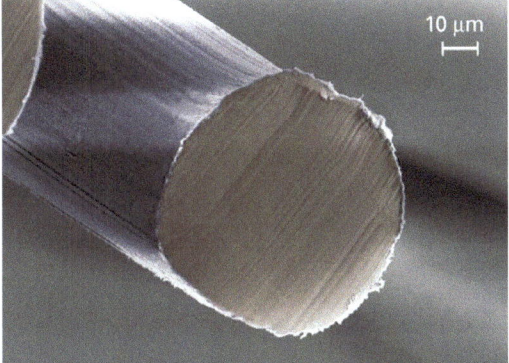

Fig. 5.71 TiMESH SEM

Fig. 5.72 TiLENE Blue

Fig. 5.73 VitaMesh

Fig. 5.74 VitaMesh Blue

laparoscopic repair (Fig. 5.73). *VitaMesh Blue* is the lighter weight version (28 g/m²) of this flat mesh and is differentiated by its blue color (Fig. 5.74). These products are singular in that they are made of condensed PP rather than the traditional PP. Regular PP mesh becomes condensed PP mesh through compression during a post-knit heat treatment. This condensing process serves to reduce mesh thickness approximately 70%. This is said to improve deliverability through increased smoothness because fiber crossover points are flattened. Improved recovery of the shape of the mesh is asserted because the knots in the mesh are flattened. This provides greater shape memory than their non-flattened PP.

The differences in the appearance of the prosthetics are easily seen in these photos. The size of the pores of these materials as well as the thickness of the product will have a significant impact on the stiffness. These factors affect the degree of scarring within the tissues. Additionally, the pore sizes vary greatly from each of these products. The lighter weight products have significantly impacted the prosthetic repair of hernias. The current thought is that, for the most part, there is less pain and a scar plate with the lightweight, larger pore meshes. In some cases, these may have become "too thin" and there are reports of mesh fracture and hernia recurrence. Generally, these are well accepted in the inguinal area but one should be sure of the strength of these products in the ventral and incisional hernia repair.

There are relatively fewer non-coated polyester mesh materials (Table 5.10). The preponderance of the polyester products that are currently available is produced in various configurations and most have some type of coating and are listed elsewhere in this chapter.

2D PET, Angimesh R2, R2-1, R2-9, and *Biomesh A2* are all fairly similar in appearance The *2D PET* and *Biomesh A2*, however, has been configured into various shapes and sizes for a variety of applications (Figs. 5.75 and 5.76). *Angimesh*

Table 5.10 Flat polyester products

2D PET, Microval, Saint-Just-Malmont, France
Angimesh R2, Angiologica, S. Martino Sicc., Italy
Angimesh R2-1, Angiologica, S. Martino Sicc., Italy
Angimesh R2-9, Angiologica, S. Martino Sicc., Italy
Biomesh A2, Cousin Biotech, Wervicq-Sud, France
CO3+, THT Bio-Science, Montpelier, France
Parietex Flat Sheet Mesh, Medtronic, Minneapolis, MN, USA
Parietex Lightweight Mesh, Medtronic, Minneapolis, MN, USA
Parietex Monofilament Macroporous Mesh, Medtronic, Minneapolis, MN, USA
SM2, THT Bio-Science, Montpelier, France
SM3, THT Bio-Science, Montpelier, France
SM3+, THT Bio-Science, Montpelier, France
Versatex, Medtronic, Minneapolis, MN, USA

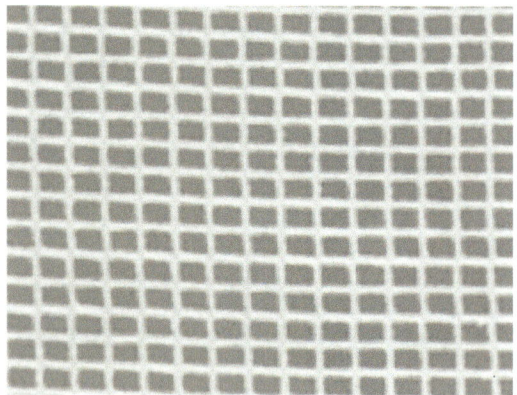

Fig. 5.76 Biomesh A2

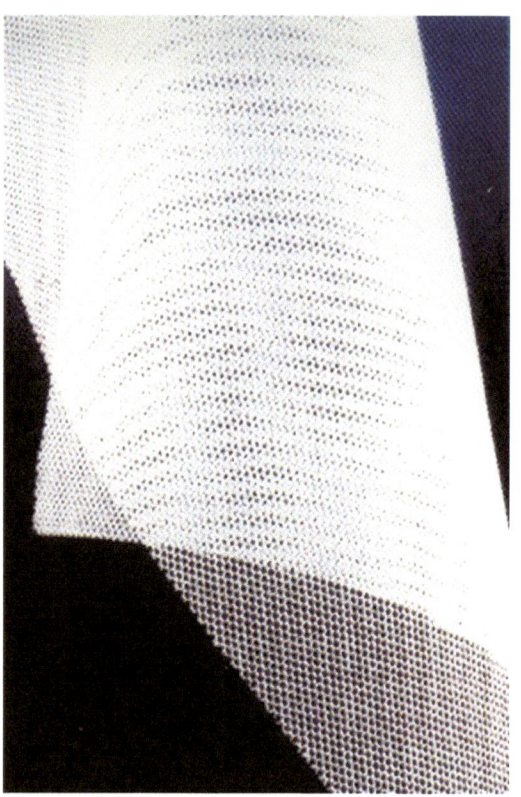

Fig. 5.77 Angimesh R2

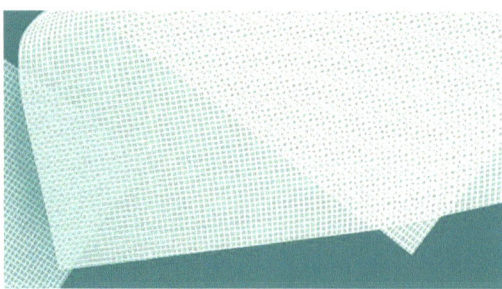

Fig. 5.75 2D PET

R2 is multifilament polyester (Fig. 5.77). *Angimesh R2-1* and *R2-9* are monofilament materials very similar in appearance and differ only in thicknesses, *R2-1* being thinner than *R2-9* (Figs. 5.78 and 5.79). *CO3+* is a rather unique material and is actually combination products that are configured in a variety of shapes and sizes. As such, it will be

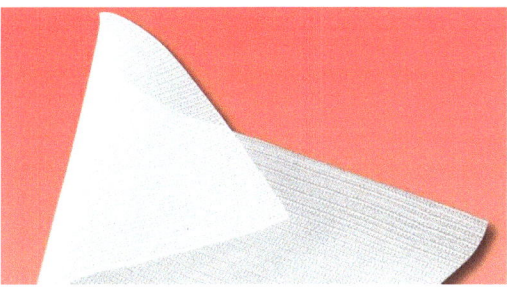

Fig. 5.78 Angimesh R2-1

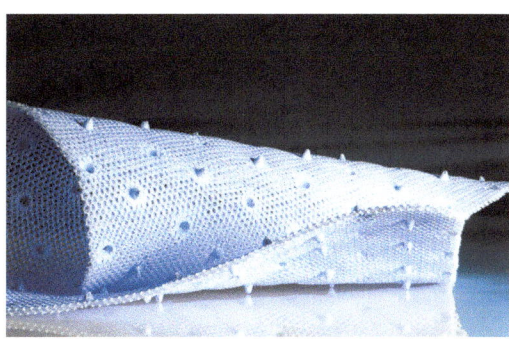

Fig. 5.80 CO3+

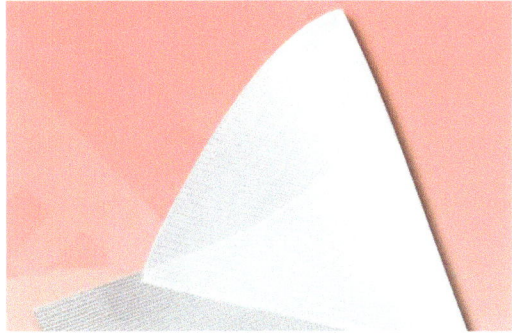

Fig. 5.79 Angimesh R2-9

Fig. 5.81 Parietex flat sheet (All rights reserved. Used with permission of Medtronic.)

mentioned later in the chapter again. It is a three-dimensional weave of polyester that has impregnated polyurethane (PUR). The differentiating factor are the knitted "grips" that are on both sides of the product (Fig. 5.80). These are designed to fixate the mesh. It can be used in open or laparoscopic surgery and for nearly all hernias.

The *Parietex Flat Sheet Mesh* is available in two- or three-dimensional weaves (Fig. 5.81). The 2D material is more rigid and is touted for laparoscopic repairs due to this fact. The 3D product is more supple and soft. *Parietex Lightweight* product is a monofilament product (Fig. 5.82). *Parietex Monofilament Macroporous* is available in a flat sheet and is a two-dimensional construct (Fig. 5.83). *SM2* is a heavyweight bidimensional weave material that is indicated for all hernia repairs (Fig. 5.84).

SM3 and *SM3+* are three-dimensional weaves of polyester (Figs. 5.85 and 5.86). Both are available in a variety of shapes and sizes and can be used in open or laparoscopic applications. *SM3* is pure polyester while the *SM3+* is polyester with

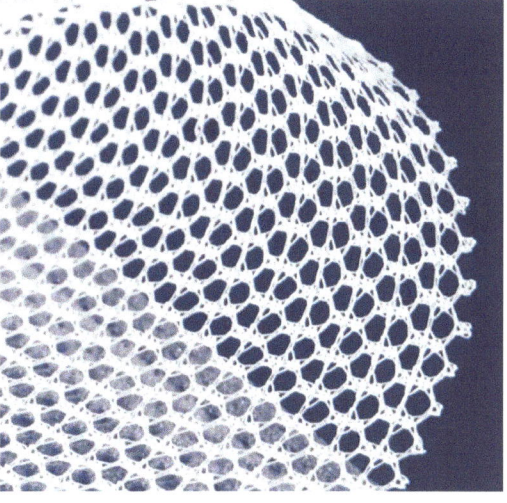

Fig. 5.82 Parietex lightweight mesh (All rights reserved. Used with permission of Medtronic.)

impregnated polyurethane and is configured in anatomical shapes. *Versatex* has a 3D construct and is macroporous (Fig. 5.87). It is a medium weight (64 g/m²) monofilament product that is designed for placement in the preperitoneal space. It also has a central teardrop.

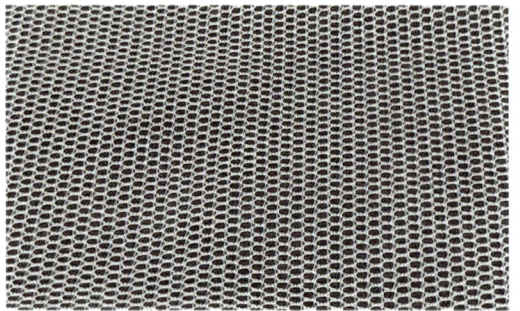

Fig. 5.83 Parietex monofilament macroporous (All rights reserved. Used with permission of Medtronic.)

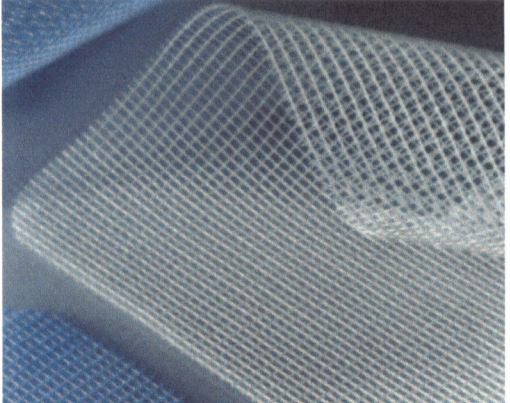

Fig. 5.84 SM2

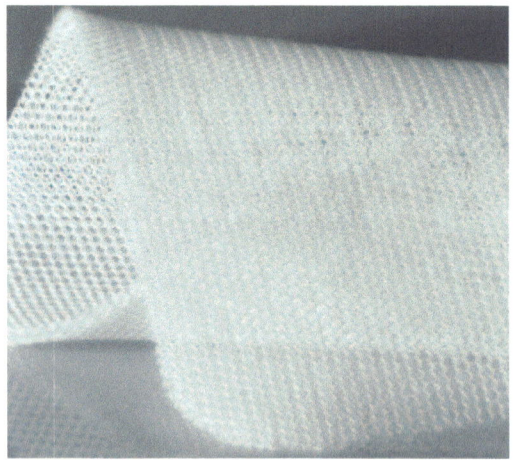

Fig. 5.85 SM3

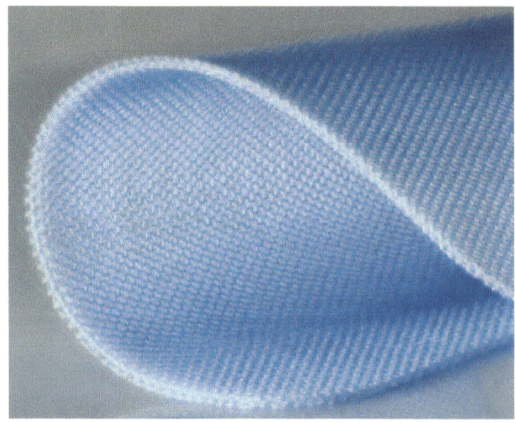

Fig. 5.86 SM3+

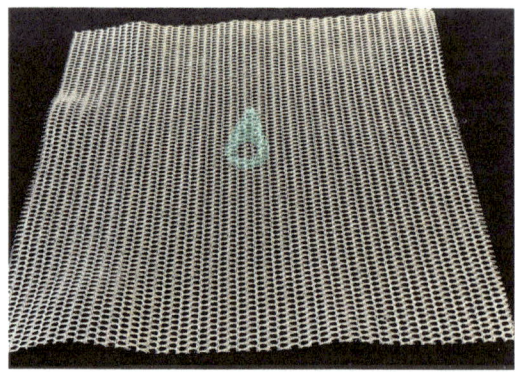

Fig. 5.87 Versatex (All rights reserved. Used with permission of Medtronic.)

Table 5.11 ePTFE products

DualMesh, W. L. Gore & Associates, Elkhart, DE, USA
DualMesh Plus, W. L. Gore &Associates, Elkhart, DE, USA
DualMesh Plus with Holes, W. L. Gore &Associates, Elkhart, DE, USA
Dulex, Davol, Inc., Warwick, RI, USA
MycroMesh, W. L. Gore &Associates, Elkhart, DE, USA
MycroMesh Plus, W. L. Gore &Associates, Elkhart, DE, USA
Soft Tissue Patch, W. L. Gore &Associates, Elkhart, DE, USA

Expanded polytetrafluoroethylene (ePTFE) prostheses have also been available in a flat sheet configuration for many years (Table 5.11). In fact, the earliest products used in the intraperitoneal space for incisional hernia repair were of ePTFE [4]. Because of their structure, they are solid and white unless an antimicrobial agent has been added.

The current DualMesh products are very similar in construction and are one of the oldest "tissue-separating" products (Fig. 5.88). These all have two distinctly different surfaces. One side is very smooth and has interstices of three microns while the other has the appearance of corduroy with an approximate "ridge to ridge" distance of 1500 µm. This prosthesis is designed for use in the intraperitoneal space. The smooth side must therefore be placed facing the viscera as this minimizes the potential for adhesion formation. The rough surface is applied to the abdominal wall so that maximum parietal tissue penetration will occur. *DualMesh* is available in one thickness, 1 mm. It is available with or without the impregnation of silver and chlorhexidine as *DualMesh PLUS* (Fig. 5.89). The 2-mm product is only available as DualMesh Plus with the antimicrobial agents within it. These two antimicrobial agents are added to decrease the risk of infection and, because of the silver, impart a brown color to the "PLUS" products. At this time, these products are the only permanent materials impregnated with any type of any antimicrobial or bactericidal agents. *DualMesh PLUS with Holes* (Fig. 5.90) is of the same construction as that of the DualMesh. The penetration of the holes requires that this product be of 1.5 mm in thickness. The concept of the addition of these perforations is that there may be greater penetration of the fibroblasts and other cells across the material. Additionally, seroma formation might be diminished.

Dulex is manufactured of laminated ePTFE and is available in 1 mm or 2 mm thick (Fig. 5.91). One surface of the material is studded with numerous outcroppings as seen on the scanning electron microscopic view that are approximately 400 microns apart. This gives the product the gross appearance of sandpaper. The intent of this surface is to provide for greater fibroblastic attachment and subsequent greater collagen

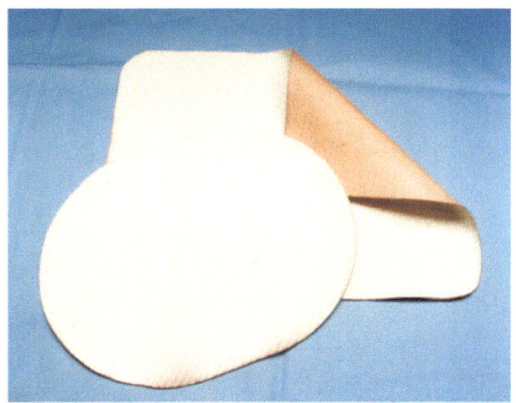

Fig. 5.90 DualMesh PLUS with holes

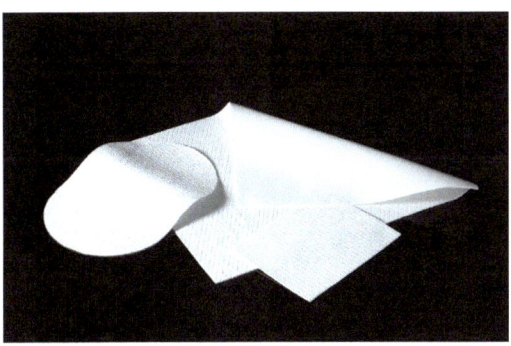

Fig. 5.88 DualMesh

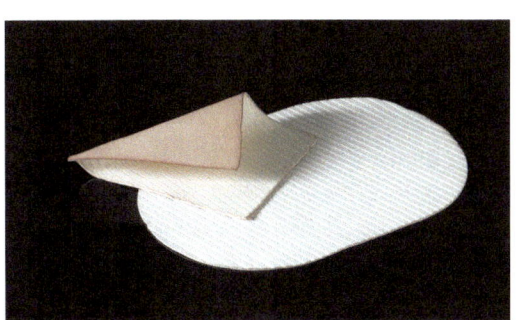

Fig. 5.89 DualMesh PLUS

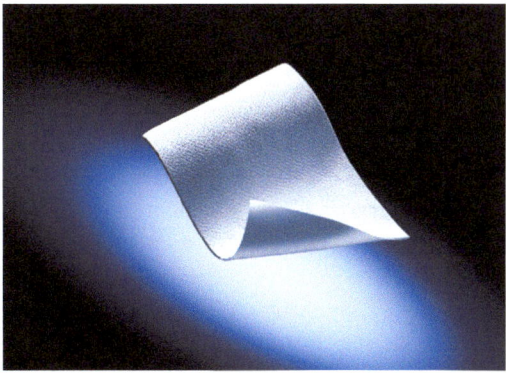

Fig. 5.91 Dulex

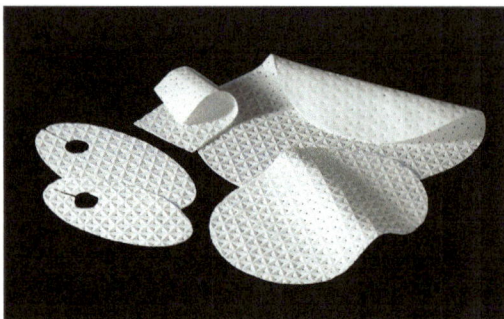

Fig. 5.92 MycroMesh

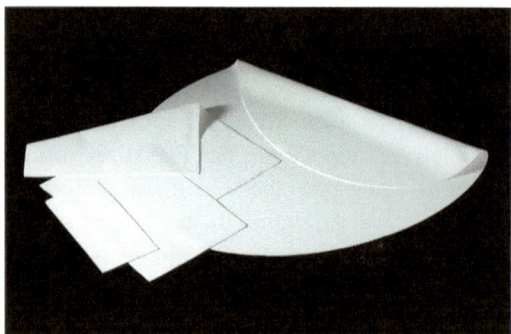

Fig. 5.94 Soft tissue patch

Table 5.12 Miscellaneous flat mesh products

Inomesh, Secqure/Medlinx Acacia, Singapore
Mosquito netting, numerous manufacturers
MotifMESH, Proxy Biomedical Ltd., Galway, Ireland
Omyra, B. Braun Melsungen AG, Melsungen, Germany
Rebound HRD V, ARB Medical, Minneapolis, MN, USA
TiO₂ Mesh, Bayreuth, Germany

Fig. 5.93 MycroMesh PLUS

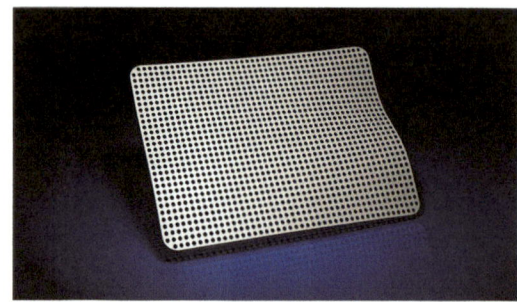

Fig. 5.95 InoMesh

deposition on this parietal surface. When used in the intraperitoneal fashion, the smooth surface should contact the intestine.

MycroMesh is also a dual-sided perforated prosthetic with one surface of three microns and the other of 17–22 µm (Fig. 5.92). The latter surface is textured. Although only 1 mm, this material is perforated for reasons similar to that of the DualMesh Plus with holes. *MycroMesh PLUS* is impregnated with the antimicrobials silver and chlorhexidine (Fig. 5.93). Neither of these products is designed for intraperitoneal placement.

Soft Tissue Patch is the earliest implants of these ePTFE products and was the product utilized in the very first laparoscopic incisional hernia repair (Fig. 5.94) [4]. The variety of available configurations of this product has increased over

the last several years. Its use, however, has waned because of the development of the other products that are listed in Table 5.11. Like the *MycroMesh*, it should not contact any viscera when applied.

Miscellaneous Flat Products

There are ranges of materials that do not fit into the exact categories above (Table 5.12). For instance, *Inomesh* is a product made of PVDF with laser cut holes (Fig. 5.95). *MotifMESH* and *Omyra* are identical in design and concept

(Figs. 5.96 and 5.97). There are made of condensed PTFE (cPTFE) and designed for use in contact with the intestine. The PTFE is laminated and then condensed with a heated compression process. The nonporous material is then laser micromachined to create the macroporous structure of the final product. They claim to be "a bacterial resistant anti-adhesive mesh."

Rebound HRD V is a unique material in that it is PP that has a ring of nitinol to stiffen the product and is available as an oval shape for umbilical hernia repair (Fig. 5.98). *TiO₂Mesh* is a titanized PP is that of (Fig. 5.99). It is lightweight (47 g/m²), large pore (2.8 mm), and has blue orientation strips. It is stated to be hydrophilic so that there is an apparent "stickiness" to the product, which eases intraoperative handling.

This chapter would be remiss if it did not include the use of mosquito netting that has been used in the repair of inguinal hernias. This has

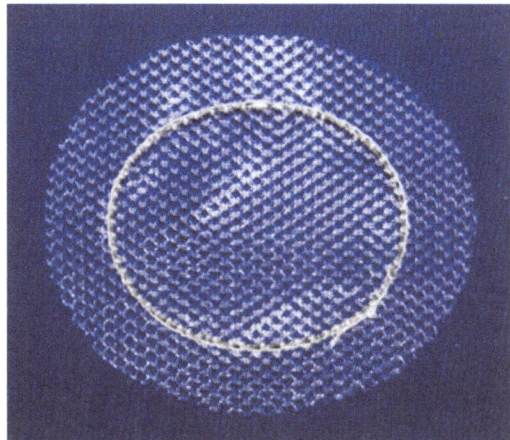

Fig. 5.98 Rebound HRD V

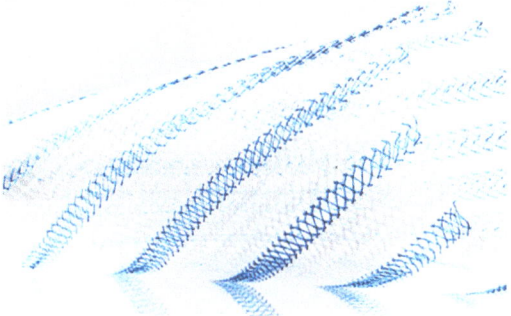

Fig. 5.99 TiO₂ mesh

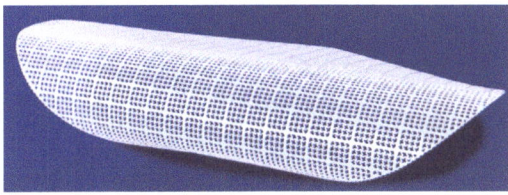

Fig. 5.96 MotifMESH

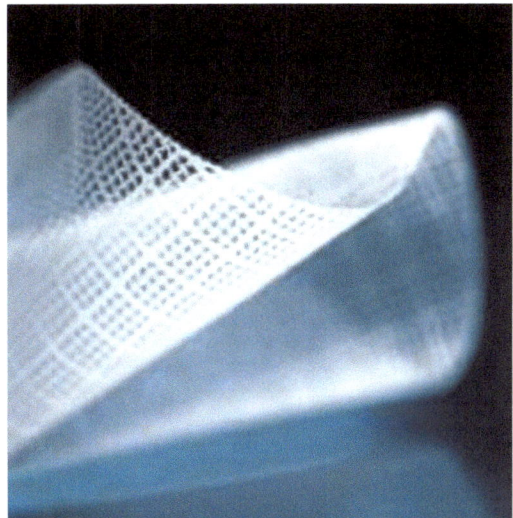

Fig. 5.97 Omyra mesh

been reported in the past in underserved countries. It appears that if this material is acceptable for use in areas of the world where the other products described in this chapter are either unavailable or are too expensive [9, 10]. In fact, recent evidence has shown there is little difference in adverse events with this or the traditional commercial mesh products [11]. This is added to this chapter because of the possibility that it might be used for some type of incisional hernia repair in the future.

Combination Flat Synthetic Prosthetics

This grouping of these products is made because there is a permanent portion of these materials and an absorbable component incorporated into the product that is not meant to be a barrier coating. These prostheses are generally not meant to contact any viscera and do not possess a specific shape (Table 5.13).

Adhesix, Parietene ProGrip, and *Parietex ProGrip* all have self-attaching portions of the prosthesis so that once placed onto the tissue surface, they will fixate themselves. The permanent portions of Adhesix and Parietene ProGrip are made of PP while the Parietex ProGrip is POL. *Adhesix* has a coating on one side that is made of polyvinylpyrrolidone and polyethylene glycol. This coating turns into an adhesive gel when it comes into contact with both heat and humidity (Fig. 5.100). The latter two products have absorbable polylactic acid microgrips on one surface. *Parietex ProGrip Laparoscopic* is a flat sheet of polyester that also

has microgrips of polylactic acid that last >18 months (Fig. 5.101). It differs from the other ProGrip products in that it has a green portion to aid in orientation of the mesh. There is a light coating of collagen which lessens the "grip' strength to make manipulation during laparoscopic use easier.

Easy Prosthesis Partially Absorbable is a partially absorbable product (Fig. 5.102). It is a combination of PP and poly(glycolide-co-caprolactone) [PGCL] monofilaments. The PGCL portion will be completely absorbed within 90–120 days. It is available in two versions, both of which have a PP weight of 30 g/m^2, which is the final weight of the material after degradation of the absorbable material. The difference lies in the weight of the PGCL, which are 30 g/m^2 in the *PAF* material and 60 g/m^2 in the *PAS* product. The *4D Ventral* is a flat sheet and differs from the 4D mesh in that it is 40% PP and 60% PLLA (Fig. 5.103).

Table 5.13 Combination products

Adhesix, Davol, Inc., Warwick, RI, USA
Easy Prosthesis Partially Absorbable PAF, TransEasy Medical Tech.Co.Ltd., Beijing, China
Easy Prosthesis Partially Absorbable PAS, TransEasy Medical Tech.Co.Ltd., Beijing, China
4D Mesh Ventral, Cousin Biotech, Wervicq-Sud, France
Parietene ProGrip, Medtronic, Minneapolis, MN, USA
Parietex ProGrip, Medtronic, Minneapolis, MN, USA
Parietex ProGrip Laparoscopic, Medtronic, Minneapolis, MN, USA
TiMESH, GfE Medizintechnik, Nuremburg, Germany
Vypro, Ethicon, Inc., Somerville, NJ, USA
Ultrapro, Ethicon, Inc., Somerville, NJ, USA
Ultrapro Advanced, Ethicon, Inc., Somerville, NJ, USA

Fig. 5.101 Parietex ProGrip laparoscopic (All rights reserved. Used with permission of Medtronic.)

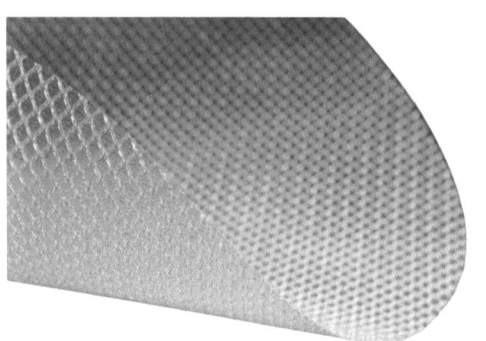

Fig. 5.100 Adhesix

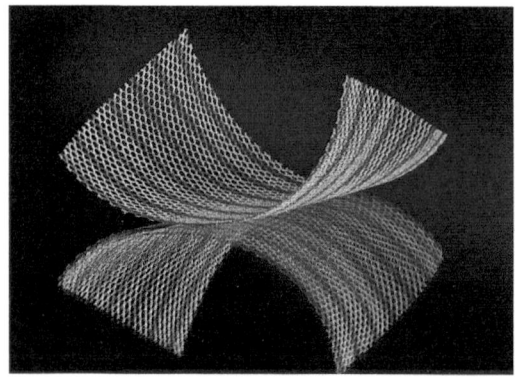

Fig. 5.102 Easy Prothes partially absorbable

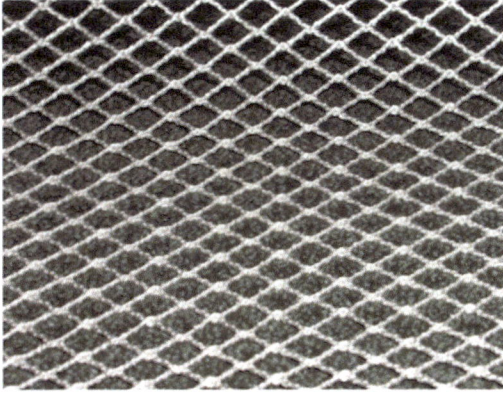

Fig. 5.103 4D Ventral

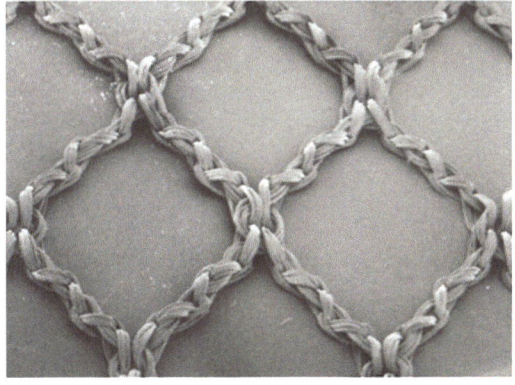

Fig. 5.104 Vypro (Image courtesy of Ethicon, Inc.)

TiMESH has been previously described above and is one of the few products in this section that can be placed against the viscera (Figs. 5.69 and 5.70). *Vypro is* actually a combination of PP and the absorbable polymer polyglactin (Fig. 5.104). The combination of these materials results in a very pliable and malleable material that should only be used in the preperitoneal position. Once

the polyglactin has been absorbed, the PP that remains has very large interstices into which the fibroblasts and collagen are deposited. The aim of this product is the improvement in the abdominal wall compliance that is more normal in function because of the very lightweight PP that remains. *Ultrapro* mesh is a similar concept and is manufactured from approximately equal parts of the absorbable poliglecaprone-25 monofilament fiber and the nonabsorbable lightweight PP (Fig. 5.105). A portion of the PP is dyed. The absorbable portion is essentially absorbed by 84 days. *Ultrapro Advanced* is similar to the former product but is designed to allow for more stretch of the abdominal wall, allowing a 2:1 stretch (Fig. 5.106). It stretches to the greatest degree perpendicular to the blue stripes.

Prostheses with an Absorbable Barrier Component

The original impetus behind the development of these products was the popularity of the laparoscopic intraperitoneal placement of mesh. In general, however, all of these prosthetic devices can or have been used in both open and laparoscopic incisional hernioplasties. All of these have the common purpose to repair the hernia and prevent the development of adhesions with the attendant complications associated with this result of the healing

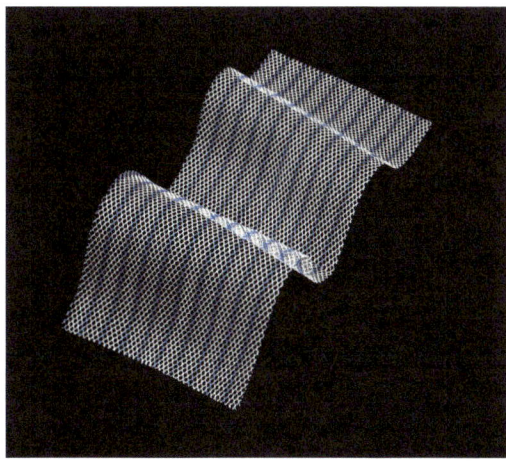

Fig. 5.105 Ultrapro flat mesh (Image courtesy of Ethicon, Inc.)

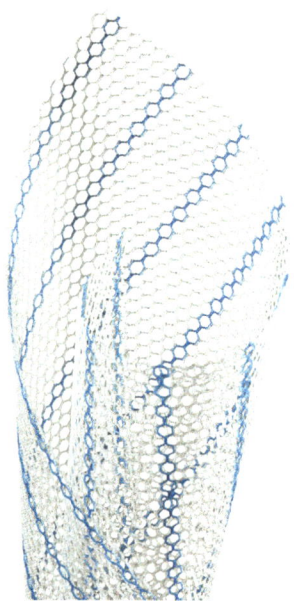

Fig. 5.106 Ultrapro Advanced (Image courtesy of Ethicon, Inc.)

Table 5.14 Combination prostheses with an absorbable barrier

Adhesix, Davol, Inc., Warwick, RI, USA
C-QUR Mosiac, Getinge Group, Wayne, NJ, USA
Easy Pro Composite Mesh, TransEasy Medical Tech. Co.Ltd., Beijing, China
Parietene Composite, Medtronic, Minneapolis, MN, USA
Parietex Optimized Composite (PCOx), Medtronic, Minneapolis, MN, USA
Parietene DS, Medtronic, Minneapolis, MN, USA
Parietene ProGrip, Medtronic, Minneapolis, MN, USA
Parietex ProGrip, Medtronic, Minneapolis, MN, USA
Proceed, Ethicon, Inc., Somerville, NJ, USA
SepraMesh IP, Davol, Inc., Warwick, RI, USA
Symbotex, Medtronic, Minneapolis, MN, USA
Ventralight ST, Davol, Inc., Warwick, RI, USA
Ventralex ST, Davol, Inc., Warwick, RI, USA
Ventrio ST, Davol, Inc., Warwick, RI, USA

processes. These are generally referred to as "tissue-separating" meshes as they create an absorbable barrier between the permanent product and the viscera (Table 5.14). They are available in a variety of shapes and sizes, which are too many to enumerate here. The reader is referred to the individual company for further information.

The resorption of that nonpermanent substance leaves a permanent layer of mesh that will incorporate into the tissues of the patient. The controversial part of this idea is the fact that the problems that are related to the development of adhesions following the implantation of a synthetic biomaterial do not become manifest for many years postimplantation. Therefore, the late effects of these products will necessitate many years of follow-up to validate these claims. At the present time, however, these meshes do seem to live up to their expectations regarding adhesion development. There have been some central failures due to materials that were too lightweight and/or macroporous are no longer available.

Adhesix can be used in the preperitoneal position, the retrorectus space or as an onlay but it is not designed for use in with contact with the viscera (Fig. 5.100). *C-QUR Mosiac* is made of a lightweight Prolite mesh onto which Omega-3 Fatty Acid (O3FA) has been coated onto the product (Fig. 5.107). These fatty acids are in a cross-linked gel that covers both sides of the material and impart a characteristic dark yellow color. O3FA will absorb over a period of 3–6 months. It is to be used when tissue-separating capabilities are required in the repair of hernias. *Easy Pro Composite Mesh* is constructed of lightweight PPM with a barrier coating of poly-lactide-co-caprolactone (Fig. 5.108). It is indicated for intraperitoneal usage. It has an "F" on the visceral surface to identify the orientation toward the intestine.

Parietene Composite is PP coated with the hydrophilic collagen and other substances that are

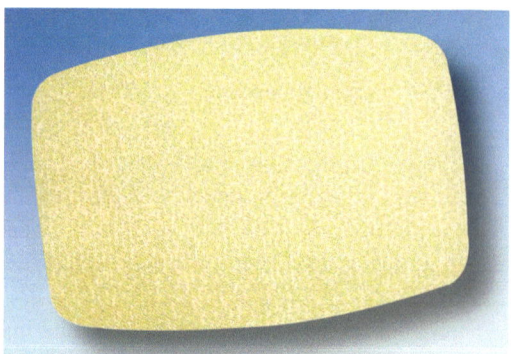

Fig. 5.107 C-Qur Mosiac

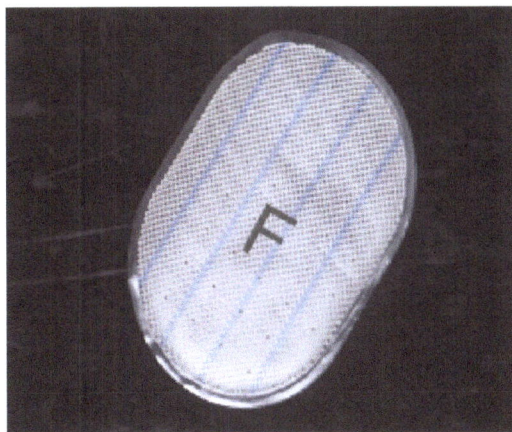

Fig. 5.108 EasyPro composite

Fig. 5.109 Parietex Optimized Composite (PCOx) (All rights reserved. Used with permission of Medtronic.)

used in the better-known Parietex Composite discussed below. It has an incorporated hydrophilic layer of a mixture of oxidized Type I atelocollagen, polyethylene glycol, and glycerol, which is absorbable. *Parietex Optimized Composite (PCOx)* is a POL biomaterial that also has this barrier coating (Fig. 5.109). It can be purchased with the *AccuMesh Positioning System* (Fig. 5.110). *Parietene DS* is a dual-sided product that has Paritene macroporous PP that is coated on one side with glycolide, caprolactone, trimethylene carbonate, and lactose. This barrier coating is essentially degraded within 105 days. There is a violet marking to help position the mesh. There are two preplaced sutures made of a stereoisomer of PP and polyethylene that are needed to differentiate the sides of the product and to be used for transparietal fixation. *Parietene ProGrip* and *Parietex ProGrip* also differ in that

the former is of PP and the latter is of POL. Both have the polylactic acid grippers (described earlier in this chapter) so that they potentially do not need fixation. The coating on these products is very minimal, so it is not recommended that these products should contact the viscera.

Proceed is composed of an oxidized regenerated cellulose (ORC) fabric and Prolene Soft Mesh which is encapsulated by a polydioxanone polymer that holds this together (Fig. 5.111). The fabric acts as a barrier to separate the PP from the tissue. The ORC is absorbed within 4 weeks. It should be noted that the instructions for use state "Proceed Mesh has an ORC component that should not be used in the presence of uncontrolled and/or active bleeding as fibrinous exudates may increase the chance of adhesion formation."

SepraMesh IP is a single layer of heavy weight polypropylene and is covered by barrier that is a combination of carboxymethylcellulose and hyaluronic acid (Fig. 5.112). It is bound together with

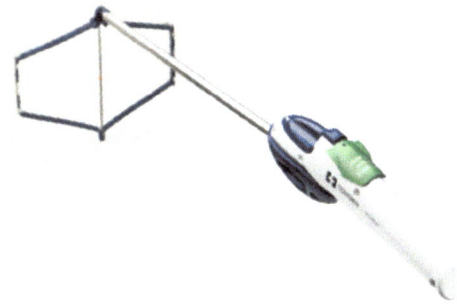

Fig. 5.110 AccuMesh positioning system (All rights reserved. Used with permission of Medtronic.)

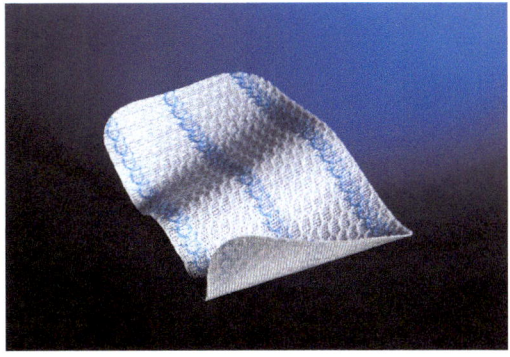

Fig. 5.111 Proceed (Image courtesy of Ethicon, Inc.)

polyglycolic acid fibers and a hydrogel. This product requires brief immersion into saline solution prior to its use to activate the gel. The hydrogel swells following implantation to cover the fixation devices that are used. This portion of the product is stated to last approximately 4 weeks, at which point, it has been resorbed. There is a lighter weight version that is Ventralight ST (Fig. 5.113). The "Sepra" technology has been extended to the original Ventralex and Ventrio products (Table 5.15). The ePTFE surface

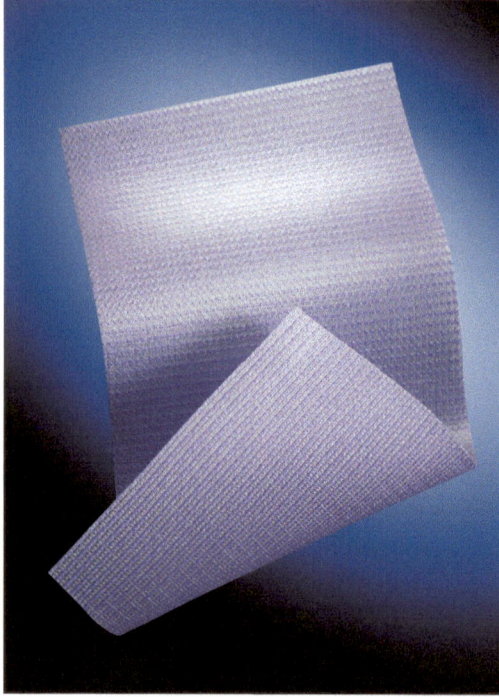

Fig. 5.112 SepraMesh IP

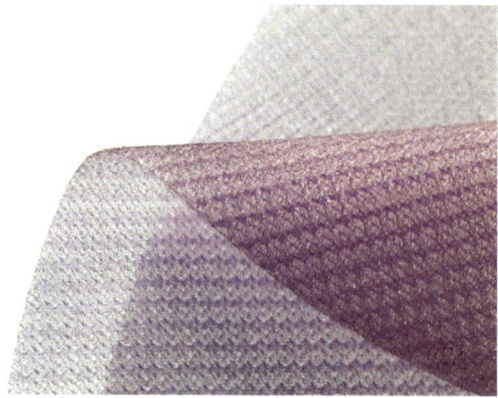

Fig. 5.113 Ventralight ST

Table 5.15 Combination prostheses with a permanent barrier

ClearMesh Composite (CMC), Di.pro Medical Devices, Torino, Italy
CO3+, THT-Bio-Science, Montpelier, France
Combi Mesh Plus, Angiologica, S. Martino Sicc., Italy
Composix E/X Mesh, Davol, Inc., Warwick, RI, USA
Composix L/P Mesh, Davol, Inc., Warwick, RI, USA
Composix L/P Mesh with ECHO PS, Davol, Inc., Warwick, RI, USA
DualMesh, W. L. Gore & Associates, Elkhart, DE, USA
DualMesh Plus, W. L. Gore &Associates, Elkhart, DE, USA
DualMesh Plus with Holes, W. L. Gore &Associates, Elkhart, DE, USA
Dulex, Davol, Inc., Warwick, RI, USA
DynaMesh IPOM, FEG Textiltechnik mbH, Aachen, Germany
Intra, Microval, Saint-Just-Malmont, France
IntraMesh T1, Cousin Biotech, Wervicq-Sud, France
IS 180, THT Bio-Science, Montpelier, France
Omyra Mesh, B. Braun Melsungen AG, Melsungen, Germany
MotifMESH, Proxy Biomedical Ltd., Galway, Ireland
MycroMesh, W. L. Gore &Associates, Elkhart, DE, USA
MycroMesh Plus, W. L. Gore &Associates, Elkhart, DE, USA
Prefix, THT Bio-Science, Montpelier, France
Plurimesh (PCMC), Di.pro Medical Devices, Torino, Italy
Rebound HRD V, ARB Medical, Minneapolis, MN, USA
RELIMESH, HerniaMesh, Torino, Italy
SMH2+, THT Bio-Science, Montpelier, France
SM3+, THT Bio-Science, Montpelier, France
Soft Tissue Patch, W. L. Gore &Associates, Elkhart, DE, USA
SurgiMesh XB, Aspide Medical, St. Etienne, France
TiMesh, GfE Medizintechnik, Nuremburg, Germany
TiO₂ Mesh, Bayreuth, Germany
Umbilical - CMC, Di.pro Medical Devices, Torino, Italy
Ventralex, Davol, Inc., Warwick, RI, USA
Ventrio Hernia Patch, Davol, Inc., Warwick, RI, USA
Ventrio-S, THT Bio-Science, Montpelier, France

has been replaced with the tissue-separating material that is used on the SepraMesh IP and Ventralight ST prostheses. These products are called *Ventralex ST* and *Ventrio ST* (Figs. 5.114

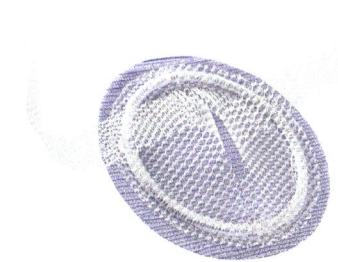

Fig. 5.114 Ventralex ST

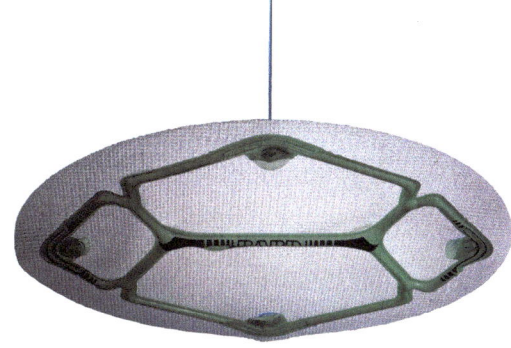

Fig. 5.116 Ventralight ST with Echo PS

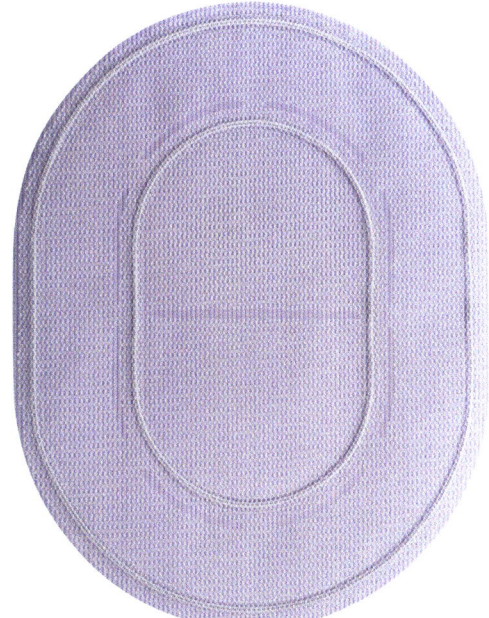

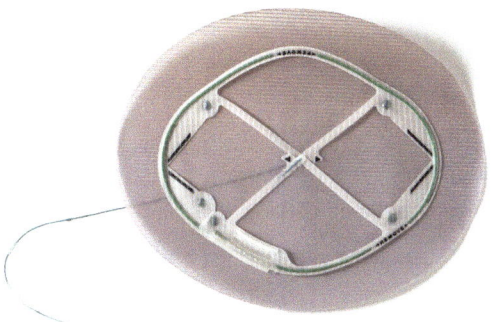

Fig. 5.117 Ventralight ST with Echo 2

Fig. 5.115 Ventrio ST

and 5.115). While the former product was originally designed for use in open repair, it has found use in the laparoscopic repair of smaller ventral and incisional hernias. *Ventralex ST* is also available with the *ECHO PS*, which is a positioning aid (Fig. 5.116). It is a balloon that is inflated to stiffen the material that effectively makes fixation much easier. There will be an improved version that is able to stiffen the product with nitinol wire (rather than the balloon) and uses a central hoisting suture rather than the tubing to inflate a balloon (Fig. 5.117). *Symbotex* is a polyester material that is lighter in weight

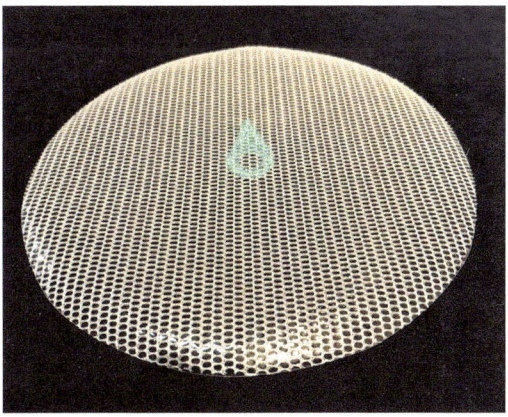

Fig. 5.118 Symbotex (All rights reserved. Used with permission of Medtronic.)

than the Parietex PCO_x (Fig. 5.118). It has the same barrier material as the PCO_x product described above (i.e., Type I atelocollagen, polyethylene glycol, and glycerol). The green marker is 2D polyester.

Combination Permanent Materials for Incisional and Ventral Hernioplasty

These products are a combination of a single product that is manufactured in two different forms or, more commonly, a combination of two different products (Table 5.15). The method of fixation of these different materials differs for each manufacturer. There are some that have been described earlier in this chapter that are single products (ePTFE, cPTFE, or PVDF) and are not described again here (Tables 5.11 and 5.12). What is consistent in all of the prostheses is the presence of a permanent barrier to resist adhesion formation while allowing for ingrowth on the parietal side of these meshes to repair a hernia effectively.

CO3+ has been described in the flat mesh section (Fig. 5.80). It is a combination of POL and PUR with grips. *ClearMesh Composite (CMC)* is a pure PP mesh (Fig. 5.119). There is a textured side that is composed of a single filament macroporous weave and a nonadhesive side that is composed of a nonporous smooth PP film. It is for use in the intraperitoneal space. It is further designated as *CMC 2P*, which is elliptical in shape, and the *CMC 2P-C*, which is round. *Plurimesh (PCMC)* is a similar concept as the CMC except that it is designed for incisional or parastomal hernia repair (Fig. 5.120). It has sewn seams that can be used to cut the mesh to conform to the needs of the hernia treated. *Combi Mesh Plus* is a combination of PP and polyurethrane to allow usage intrabdominally (Fig. 5.121). There is an

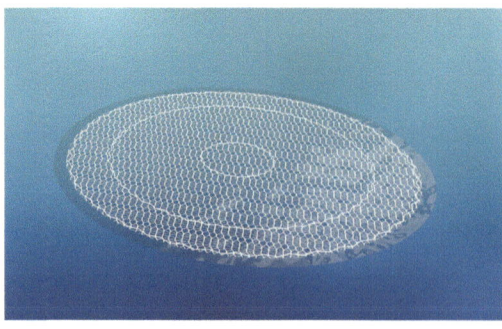

Fig. 5.119 ClearMesh composite

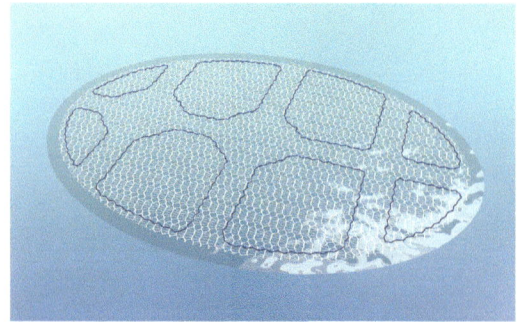

Fig. 5.120 Plurimesh

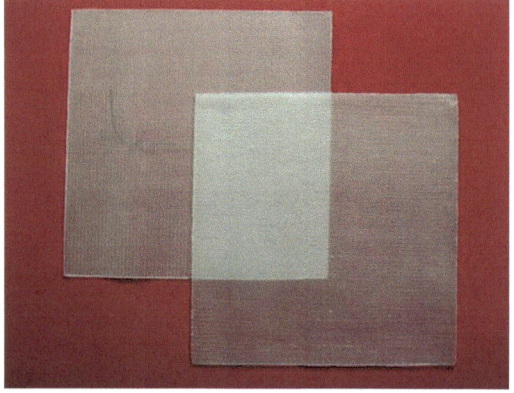

Fig. 5.121 Combi Mesh Plus

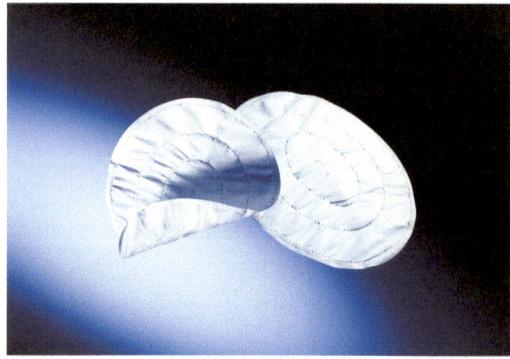

Fig. 5.122 Composix E/X

attached suture to delineate the parietal surface. The polyurethane layer faces the viscera. *Composix E/X Mesh* is flat Bard mesh on one side and ePTFE on the other side (Fig. 5.122). The edge of the perimeter of the elliptically shaped product is sealed to prevent contact of viscera to the PP. It is a low profile mesh. *Composix L/P* is very similar to the Composix E/X except that the former uses the lighter Bard Soft Mesh rather than the Bard mesh (Fig. 5.123). It is specifically designed for laparoscopic usage and can be used with a supplied introduction tool. The two mesh layers are sutured together with ePTFE suture. The Composix L/P is also available with the ECHO PS (Fig. 5.124). The green balloon shown in the figure will be inflated to firm up the mesh to allow for accurate positioning and fixation. There is an attached blue tubing on the opposite side that is not seen in the figure that is pulled through the abdominal wall to center the mesh. It is then cut and attached to a syringe that is used to inflate the balloon. Once fixation is completed, the balloon is deflated and removed.

DynaMesh IPOM is a similar PP weave as the DynaMesh described earlier in this chapter but it is slightly lighter than the latter product (Fig. 5.125). This version is intertwined with monofilament polyvinylidene fluoride (PVDF) on one surface. Because of this PVDF tissue-separating component it can be placed onto the viscera. The suture noted in the figure signifies which side should be placed against the abdominal wall, as it is impossible to be certain with the naked eye which side should go up. *Intra* mesh is a combination of nonwoven PP on one side with another layer of silicone on the other as a tissue-separating material (Fig. 5.126). It is one of the few materials available with this silicone barrier. This side is marked with a cross and "intra side" in black silicone ink. *IntraMesh T1* is similar to the Composix product line in that it is composed of one layer of PP and a second layer of ePTFE (Fig. 5.127). It is the only material that possesses lines on the product to delineate the midportions of each side to ease positioning. Cousin Biotech also sells a "mesh roller" which is a device to aid in the rolling of these materials to ease insertion via a trocar. *IS 180* is

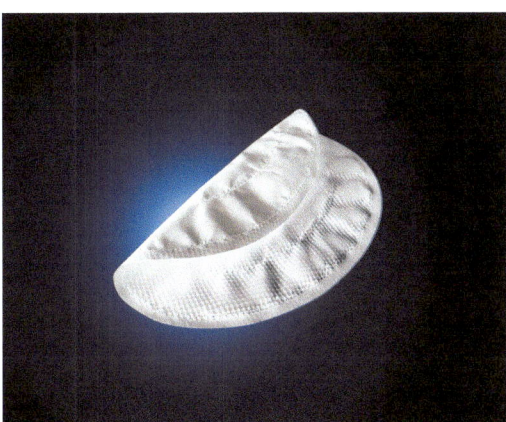

Fig. 5.123 Composix L/P

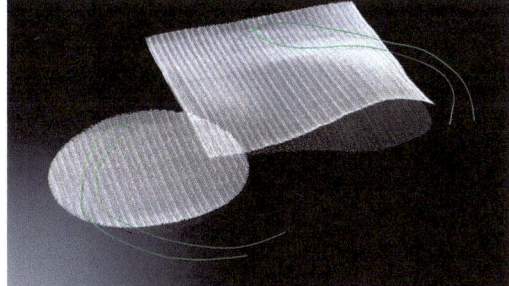

Fig. 5.125 DynaMesh IPOM

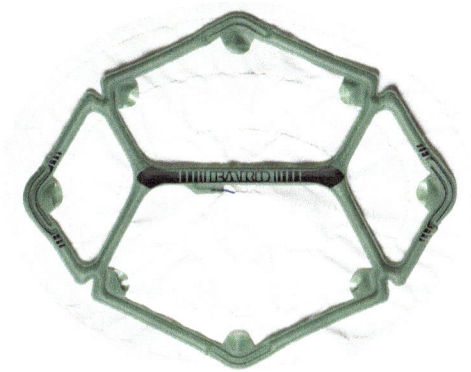

Fig. 5.124 Composix L/P mesh with Echo PS

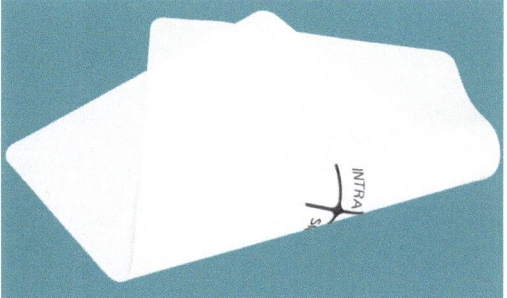

Fig. 5.126 IntraMesh

part of the Intra-Swing composite family, which is a macroperforated three-dimensional POL that has a coating of tissue-separating PUR on one surface (Fig. 5.128). It is configured in a variety of shapes with or without PP sutures to aid in fixation. The company also has an available *Easy-Catch EC* device to be used for introduction of the material into the abdominal cavity. *Prefix* is similar in concept to the IS 180 but, as shown in the photo, there are preplaced sutures to allow for positioning of the product (Fig. 5.129). It is one of the few products that include pre-attached sutures with straight needles on them.

Rebound HRD V has previously been described in miscellaneous flat mesh section above

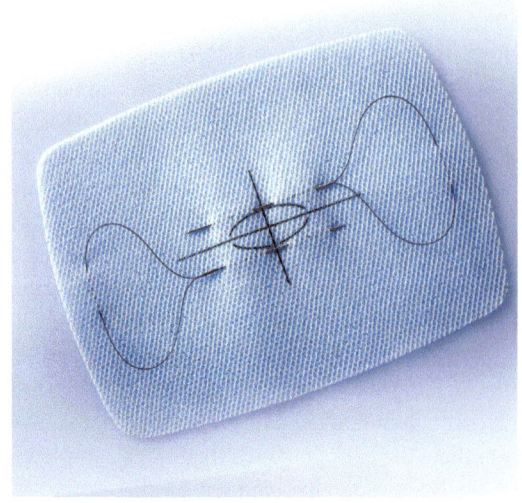

Fig. 5.129 Prefix

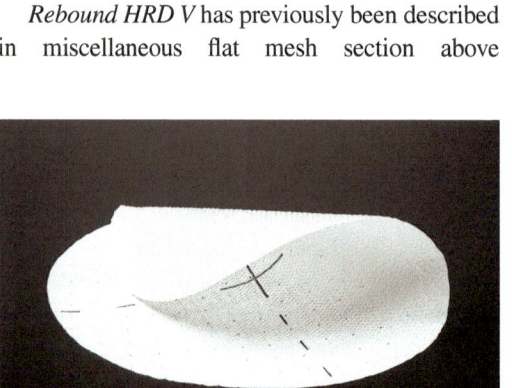

Fig. 5.127 IntraMesh T1

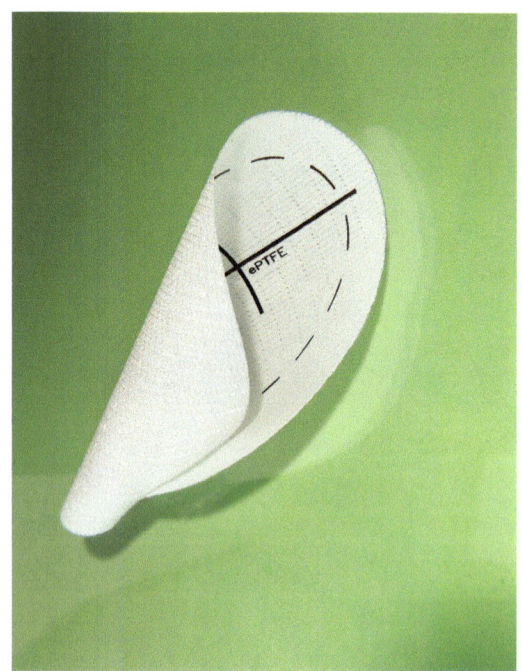

Fig. 5.130 RELIMESH

(Fig. 5.98). It is designed for use in the preperitoneal space. *RELIMESH* is another product that incorporates the PP on one surface and ePTFE on the other to allow placement against the viscera (Fig. 5.130). It is a lighter weight product compared to other HerniaMesh products. Because of this, it can be rolled for insertion via a trocar. It is

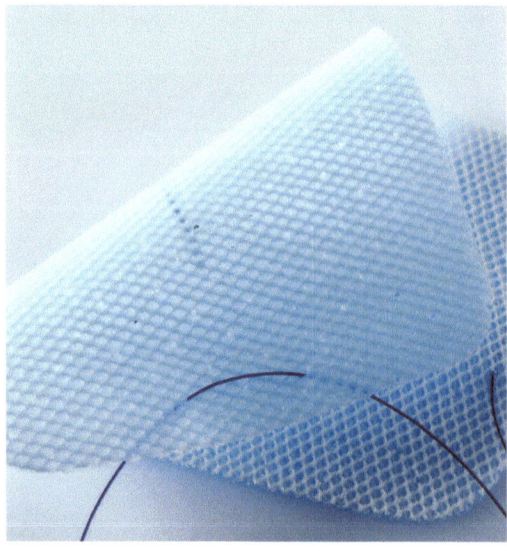

Fig. 5.128 IS 180

marked to aid in positioning and fixation. *SMH2+* is PP and PUR and is available for ventral and incisional hernia repair even though the shape in the figure is rather rounded (Fig. 5.131). *SM3+* has been described in the flat mesh section of the chapter and has also been noted in other sections (Fig. 5.86). It is made of polyester and impregnated polyurethane and can be used in open or laparoscopic methods.

SurgiMesh XB has a nonwoven, non-knitted structure as does the SurgiMesh WN described earlier (Fig. 5.132). It has an additional layer of silicone to allow contact with the viscera and is microperforated. This product is available in different shapes. There is a circular one that has an attached suture as a positioning aid (Tintra C). *TiMesh* is the same material that has been described in several locations within this chapter

(Fig. 5.70). The titanized PPM can be used in the intraperitoneal location (per the manufacturer). Another titanized PPM is that of *TiO₂Mesh* (Fig. 5.99). This is described in the Miscellaneous Flat Mesh section above.

Ventralex is a self-expanding PP device (because of the outer ring of PDO) that has ePTFE on one side to allow placement adjacent to viscera (Fig. 5.133). It is round but smaller than the larger products such as the Composix products described above. It is intended for use in the smaller defects of the abdominal wall such as trocar or umbilical hernias. Two long straps are attached that can be used for fixation to the fascia. They are very long as this product can be inserted through a laparoscopic trocar to aid in the prevention of trocar hernias. The *Ventrio Hernia Patch* is comprised of two layers of PP that are stitched to an ePTFE layer as the tissue-separating component (Fig. 5.134). Within the PP surface there are

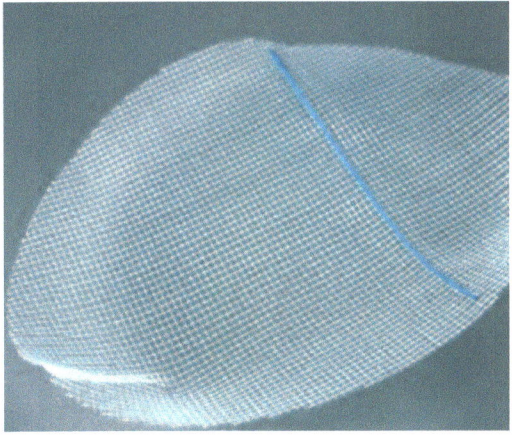

Fig. 5.131 SMH2+

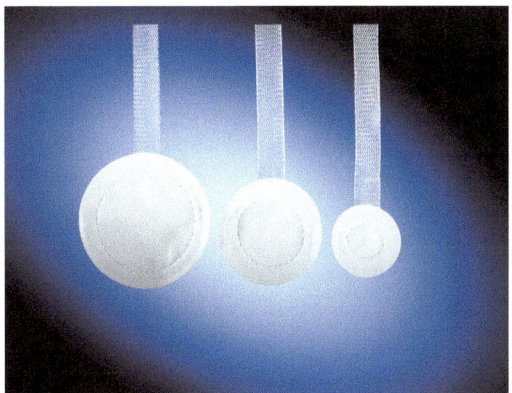

Fig. 5.133 Ventralex

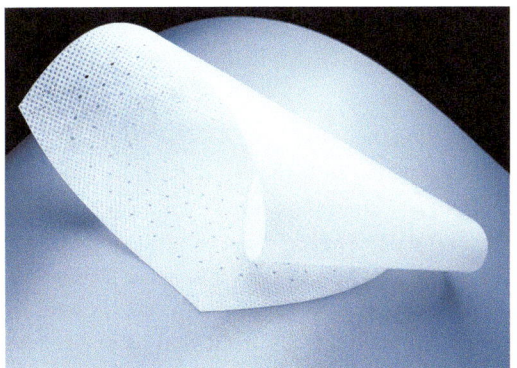

Fig. 5.132 Surgimesh XB

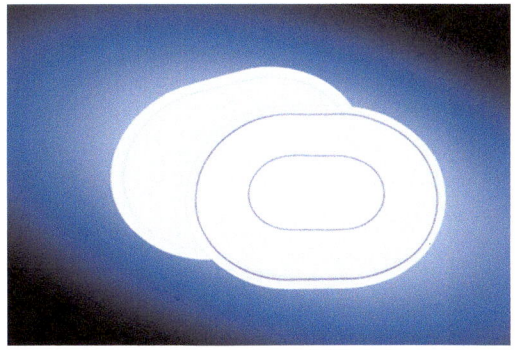

Fig. 5.134 Ventrio Hernia Patch

"tubes" that house the absorbable polydioxanone (PDO) monofilament rings to give the mesh rigidity to aid in positioning and fixation. The purple PDO ring is absorbed within 6–8 months.

Stomal Products

The development of a hernia wherever a stoma is created has been the challenge in the life of all patients with some type of an ostomy. Traditionally, relocation or primary closure was used to repair these hernias; it is now recognized that the result is failure in most cases. Consequently, the use of a prosthetic material has become nearly standard to repair these hernias. In fact, recent trends indicate that the use of a mesh of some type when the stoma is created may be the preferred option. Prevention has become the new effort in mesh construction. Many of these options involve the use of one of the biologic, synthetic absorbable or permanent products described earlier in this chapter. These will not be rediscussed. As with many of the other products in this chapter, these can generally be used with the open or laparoscopic technique. The materials listed in Table 5.16 are specifically designed for stomal hernia repair.

Colostomy Mesh is a single layer PP product (Fig. 5.135). It has a five-centimeter hole in the center of the material through which the intestine can be placed during stomal creation. Of course, the mesh can be cut if this product is used to repair a parastomal hernia. It is available in a "rigid" and a "semi-rigid" construction.

DynaMesh-IPST, like its parent material, is made of both PVDF and PP (Fig. 5.136). It is pre-shaped and three-dimensional. *Parietex*

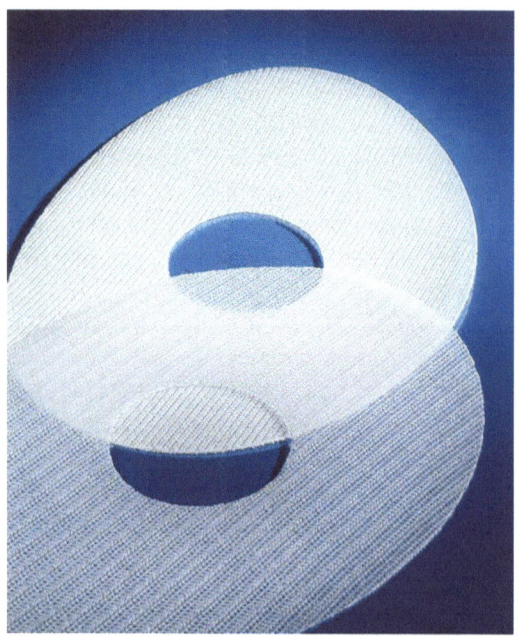

Fig. 5.135 Colostomy mesh

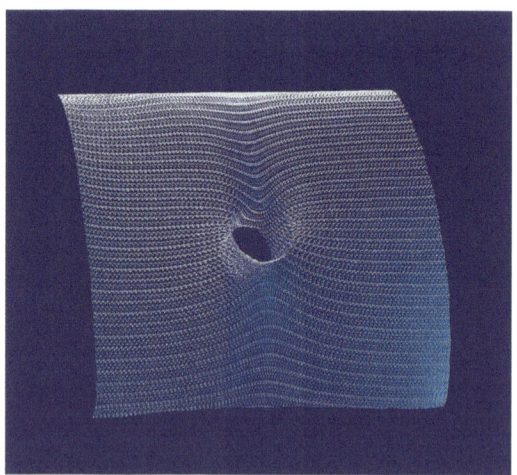

Fig. 5.136 DynaMesh IPST

Table 5.16 Stomal prostheses

Colostomy Mesh, HerniaMesh, Torino, Italy
DynaMesh-IPST, FEG Textiltechnik mbH, Aachen, Germany
Parietex Composite Parastomal Mesh, Medtronic, Minneapolis, MN
Plurimesh (PCMC), Di.pro Medical Devices, Torino, Italy
TiLENE Guard, GfE Medizintechnik, Nuremburg, Germany

Composite Parastomal Mesh is of the same material as that described previously. This is supplied in two sizes and is available with a hole with an available opening of 3.5 cm or 5.0 cm (Fig. 5.137). It is also supplied without a hole and can be configured as required (Fig. 5.138). *Polyvalent Clear Mesh Composite (PCMC)* has already been described for incisional and ventral hernia repair. It can also be used for parastomal hernia repair

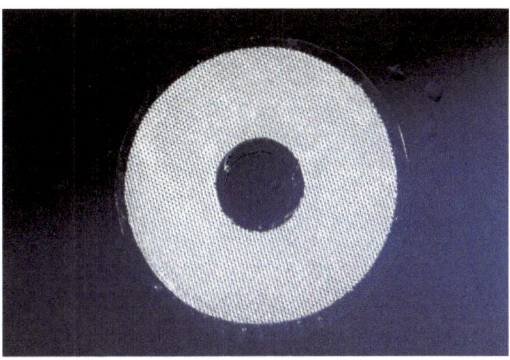

Fig. 5.137 Parietex Parastomal with hole (All rights reserved. Used with permission of Medtronic.)

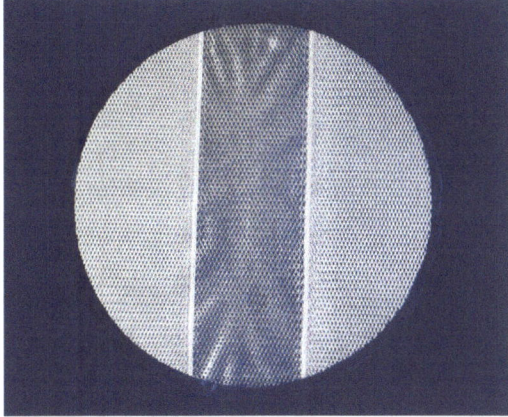

Fig. 5.138 Parietex Parastomal without hole (All rights reserved. Used with permission of Medtronic.)

(Fig. 5.120). It is supplied in such a manner that it can be cut to confirm to whatever the size the surgeon chooses.

TiLENE Guard is of titanized PP (Fig. 5.139). It is supplied with a flap, which is closed after the intestine is placed through the central hole. It is supplied in the light and dual-weight (light and medium) meshes. There is a set, which contains *TiLENE* mesh that is to be applied as a "sandwich" technique to repair or prevent herniation through the stoma location.

Fixation Devices

Fixation devices became prevalent early in the development of the laparoscopic repair of hernias. They are mostly available as 5 mm versions

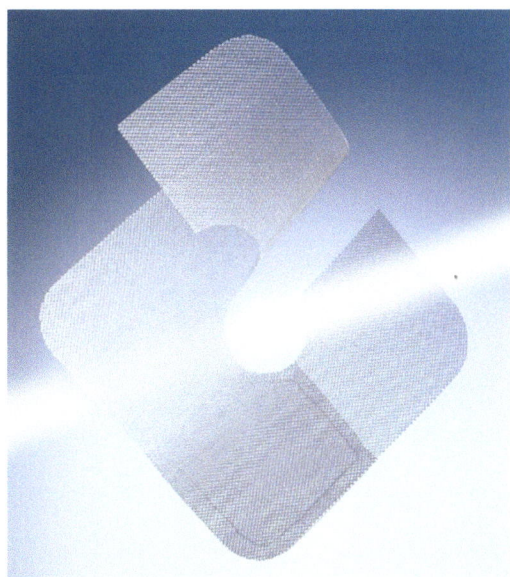

Fig. 5.139 TiLENE guard

Table 5.17 Fixation devices for hernia repair (an asterick indicates absorbable fasteners)

AbsorbaTack*, Medtronic, Minneapolis, MN, USA
CapSure, Davol, Inc., Warwick, RI, USA
DegraTack*, TransEasy Medical Tech.Co.Ltd., Beijing, China
Endo Universal Stapler, Medtronic, Minneapolis, MN, USA
FasTouch, Via Surgical, Tel Aviv, Israel
iMesh Tacker*, *Corregio (RE), Italy*
Multifire Endo Hernia Stapler, Medtronic, Minneapolis, MN, USA
Multifire VersaTack Stapler, Medtronic, Minneapolis, MN, USA
Optifix*, Davol. Inc., Warwick, RI, USA
PermaFix, Davol, Inc., Warwick, RI, USA
ProTack, Medtronic, Minneapolis, MN, USA
ReliaTack*, Medtronic, Minneapolis, MN, USA
SecureStrap*, Ethicon Inc., Somerville, NJ, USA
SorbaFix*, Davol, Inc., Warwick, RI, USA
Spire' it, Microval, Saint-Just-Malmont, France
Tacker, Medtronic Minneapolis, MN, USA
TiTack, TransEasy Medical Tech.Co.Ltd., Beijing, China

as these have become the most popular. Currently, there are a variety of these devices that one may choose to fixate the meshes placed in hernia repair (Table 5.17). Surgeon preference, mesh selection, and whether permanent or absorbable fixation is

Fastener Comparison

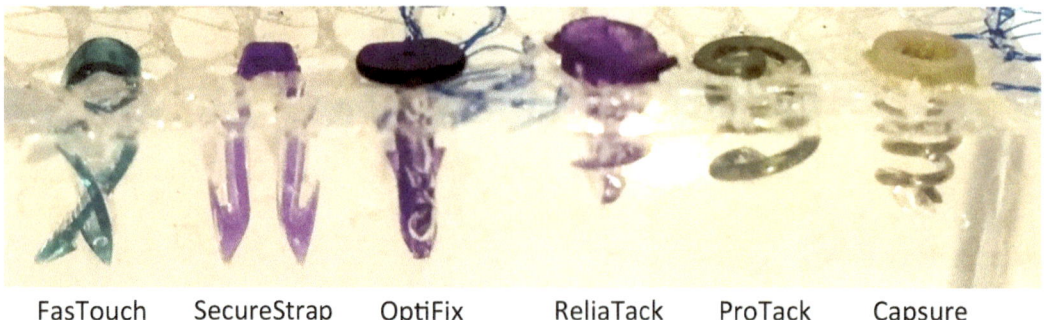

| FasTouch | SecureStrap | OptiFix | ReliaTack | ProTack | Capsure |

Fig. 5.140 Tack comparison

Fig. 5.141 Absorbatack (All rights reserved. Used with permission of Medtronic.)

needed will dictate the product decision. One should consider the configuration of the head of these fasteners and the total length of these fasteners, as the depth of penetration will be dependent upon the thickness of the mesh used to repair the hernia (Fig. 5.140). For example, a 5-mm fastener will provide no more of tissue penetration than 4 mm when used with 1 mm prosthesis. The reader is referred to the specific manufacturer of these products for more information.

AbsorbaTack is a 5 mm fixation device and provides an absorbable synthetic polyester copolymer screw-like fastener derived from PGLA (Fig. 5.141). The fastener itself measures 5.1 mm in length. The laparoscopic version is available with either 15 or 30 tacks. The tacks are significantly absorbed within 3–5 months with complete absorption within 1 year. *CapSure* is a permanent product, which has a smooth polyetheretherketone (PEEK) cap and screw threads that are made of 316L stainless steel (Fig. 5.142). The *DegraTack* is an absorbable screw-like tack

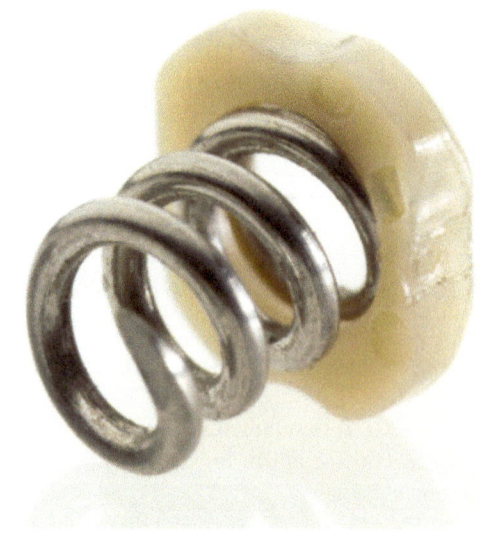

Fig. 5.142 CapSure

and is also made of polylactide-co-glycolide (PGLA), which is totally degraded in 12 months (Fig. 5.143). The iMesh tack is another PGLA device (Fig. 5.144). It has a depth of purchase of 5.2 mm. It has a large variety of loads of 10, 15, 20, 25, 30, or 38 tacks. The tip of the delivery device can articulate up to 60°.

FasTouch is a unique 5-mm device that does not employ any of the screw-like fasteners listed in this section but instead delivers a suture-like closed "locked" loop (Figs. 5.145 and 5.146). It can be reloaded with either a 10 or 25 reload. Its

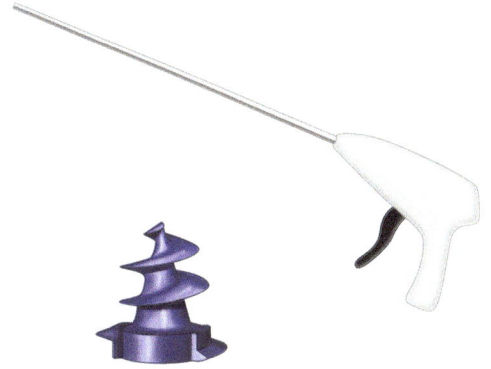

Fig. 5.143 DegraTack

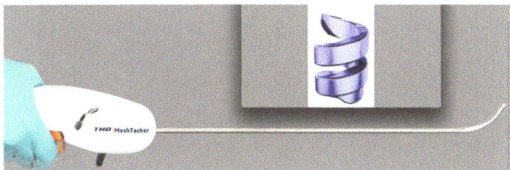

Fig. 5.144 iMesh tacker

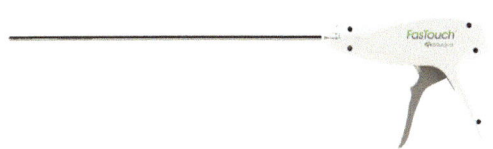

Fig. 5.145 FasTouch

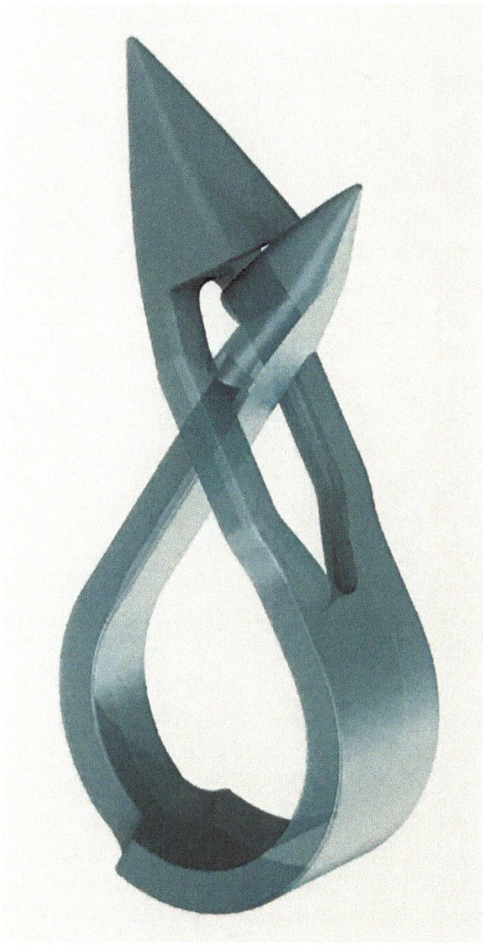

Fig. 5.146 FasTouch fastener

shape and size delivers the lowest amount of foreign body to fixate the mesh than any other available product. The permanent fastener is made of poly-carbonate-urethane (PCU). Although not available at the time of this writing, there will be an absorbable fastener soon. The *Endo Universal Stapler* is to be used via a 10 or 12 mm trocar (Fig. 5.147, middle). It can be rotated 360° and articulated up to 65%. Consequently, this device can be used in four different positions. The *MultiFire Endo Hernia Stapler* is introduced through a 12-mm trocar (Fig. 5.147, upper). Both of these devices fire "box-shaped" titanium staples that will fixate the prosthesis into which it is fired. They are both reloadable with either 4.0 mm or 4.8 mm staples (Fig. 5.147, lower). The obvious difference is that the former product will articulate up to 65° while the latter does not. The *MultiFire VersaTack Stapler* is designed for

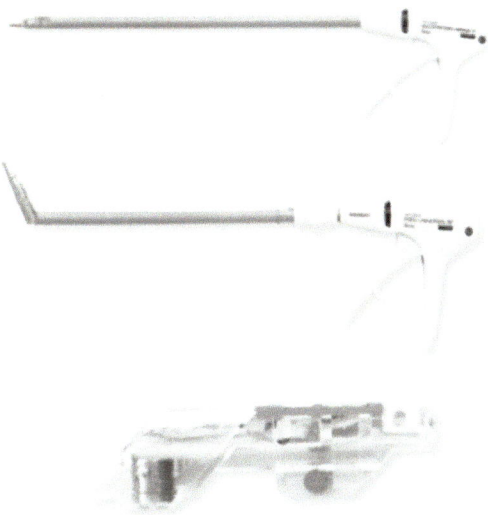

Fig. 5.147 Multifire and Endo universal staplers (All rights reserved. Used with permission of Medtronic.)

usage during open hernia repair (Fig. 5.148). It, too, can be rotated 360° and is available with either the 4.0 or 4.8 mm staples with ten staples. These staples are usually acceptable for use with MRI and NMR up to 3 T.

The *OptiFix* device delivers a poly(D,L)-lactide (PDLLA) fastener that has two barbs on the end of it and two on the shaft (Fig. 5.149). They are delivered over an introducer needle. This product is available in either a 15 or 30 shot shaft. These fasteners are fully absorbed at 16 months. *PermaFix* and *SorbaFix* each deliver the same size (6.7 mm) screw-type fasteners by an identical delivery mechanism with a pilot tip and mandrel (Fig. 5.150). Both of these fasteners are available in either 15 or 30 devices delivered via a 5 mm product. Permafix is made of a gray molded permanent (nonabsorbable) polymer. SorbaFix is made of the same purple absorbable material as OptiFix.

The *ProTack* is one of the older products that delivers a permanent titanium helical fastener by a 5 mm device (Fig. 5.151). It is available with 30 tacks. These are the easiest fixation products to visualize on a plain radiologic study. They are 3.9 mm in total length. *ReliaTack* is an articulating 5 mm device that also delivers a similar screw-like Absorbatack (Fig. 5.152). It can be

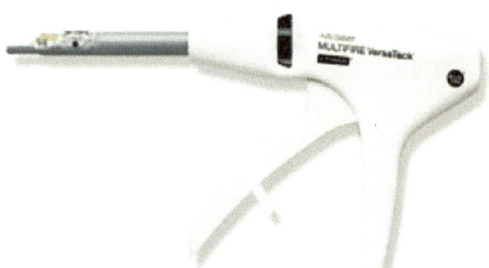

Fig. 5.148 MultiFire VersaTack

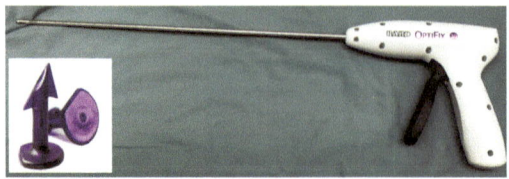

Fig. 5.149 Optifix

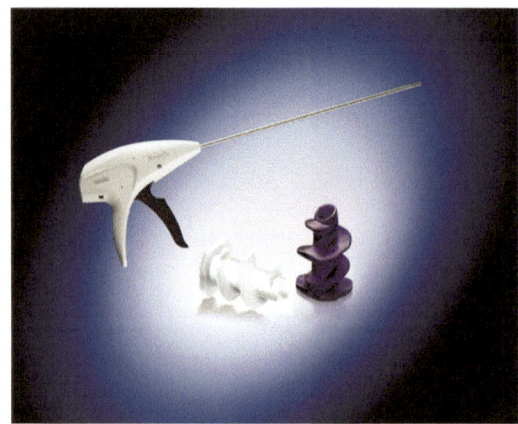

Fig. 5.150 Sorbafix and Permafix

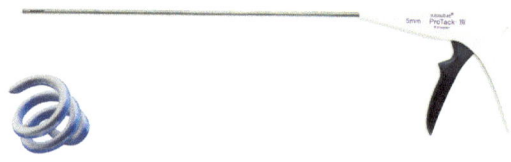

Fig. 5.151 ProTack

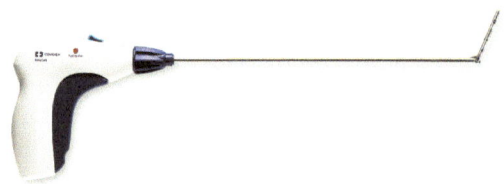

Fig. 5.152 Reliatack

reloaded with a cartridge that contains either 5 or 10 fasteners. It is supplied with either a standard 5.1 mm device or a deep tack that is 7.0 mm in length (Fig. 5.153). It is the only fastener that is available with two different tack lengths.

The *SECURESTRAP* is pre-loaded with *25* absorbable straps (Fig. 5.154). The straps are composed of a blend of polydioxanone and L(−)-lactide and glycolide dyed with D&C Violet No. 2. This product has two legs similar to the staplers and does not screw into the tissues. The ends of these straps are barbed to aid in fixation. The width between the points is 3.5 mm. The entire devices length is 6.7 mm but the distance

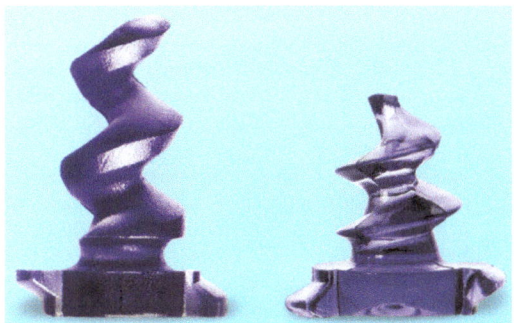

Fig. 5.153 ReliaTack standard or deep purchase tack (All rights reserved. Used with permission of Medtronic.)

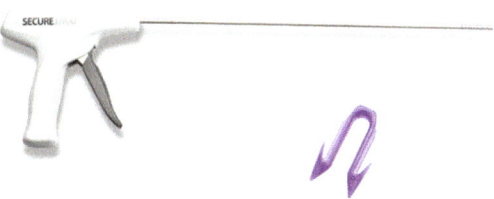

Fig. 5.154 Securestrap (Image courtesy of Ethicon, Inc.)

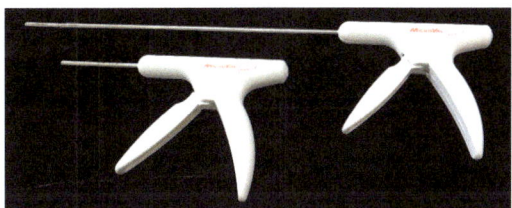

Fig. 5.155 Spire' it

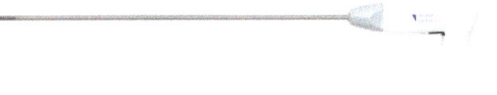

Fig. 5.156 Tacker (All rights reserved. Used with permission of Medtronic.)

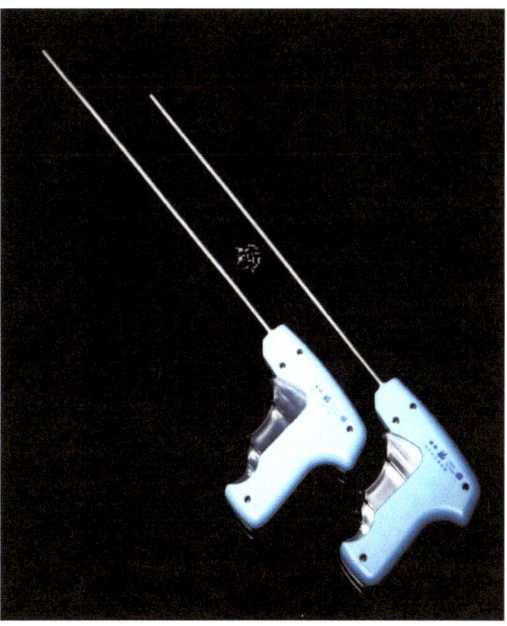

Fig. 5.157 TiTack

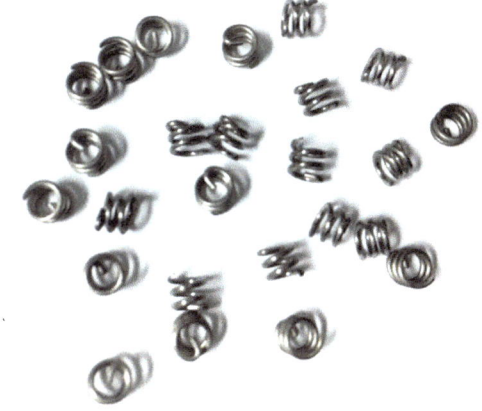

Fig. 5.158 TiTack tacks

from the inner portion of the strap to the point of fixation of the strap is 4.9 mm (i.e. the "grip"). *Spire' It* is a different device in that it is made of nitinol and advances in the shape of a ring once fully formed (Fig. 5.155). There are two turns of the ring with a final form of 4 mm. It is reloadable and is available in a 30 cm length for laparoscopic surgical applications.

The *Tacker* delivers helical titanium tacks virtually identical to the ProTack (Fig. 5.157). The *Tacker* delivers 30 tacks in the single-use device. There is an available multiuse handle of the *Tacker* that can be attached to an available tube of 20 tacks. The multiuse product has a shorter tube than the single-use product. The *TiTack* is another permanent titanium screw-like device that has a similar appearance to the devices listed above (Figs. 5.157 and 5.158).

Conclusion

The use of a prosthetic material for all hernia repairs is generally considered the standard of care unless there are extenuating circumstances. The purpose of this chapter is to identify and differentiate the products that can be used in hernioplasties. It is as complete as we could make this at this time. Undoubtedly by the time of the printing of this textbook other products will have become available. The surgeon should choose carefully.

I believe that the ideal material has not yet been developed. There are, however, many that have been described above that do function quite well for the surgeon and the patient. Perhaps in the future, the use of genetic engineering will produce a product that is based from the protein of the patient and will allow the patient to incorporate a "natural" and "native" product into the tissues without fear of infection or adhesions. A permanent solution to the quest of the perfect biomaterial may be the result.

Acknowledgements Although it is not designated on the propriety names of any of the products listed in this chapter, it should be acknowledged to the reader that all manufacturer names and products are either registered trademarks, copyrighted, or exclusive to that company. These cannot be used without the permission of the respective company.

Many of these photos were taken by myself or provided by the company itself. I wish to thank all of these companies for their permissions and invaluable assistance in putting the most accurate information into this chapter that I could not have obtained without their assistance.

References

1. Hesselink VJ, Luiiendijk RW, de Wilt JHW, Heide R. An evaluation of risk factors in incisional hernia recurrence. Surg Gynecol Obstet. 1993;176:228–34.

2. Luijendijk RW, Hop WCJ, van den Tol P, de Lange DC, Braaksma MM, IJzermans JN, Boelhouwer RU, de Vries BC, Salu MK, Wereldsma JC, Bruijninckx CM, Jeekel J. A comparison of suture repair with mesh repair for incisinoal hernia. N Engl J Med. 2000;34(6):393–8.

3. Kokotovic D, Bisgaard T, Helgstrand F. Long-term recurrence and complications with elective incisional hernia repair. JAMA Surg. 2016;316(15):1575–82.

4. LeBlanc KA, Booth WV. Laparoscopic repair of incisional abdominal hernias using expanded polytetrafluoroethylene: preliminary findings. Surg Laparosc Endosc. 1993;3:39–41.

5. Bucknall TE, Cox PJ, Ellis H. Burst abdomen and incisional hernia: a prospective study of 1129 major laparotomies. Br Med J. 1982;284:931–3.

6. Cumberland O. Ueber die Verschliessung von Bauchwunden und Brustpforten durch Bersenkte Siberdragrnetze. Zentralbl Chir. 1900;27:257.

7. Scales JT. Discussion on metals and synthetic materials in relation to soft tissues: tissue reactions to synthetic materials. Proc R Soc Med. 1953;46:647.

8. Rosen MJ, Bauer JJ, Harmaty M, Carbonell AM, Cobb WS, Matthews B, Goldblatt MI, Selzer DJ, Poulose BK, Hansson BME, Rosman C, Chao JJ, Jacobsen GR. Multicenter, prospective longitudinal study of the recurrence, surgical site infection, and quality of life after contaminated ventral hernia repair using biosynthetic absorbable mesh. Ann Surg. 2017;265:205–11.

9. Oribabor FO, Amao OA, Akanni SO, Fatidinu S. The use of nontreated mosquito-net mesh cloth for a tension free inguinal hernia repair: our experience. Niger J Surg. 2015;21(1):48–51.

10. Stephenson BM, Kingsnorth AN. Safety and sterilization of mosquito net mesh for humanitarian inguinal hernioplasty. World J Surg. 2011;35(9):1957–60.

11. Patterson T, Currie P, Patterson S, Patterson P, Meek C, McMaster R. A systematic review and meta-analysis of the postoperative adverse effects associated with mosquito net mesh in comparison to commercial hernia mesh for inguinal hernia repair in low income countries. Hernia. 2017;21:397–405.

Laparoscopic Closure of Fascial Defect

Vashisht Madabhushi and J. Scott Roth

Introduction

Nearly one in five of the two million laparotomies performed in the United States each year is complicated by an incisional hernia [1–5]. Interestingly, only 300,000 ventral and incisional hernia repairs are performed in the United States each year. Incisional hernia repairs are plagued by recurrence. Approximately 24% of open repairs end up with recurrence, which places a significant burden on the healthcare system financially [6]. Reducing the recurrence rate by only 1% can save $32 billion dollars in healthcare expenses [7]. Prior to 1993, incisional hernias were repaired exclusively through open techniques associated with significant rates of wound complications, prolonged recovery, and significant postoperative pain. Since its introduction and initial report by LeBlanc in 1993 [8], laparoscopic incisional hernia repair has slowly gained popularity as an alternative method of incisional hernia repair. In the initial case series, LeBlanc described placement of intraperitoneal mesh, covering the hernia defect without apposition of the fascial defect and subsequent fixation of the mesh with staples.

This intraperitoneal onlay mesh (IPOM) repair has proven to have decreased rates of surgical site infections (SSIs), hospital lengths of stay, and complication rates relative to open repairs. However, the rates of recurrence relative to open repairs is comparable [9].

Innovations in the techniques for laparoscopic ventral hernia repair have resulted in techniques that facilitate repair that more closely model open repairs. These techniques allow for the fascial defects and may be closed primarily with subsequent placement of an intraperitoneal mesh [10–13]. The advantages and drawbacks of defect closure at the time of laparoscopic ventral hernia repair remain controversial, without any reduction of wound complications or recurrence rates [14]. Many proponents of defect closure will cite the improved cosmetic outcomes and reduction in bulging of the abdominal wall as an advantage [12]. However, prospective randomized trials comparing techniques are lacking and available evidence is based upon retrospective studies and meta-analysis.

The recent increase in utilization of robotic platforms for hernia repair has spawned further debate regarding the value of defect closure in laparoscopic ventral hernia repair. Robotic platforms have significantly enhanced the ease by which suturing may be accomplished laparoscopically, particularly when suturing on the anterior abdominal wall. The use of robotic platforms has facilitated defect closure utilizing intracorporeal suturing techniques. Case series describing outcomes utilizing these techniques are emerging in

V. Madabhushi · J. Scott Roth (✉)
University of Kentucky, Lexington, KY, USA
e-mail: s.roth@uky.edu

© Springer International Publishing AG, part of Springer Nature 2018
K. A. LeBlanc (ed.), *Laparoscopic and Robotic Incisional Hernia Repair*,
https://doi.org/10.1007/978-3-319-90737-6_6

the literature, although there is a paucity of evidence evaluating outcomes with this approach. Nevertheless, there seems to be a growing interest among surgeons in exploring the potential advantages of the use of robotic platforms to facilitate defect closure during laparoscopic ventral hernia repair.

Techniques

Techniques for laparoscopic defect closure include both extracorporeal or intracorporeal methods. Extracorporeal defect closure typically is performed utilizing a suture passer. This is placed transcutaneously through small skin incisions on the external abdominal wall, centered over the midportion of the hernia defect. The suture is directed toward the fascial edge on one side and subsequently retrieved via the opposing fascial edge, through the same incision. At least 1 cm of fascia on either side of the edge is incorporated (Fig. 6.1). Sutures are generally placed every two to three centimeters along the entire length of the hernia defect. Once sutures are placed, pneumoperitoneum is evacuated to allow for the sutures to be secured without the tension created by pneumoperitoneum. A hemostat is utilized to release the suture from the dermis to avoid skim dimpling. While this technique is the most simplistic method of defect closure, the leakage of pneumoperitoneum can occur from the suture sites due to the suture passer entering the hernia sac. Additionally, this technique is best suited for hernias of modest size in which the suture passer can readily reach the fascial edges from a single centrally located incision. Therefore, this technique may be technically challenging in patients with a wide defect or a

relatively thick abdominal wall, due to the oblique angle at which the suture passer is introduced through the soft tissues.

Alternatively, a mattress stitch may be utilized to approximate the fascial edges. In this technique, small incisions are placed through the skin overlying the medial border of the fascia on either side of the defect. Sutures are placed utilizing a suture passer to create a horizontal mattress or figure-of-eight stitch with knots secured below the skin. Again, pneumoperitoneum is released prior to securing the knots (Fig. 6.2). This technique avoids placement of the suture passer through the hernia sac and minimizes the loss of pneumoperitoneum through the incisions. This technique also facilitates defect closure in defects of greater width as the horizontal sutures are less likely to tear through the fascia. Sutures are placed along the entire length of the hernia defect to fully close the defect.

Intracorporeal techniques for defect closure involve the placement of interrupted or running sutures placed laparoscopically to close the defect (Fig. 6.3). There are unique challenges to suturing the abdominal wall laparoscopically related to the ergonomics of laparoscopic equipment and the contour of the abdominal wall due to insufflation. Although feasible, laparoscopic intracorporeal defect closure is technically demanding and, therefore, has precluded widespread adoption. The use of barbed suture material may facilitate laparoscopic defect closure as the suture barbs lock the tissue in place with each pass of the suture. This facilitates approximation of the tissue while suturing and eliminates the need for an assistant to hold tension. Adequate visualization for this intracorporeal suturing necessitates pneumoperitoneum, which leads to increased pressure upon the closure. Reducing the pressure of pneumoperitoneum to the lowest pressure feasible, while still allowing for an adequate working space, helps to reduce the tension upon the closure. Robotic platforms have been more recently described to facilitate the placement of intracorporeal sutures to close the hernia defects [15]. The ergonomically enhanced robotic platform greatly facilitates laparoscopic suturing

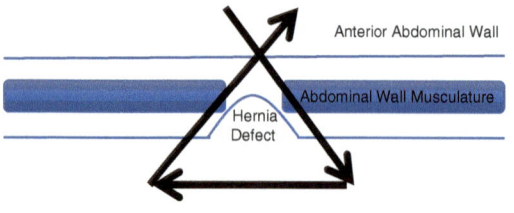

Fig. 6.1 Single-incision extracorporeal defect closure

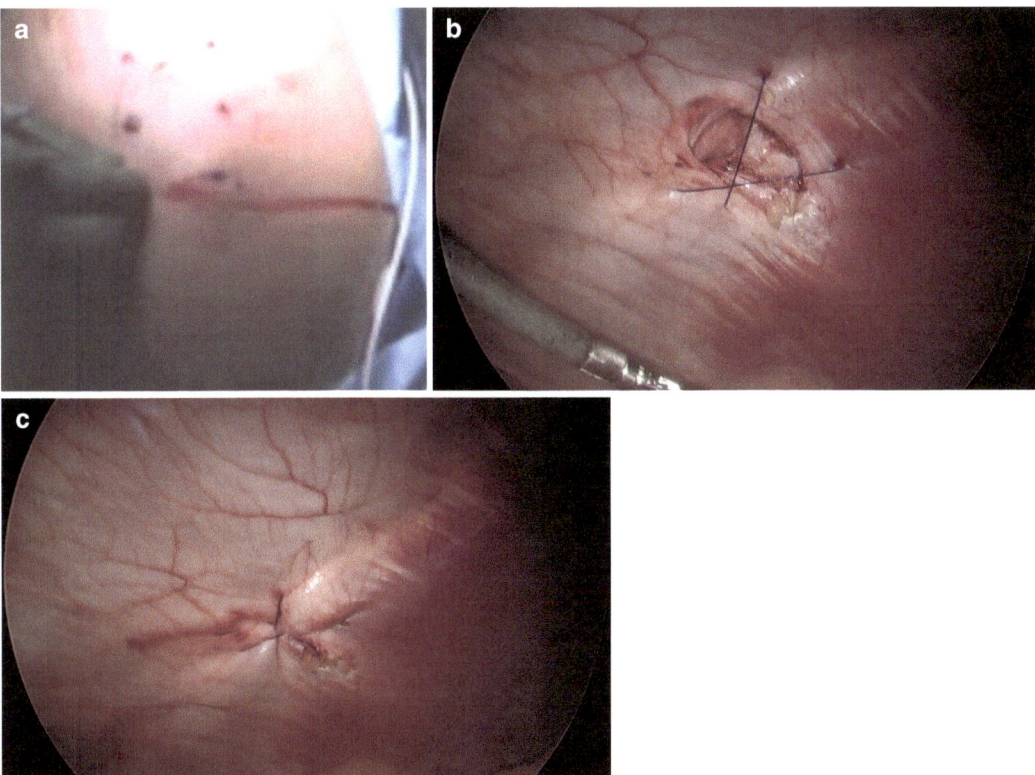

Fig. 6.2 Laparoscopic percutaneous defect closure. (**a**) Incisions in skin overlying the medial edges of the defect. (**b**) Figure-of-eight stitch with a suture passer. (**c**) Stitch secured as pneumoperitoneum is released

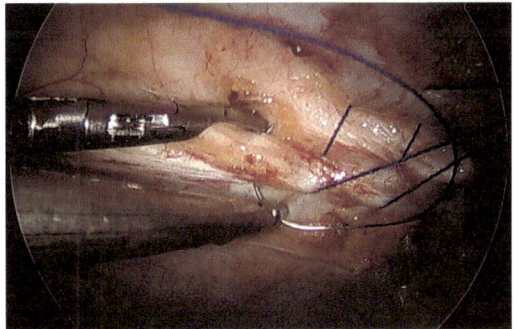

Fig. 6.3 Laparoscopic intracorporeal defect closure utilizing a barbed suture

on the anterior abdominal wall due to the increased degrees of freedom created by the articulations of the instruments.

To date there are no studies comparing outcomes between laparoscopic defect closure techniques. Trade-offs exist between technical ease, additional skin incisions, and suturing under tension. Absent comparative data, surgeon experience, and preference often guide these clinical decisions.

Recurrence

Recurrence is generally regarded as the most notable complication of incisional hernia repair. Laparoscopic incisional hernia repair has been demonstrated to have excellent clinical outcomes with few complications and low recurrence rates. In a study by Chelala et al. evaluating the recurrence rates for laparoscopic incisional hernia repair with defect closure in over 1300 patients, the rate of recurrence was found to be 4.72% at 3 years [16]. There have been several studies comparing recurrence rates between IPOM and IPOM with defect closure. Nguyen et al. performed a systematic review of the literature to evaluate the rates of recurrence with primary fascial closure compared to non-closure [17]. In this study, fascial defect closure resulted in lower recurrence rates (0–5.7% vs. 4.8–16.7%). However, the studies included within this trial were deemed low quality with a high risk of bias.

Recurrence rates following laparoscopic ventral hernia repair with and without defect closure vary between studies. In a study by Clapp et al., a statistically significant reduction of recurrence was demonstrated with defect closure relative to bridged IPOM repair (0% vs. 16.7%, $P = 0.02$) [12]. Rates of recurrence were decreased with primary fascial closure versus non-closure for incisional hernia repair (3.8% vs. 7.1%, $P = 0.27$) in a single-institutional retrospective observational study by Banerjee et al. [10]. Similarly, in a single-institute, single-surgeon study by Karpineni et al., recurrence rates were found to be 5.1% for laparoscopic incisional hernia repair with primary fascial closure compared to 5.6% for bridged IPOM repairs ($P = 0.947$). While both studies noted a reduction in recurrence rates, neither was statistically significant. Other studies have similarly failed to demonstrate a benefit to defect closure [18].

The largest study comparing outcomes between laparoscopic ventral hernia repair with defect closure and a laparoscopic repair with bridging mesh did not demonstrate any significant difference in outcomes between techniques [14]. This multicenter retrospective study compared outcomes in 97 patients who underwent primary fascial closure with 99 bridged repairs with a median of 17.5 months. There was no difference in recurrence rates, seroma formation, surgical site infection, reoperation, or readmission. Subgroup analyses were also performed evaluating outcomes based upon defect size and there again were no differences in outcomes. A propensity score analysis controlling for patient age, gender, American Society of Anesthesia score, body mass index, smoking status, and acute repair again demonstrated no difference in recurrence rates incidence of seroma or surgical site infection.

The concept of defect closure has emerged as an adjunctive technique that may be utilized dur-ing laparoscopic ventral hernia repair, despite the conflicting evidence. While the technical details of defect closure are important, it is our opinion that other technical factors associated with the repair are equally important. Appropriate techniques include adequate mesh overlap with a minimum of 5 cm of mesh overlap surrounding all hernia defects is essential. It is our practice to measure the size of hernia defects prior to defect closure and to select a mesh that allows a minimum overlap of 5 cm regardless of whether the defect is closed. Appropriate mesh fixation is similarly important to ensure the mesh does not migrate or shift prior to integration into the abdominal wall. Future controlled studies will be required to definitively resolve the question as to the benefit of closing defects.

Seroma Formation

Seroma formation is a frequent postoperative sequelae of laparoscopic incisional hernia repair. Because the fascial defect is not closed during an IPOM repair, seromas frequently develop in the hernia cavity, although most resolve spontaneously. Closure of the fascial defect may theoretically reduce seroma formation by obliterating this potential space. However, the current literature is not definitive regarding the rates of seroma between repairs with and without defect closure. Clapp et al. reported a reduced incidence of seroma reduced with the closure of the fascial defect (5.6% vs. 27.8%, $P = 0.02$), whereas Wennergren et al. reported no difference between techniques. In a meta-analysis of literature by Tandon et al., higher rates of seroma formation were demonstrated in bridged repairs (12.2% vs. 2.5%, $P < 0.0001$). But no prospective randomized trials have been published to date addressing this question.

Patient Satisfaction

A common complaint associated with laparoscopic ventral hernia repair with bridging mesh is related to laxity of the abdominal wall. This is particularly prominent in patients in which large defects are bridged with a prosthetic mesh resulting in a perceived laxity of the abdominal wall. In some situations, the mesh may eventrate into the hernia defect resulting in poor cosmetic outcomes despite the presence of a well-positioned mesh. These poor outcomes are often described as mesh eventration, bulging, laxity, or pseudo-hernia. Regardless of its name, this may result in patient dissatisfaction. The bulging of the mesh is less of a complication of an IPOM repair, but more of an inherent drawback of the laparoscopic repair with bridging mesh. However, defect size has been demonstrated to be a factor related to the degree of eventration [19]. Patients undergoing laparoscopic repair for larger defects are more likely to develop postoperative eventration of the abdominal wall. Laparoscopic defect closure may reduce the potential for eventration of the mesh into the hernia defect because of the approximation of the fascial edges. However, the permanence of the fascial closure has not been studied. In the study by Clapp et al., laparoscopic repair with defect closure was associated with a reduced incidence of mesh eventration (0.0% vs. 41.4%; $P = 0.0002$) and clinical eventration (8.3% vs. 69.4%; $P = 0.0001$) [14] compared to bridged repair with a 24-month follow-up duration. In this same study, among case-controlled patients, patient satisfaction scores (8.8 ± 0.4 vs. 7.0 ± 0.5; $P = 0.008$), cosmetic satisfaction scores (8.8 ± 0.4 vs. 7.0 ± 0.6; $P = 0.01$), and AAS functional status scores (79.1 ± 1.9 vs. 71.3 ± 2.3; $P = 0.002$) were higher in the patients who underwent defect closure. Although compelling, the limited data evaluating patient satisfaction following laparoscopic hernia repair with defect closure limits the ability to make definitive conclusions. Future studies specifically addressing quality of life following laparoscopic ventral hernia repair with defect closure are needed.

Conclusion

The role of fascial defect closure during a laparoscopic incisional hernia repair is controversial. As of this time, there are no published prospective randomized trials addressing this topic. Potential benefits of defect closure include a reduction in the incidence of seroma and eventration and improved patient satisfaction, comparable recurrence rates and infrequent complications or drawbacks associated with defect closure. Considering the minimal increased risk and limited evidence, we feel that closure of the defect is a reasonable alternative to repair with a bridging mesh. Well-designed prospective trials are required to fully elucidate the potential benefits and drawbacks of a strategy of defect closure during laparoscopic ventral hernia repair.

References

1. Wechter ME, Pearlman MD, Hartmann KE. Reclosure of the disrupted laparotomy wound. Obstet Gynecol. 2005;106:376–83. https://doi.org/10.1097/01. aog.0000171114.75338.06.
2. Cengiz Y, Israelsson LA. Incisional hernias in midline incisions: an eight-year follow up. Hernia. 1998;2:175–7. https://doi.org/10.1007/bf01569142.
3. Mudge M, Hughes LE. Incisional hernia: a 10 year prospective study of incidence and attitudes. Br J Surg. 1985;72:70–1. https://doi.org/10.1002/bjs.1800720127.
4. Pans A, Elen P, Dewé W, Desaive C. Long-term results of polyglactin mesh for the prevention of incisional hernias in obese patients. World J Surg. 1998;22:479–83. https://doi.org/10.1007/s002689900420.
5. Trimbos JB. A randomized clinical trial comparing two methods of fascia closure following midline laparotomy. Arch Surg. 1992;127:1232. https://doi.org/10.1001/archsurg.1992.01420100094016.
6. Luijendijk RW. A comparison of suture repair with mesh repair for incisional hernia. N Engl J Med. 2000;343:392–8.
7. Poulose BK, Shelton J, Phillips S, Moore D, Nealon W, Penson D, et al. Epidemiology and cost of ventral hernia repair: making the case for hernia research. Hernia. 2011;16(2):179–83.
8. LeBlanc KA, Booth WV. Laparoscopic repair of incisional abdominal hernias using expanded polytetrafluoroethylene: preliminary findings. Surg Laparosc Endosc. 1993;3(1):39–41.
9. Itani KMF, Hur K, Kim LT, Anthony T, Berger DH, Reda D, Neumayer L. Veterans Affairs Ventral Incisional Hernia Investigators. Comparison of laparoscopic and open repair with mesh for the treatment of ventral incisional hernia a randomized trial. Arch Surg. 2010;145(4):322–8. https://doi.org/10.1001/archsurg.2010.18.

10. Banerjee A, Beck C, Narula VK, Linn J, Noria S, Zagol B, et al. Laparoscopic ventral hernia repair: does primary repair in addition to placement of mesh decrease recurrence? Surg Endosc. 2011;26(5):1264–8.
11. Tandon A, Pathak S, Lyons NJR, Nunes QM, Daniels IR, Smart NJ. Meta-analysis of closure of the fascial defect during laparoscopic incisional and ventral hernia repair. Br J Surg. 2016;103(12):1598–607.
12. Clapp M, Awad S, Subramanian A, Liang M. Transcutaneous closure of central defects (TCCD) in laparoscopic ventral hernia repairs (LVHR). J Surg Res. 2012;172(2):286–7.
13. Suwa K, Okamoto T, Yanaga K. Closure versus non-closure of fascial defects in laparoscopic ventral and incisional hernia repairs: a review of the literature. Surg Today. 2015;46(7):764–73.
14. Wennergren JE, Askenasy EP, Greenberg JA, Holihan J, Keith J, Liang MK, et al. Laparoscopic ventral hernia repair with primary fascial closure versus bridged repair: a risk-adjusted comparative study. Surg Endosc. 2015;30(8):3231–8.
15. Allison N, Tieu K, Snyder B, Pigazzi A, Wilson E. Technical feasibility of robot-assisted ventral hernia repair. World J Surg. 2011;36(2):447–52.
16. Chelala E, Baraké H, Estievenart J, Dessily M, Charara F, Allé JL. Long-term outcomes of 1326 laparoscopic incisional and ventral hernia repair with the routine suturing concept: a single institution experience. Hernia. 2015;20(1):101–10.
17. Nguyen DH, Nguyen MT, Askenasy EP, Kao LS, Liang MK. Primary fascial closure with laparoscopic ventral hernia repair: systematic review. World J Surg. 2014;38(12):3097–104.
18. Zeichen MS, Lujan HJ, Mata WN, Maciel VH, Lee D, Jorge I, Plasencia G, Gomez E, Hernandez AM. Closure versus non-closure of hernia defect during laparoscopic. ventral hernia repair with mesh. Hernia. 2013;17(5):589–96.
19. Carter SA, Hicks SC, Brahmbhatt R, Liang MK. Recurrence and pseudorecurrence after laparoscopic ventral hernia repair: predictors and patient-focused outcomes. Am Surg. 2014;80(2):138–48.

Recommended Reading

Karipineni F, Joshi P, Parsikia A, Dhir T, Joshi A. Laparoscopic-assisted ventral hernia repair: primary fascial repair with polyester mesh versus polyester mesh alone. Am Surg. 2016;82(3):236–42.

Light D, Bawa S. Trans-fascial closure in laparoscopic ventral hernia repair. Surg Endosc. 2016;30(12):5228–31.

Misiakos EP, Patapis P, Zavras N, Tzanetis P, Machairas A. Current trends in laparoscopic ventral hernia repair. J Soc Laparoendosc Surg. 2015;19(3):e2015.00048.

Tayar C, Karoui M, Cherqui D, Fagniez PL. Robot-assisted laparoscopic mesh repair of incisional hernias with exclusive intracorporeal suturing: a pilot study. Surg Endosc. 2007;21(10):1786–9.

Intraoperative Considerations for Laparoscopy

David Earle

Introduction

The laparoscopic approach for ventral hernia repair began over 20 years ago with the first published report in 1993 by Karl LeBlanc in Baton Rouge, Louisiana [1]. Despite its equivalent cost and hospital resource utilization [2], and patient benefits over open repair [3], the laparoscopic technique is still utilized in only about 20% of all ventral hernia repairs [4, 5]. Given the benefits to patients, logic would dictate that the relative lack of utilization is mostly due to technical difficulty and gaps in laparoscopic skill acquisition necessary for the adhesiolysis, mesh placement, and mesh fixation. There has been recent interest in utilizing a robotic-assisted surgical device (RASD) for laparoscopic ventral hernia repair (LVHR), the details of which will be covered elsewhere in this book. These relatively new tools for LVHR may allow increased adoption of the laparoscopic approach, but it is important to note that the fundamentals of the laparoscopic approach should not be changed without scrutiny and informed consent. These fundamental principles include known risk factors for recurrence, such as utilizing an adequate size mesh with appropriate strength and fixation, all of which become increasingly important as the size of the hernia defect and number of previous failed repairs increases.

Another important and fundamental aspect of LVHR is utilizing the most appropriate technique, a decision that can sometimes be difficult to make. Use of an algorithm, such as that listed below, can be helpful in deciding whether or not to utilize a laparoscopic approach.

Algorithm for ventral hernia repair

1. Explicitly identify the patient's goals of repair (e.g., symptom relief, abdominal wall contour issues).
2. Align the patient goals with the health care team (keep goals realistic).
3. Consider the clinical scenario (emergent, urgent, elective).
4. Consider the patient's history (medical conditions, previous hernia repairs, postoperative complications, types of typical activities, etc.)
5. Consider the details of the hernia (defect and sac size, location, overlying skin changes).
6. Choose a repair technique that will most likely meet the above goals (open, laparoscopic, hybrid, myofascial flap of the trunk, etc.)
7. Choose a prosthetic most appropriate for the technique (intra/extraperitoneal design, proper strength if bridging, etc.)

D. Earle
Tufts University School of Medicine,
Boston, MA, USA

© Springer International Publishing AG, part of Springer Nature 2018
K. A. LeBlanc (ed.), *Laparoscopic and Robotic Incisional Hernia Repair*,
https://doi.org/10.1007/978-3-319-90737-6_7

Access

For laparoscopic surgery in general, existing data do not support one method of trocar insertion over another [6]. Initial access for LVHR should generally be performed under direct visualization, although the existing data suggest a Veress needle can be safely placed away from old incisions with proper training and experience [7]. Direct visualization techniques include open techniques or use of an optical entry trocar. In general, the first port should be placed as far from previous scars and the hernia defect as possible [8].

The secondary ports used for the working instruments and scope should also be placed as far from the hernia as possible, in order to allow for adequate working space, visualization of the defect, and repair of the defect. Once the primary port has been placed, secondary ports should be placed under direct vision to avoid unrecognized visceral injury.

Occasionally, adhesions are covering the area of the desired location of the secondary ports, requiring that some adhesiolysis before placing them. One strategy for this is to utilize a 10–12 mm port as the first port, and operate through this port to take down enough adhesions to allow a secondary port to be placed. This can be accomplished by using the scope itself to brush the adhesions down, or using a 5 mm instrument adjacent to a 5 mm scope, both placed through the same port. Standard ports with mechanical seals to maintain pneumoperitoneum can be used, but the technique is enhanced with use of the AirSeal™ port (ConMed, Utica, NY), which does not use a mechanical seal, and will maintain pneumoperitoneum and thus operative exposure when utilizing two separate instruments through a single port.

Another access strategy utilizes an open technique for the initial port placement that is somewhat closer to the hernia or previous scars. In addition to initial access, this port can then be used for subsequent mesh insertion. Its location relatively close to the defect will ultimately be covered with the mesh, eliminating the need for fascial closure, provided the port site is not too close to the edge of the mesh. This strategy could also be accomplished by performing the adhesiolysis first, utilizing all 5 mm ports, then placing a secondary 10–12 mm port within the boundaries of where the mesh will be placed, or through the hernia defect itself. If the skin overlying the hernia sac will be used for port and/or mesh placement, consider closing the skin well in order to prevent leakage of seroma fluid, as seromas within the hernia sac are common after LVHR [9].

Three ports on one side of the abdominal wall are most commonly utilized. For midline hernias, I usually place the first port in the left upper quadrant, and the two working ports evenly spaced inferior to this. With increasing area covered by adhesions, and larger defects/mesh, it is more common and necessary to also place ports on the opposite side of the abdomen. Usually two additional ports are necessary, however, if the defect and/or mesh is large enough, a third port will be placed on the opposite side as well (Fig. 7.1). These additional ports are frequently used for not only dissection, but mesh fixation as well. In my

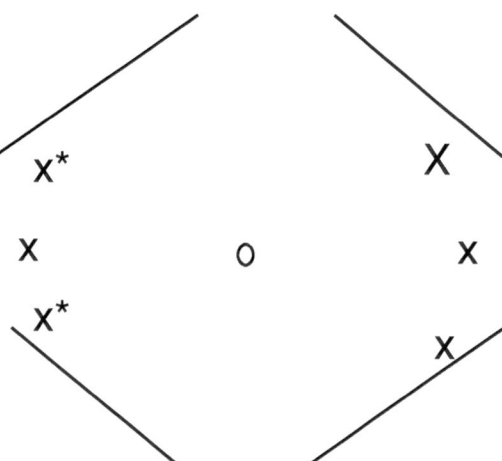

Fig. 7.1 Typical port placement for laparoscopic ventral hernia repair. The ports on the patient's left side are often the only ports necessary. Additional 1–3 ports placed on the patient's right side are necessary for larger defects and larger mesh sizes. $X = 10–12$ mm, $x = 5$ mm, * = For cases requiring right sided ports, 1–3 ports are utilized depending on the tasks required. Most commonly, two extra ports are used

practice, I still see patients with recently repaired recurrent hernias, where the mesh was displaced towards the side of the abdomen opposite from the port sites, thereby leaving the defect edge in close proximity to the mesh edge on the ipsilateral side. Simply placing ports on the opposite side of the abdomen would be anticipated to allow for use of a larger mesh, more accurate placement, and better fixation, thus reducing the risk of hernia recurrence.

Lysis of Adhesions

This portion of the operation can be one of the more challenging aspects to a laparoscopic approach for ventral hernia repair. In general, there are two types of adhesions I consider— acquired and anatomic. Acquired adhesions develop after previous surgical procedures, trauma, or some type of intra-abdominal inflammatory process. Anatomic adhesions are naturally occurring peritoneal ligaments, such as the umbilical and falciform ligaments.

It is important that a wide area surrounding the hernia is freed from adhesions in order to assess the presence of additional, unsuspected hernia defects, and have a wide enough area to place an appropriately sized mesh adjacent to the abdominal wall. Indeed, this usually mandates lysing all of the adhesions from the anterior abdominal wall, particularly for midline hernias. Even primary midline hernia defects are adjacent to the umbilical and falciform ligaments, which in my opinion should be taken down prior to mesh placement. When taking these ligaments down, I begin near the umbilicus, and proceed caudad and cephalad, leaving the ligaments attached where they are thickest, typically over the bladder inferiorly, and at the ligamentum teres superiorly. Inferiorly, this dissection is often carried out all the way to the symphysis pubis, exposing Cooper's ligaments bilaterally. Superiorly, the dissection is carried out to, or above the xiphoid process, depending on the proximity of the hernia defect to the xiphoid. The extraperitoneal fat is mobilized as closely as possible to the lateral attachments to minimize the amount of fat between the mesh and the abdominal wall. In contrast to acquired adhesions, where an energy source is used carefully, and sparingly, there is less risk of inadvertent thermal injury when taking down the umbilical and falciform ligaments, and thus a more liberal use of an energy source is typically utilized. The exception to this is near the urinary bladder. It is often helpful to place a three-way bladder catheter preoperatively, and use this to instill sterile water or saline into the bladder, thus making the borders easy to visualize, and help avoid inadvertent injury.

Acquired adhesions are taken down with both blunt and sharp dissection, with sparing use of an energy source for hemostasis. Good visualization is critical, and for the more dense adhesions, precise fine motor control of the instrument tips is mandatory. It is important to recognize that as the further the laparoscopic instrument is placed into the port, the fulcrum on the instrument shaft moves towards the handle, resulting in more difficult fine motor control of the instrument tip [10].

The solutions to this are to employ a longer instrument, use two hands on the instrument to steady the tip, and/or place another port closer to the target. For example, while using non-energized scissors to lyse adhesions that are becoming increasingly far away from the ports, there will occasionally be a need to grasp the tissue adherent to the abdominal wall at a safe location, lock the grasper, and have an assistant apply gentle traction. Two hands are then placed on a longer scissor to improve fine motor control of the scissor tip, and the adhesiolysis can be completed in this area. It is also important to note that adhesions that are very close to the port site can also cause problems with fine motor control, particularly because they are often done at an odd angle to the viewing scope, sometimes even with a mirror image view.

The use of an energy source during adhesiolysis is quite acceptable, but fundamental knowledge of the energy type being used will help mitigate the risk associated with its use [11]. For example, an ultrasonic energy device is commonly used for this purpose, but the heat

Table 7.1 Adhesiolysis—factors that increase risk and difficulty level, and helpful tips for management of these scenarios

	Clinical scenario	Mitigation strategies
Increased density	Discovered intraoperatively	Improve fine motor control by using two hands, adjusting port sites, utilizing assistant for retraction
		Avoid energy source near critical structures
		Use sharp scissors
Difficult location		
Close to initial port site insertion	Discovered intraoperatively	Use a sweeping motion of the scope to take down flimsy adhesions under direct vision
		Use scope and scissors and/or grasper through the same port to get started. AirSeal™ port particularly useful in this scenario
Anterior portion of anterior abdominal wall	Suggested preoperatively: Irreducible hernia contents, Small defect, large hernia sac	Adjust ports (number and/or location) as necessary to improve retraction. Use of extra ports and an assistant to retract may also be helpful
	Discovered intraoperatively: Parastomal hernia (especially bowel leading to stoma)	Avoid energy source near bowel
		Utilize an open incision at or near the area of dense adhesions, avoiding or resecting areas of poor skin quality
		Open defect laparoscopically to allow better access to adhesions
Adjacent to critical structures (GI tract, urinary bladder, diaphragm, iliac vessels)	Discovered intraoperatively, previous prostatectomy or lower midline incision (concern for urinary bladder adhesions)	Improve fine motor control by using two hands, adjusting port sites, utilizing assistant for retraction
		Avoid energy source if near a critical structure
		Use sharp scissors
		If urinary bladder is a concern, place a 3-way catheter preoperatively, and use this to instill sterile water or saline to fill up the bladder to identify the borders, which are typically covered in fat

associated with its use should not be underestimated. A short period of cooling after use, but before handling sensitive tissue, such as the GI tract, will help avoid thermal injury to the bowel. If there were a concern regarding a thermal injury to the bowel, one should strongly consider some sort of imbricating sutures over the suspected area of injury.

Adhesions that are flimsy and do not involve bowel are less risky compared to adhesions that are dense and involve bowel. Therefore, the surgeon should adjust their ergonomics, use of energy, and visualization of the operative field according to the relative risk and difficulty of the adhesions.

One scenario where adhesions are notoriously difficult is when they are between the anterior aspect of the abdominal wall and the viscera (within the hernia sac), especially with a relatively small defect. Laparoscopic access to these adhesions is limited due to the intraperitoneal approach, a situation frequently encountered with large hernia sacs and parastomal hernias. These technically challenging situations sometime necessitate the placement of ports on the opposite side of the abdomen, or a hybrid open approach, with an incision placed near the area of difficulty. Again, use of an energy source in close proximity to critical structures, such as the GI or GU tract should be used with an abundance of caution. Table 7.1 lists the clinical scenarios and mitigation strategies for difficult adhesiolysis.

Measuring the Defect

Noting the size and location of the defect, as well as its shape, will help determine the most appropriate size and shape of the mesh, and whether or not the defect is amenable to closure. There are many techniques available for this, with no data showing superiority of one method over another. An important principle however is to recognize that measurements taken on the outside of the abdomen, on the skin, will be larger than those taken from the inside of the abdominal cavity. This discrepancy is usually 1–2 cm, but increases with obesity, larger hernia sacs, and when the peritoneal cavity is fully insufflated. When measuring the defect from the inside of the abdominal cavity, it is important to measure the widest location of the defect in the vertical and transverse direction without skewing the axis. This can be accomplished by using spinal needles placed at the 12 and 6 o'clock, then 3 and 9 o'clock positions while measuring the defect dimensions from the inside with a suture, umbilical tape, or ruler.

Regardless of the method of defect measurement, the size and location of the defect should be documented in the operative note [7].

Closing the Defect

If one were to consider just the physics of covering a defect with a mesh, it is obvious that the pressure exerted on the mesh would increase as the mesh:defect ratio increases. As this ratio increases, the strength of the mesh and fixation become increasingly important. Therefore, closing the defect should decrease the pressure exerted on the mesh, and reduce the importance of the mesh and fixation strength. By way of examples, a 1 cm diameter defect at the umbilicus covered by a 20 × 30 cm mesh would render fixation strength almost irrelevant, whereas a 10 × 10 cm defect patched with a 10 × 10 cm mesh would be highly dependent on fixation strength in order to prevent recurrence. These extreme examples illustrate the changes in force experienced by the mesh based on the ratio of mesh:defect size.

Complicating intraoperative defect size however, with or without closure, is that it is not predictive of whether all or a portion of the defect closure will fail. Further, the variable contribution of tissue ingrowth in terms of fixation strength is also unpredictable. Therefore, it is probably best to minimize the contribution of defect closure and tissue ingrowth in terms of estimating the mesh:defect ratio, and size the mesh as though the defect was not closed, and tissue ingrowth was minimal. Clinically, defect closure has been seen to have variable influence on the outcomes of LVHR [12–14]. The ultimate application of this knowledge will be utilized by the surgeon, intraoperatively, keeping in mind the patient's goals and tolerance for risk in certain scenarios. This general concept of mesh:defect ratio as it relates to known risk factors for recurrence is illustrated in Fig. 7.2.

Choosing a Mesh

While a detailed explanation of mesh properties is not the goal of this chapter, I will highlight some important features that may help surgeons in their mesh choices. There are many properties of hernia prosthetics. Among these, strength is probably the most important. Surgeons and manufacturers frequently refer to weight as a surrogate for strength. While this this is a reasonable approach, lack of context and standard definitions present many pitfalls. The most common way to express the weight of a hernia mesh is in g/m^2. When comparing prosthetics, the weight/area metric is valid, as long as the mesh is composed of material with similar density. Many prosthetics however are made from different polymers, with different densities, and some contain absorbable components and permanent components. The permanent component is probably the most important in terms of hernia recurrence. Consider the recent manufacturer recall of PhysioMesh™ (Ethicon, Inc. Cincinnati, OH) [15], where the weight of the permanent polypropylene is only 28 g/m^2. This mesh was experiencing failures in strength, and was pulled from the market due to real world data from European her-

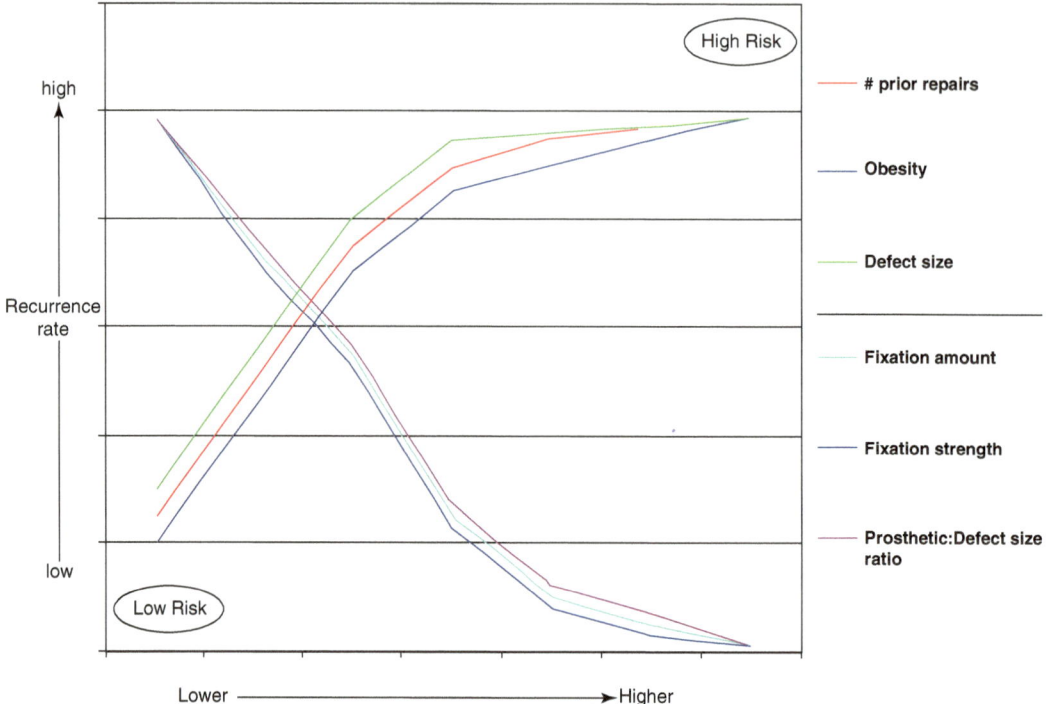

Fig. 7.2 Known risk factors for recurrence are plotted along the X axis, and anticipated risk of recurrence is plotted along the Y axis. As the risk factors (# of prior repairs, obesity, defect size) increase in total number present and individual values, recurrence rates are expected to increase. Recurrence rates are expected to decrease, with increasing fixation amount, strength, and mesh:defect ratio. In situations where risk factors are high (right upper quadrant of the graph), increasing fixation amount and strength, and mesh:defect ratio will become more important if recurrence is to be avoided. In low risk scenarios (left lower quadrant of graph), fixation and mesh size become less important. There are no absolute values, as it is the relative risk that is important to help guide the surgeon in mesh and fixation choices

nia registries. Compare this to the Marlex™ and Prolene™ mesh at around 95 g/m², and currently popular "lightweight" mesh, such as Bard's Soft Mesh™, Ethicon's Prolene Soft™, and Atrium's ProLite Ultra™, all at around 45–50 g/m², prosthetics known to perform well in a variety of situations where bridging may be required [16]. Because strength data is not universally available or obtained in a consistent manner, it is not easily comparable. However, bridging a defect with increasingly lower weight polypropylene mesh will be more likely to fail as the size of the defect increases. And because these may not be linear relationships, patient characteristics are variable and host tissue response is unpredictable, there is no cutoff point where one size/strength mesh should be used for a particular sized defect. So without a specific size and strength cutoff for the

defect and mesh, respectively, it remains logical to *avoid scenarios where large defects are bridged with ultra-lightweight mesh*, particularly in obese patients [17].

Mesh Insertion and Placement

Inserting a large mesh through a small incision can be difficult. Usually, the larger and stiffer the mesh, the more difficult it is to place in the peritoneal cavity. Larger prosthetics typically require placement through the port site after the port has been removed. It is useful to pull the mesh in, rather than try to push it through the port and/or port site. To pull the mesh through, insert an appropriate locking grasper backwards through the 10–12 mm port, then remove the port which will leave the instrument tip protruding from the port site. The mesh can then be grasped and pulled in. Reestablishment of the pneumoperitoneum is recommended before releasing the mesh and readjusting the grasper, so it can be done under direct vision. Smaller sizes of mesh can often be placed through the port itself. One must be careful and avoid the use of an excessive amount of force, as the subsequent release through the port could cause the instrument tip to enter uncontrolled into the peritoneal cavity, and unintentionally damage intra-abdominal organs.

Once the mesh has been inserted into the abdomen, it must be accurately placed on the anterior abdominal wall. Placement of a suture in the center of the mesh prior to insertion can be done, then the suture pulled through the skin in the center of the coverage area, and held in place while the mesh is fixed to the abdominal wall. Once fixation is accomplished, the suture can be removed [18].

Preplacement of sutures at the cardinal points (12, 3, 6, and 9 o'clock positions) is a frequently used technique. Some place the sutures at the corners of the mesh, but the corners are not typically at the location of the mesh closest to the defect, where stronger fixation is desired. These are then pulled out through corresponding stab incisions, then lifted to bring the mesh up to the abdominal wall, covering the defect. They can then be held or tied while additional fixation is placed as appropriate.

There are two devices currently available to assist with mesh placement. The AccuMesh™ device (Medtronic, Minneapolis, MN) can help with both insertion and placement, and utilizes a collapsible frame on which the mesh is fixed with releasable hooks. With the frame collapsed and the mesh rolled, it is inserted into the peritoneal cavity. The frame is then opened, which spreads out the mesh. The frame/mesh can be adjusted with the articulating shaft (four degrees of freedom), and held in the proper orientation on the abdominal wall while the mesh is fixed to the abdominal wall with a mechanical fixation device and/or sutures. The device is then released from the mesh by pulling a lever on the handle, and removed. Additional sutures can then be placed

as appropriate. The Echo PS™ device (CR Bard; Warwick, RI) utilizes two parts. A mesh rolling device aids in insertion, and a balloon frame that is attached to the mesh is then inflated after retrieving the tubing and pulling it through the center of the coverage area, typically the center of the defect, which places the mesh flush against to the abdominal wall. The device/mesh is held taut while a mechanical fixation device and/or sutures are used to attach the mesh to the abdominal wall. The frame is then deflated and removed by simply pulling it out through a cannula with a grasper. Additional full thickness sutures are then placed where appropriate. These devices are depicted in Fig. 7.3. Most recently released is a new expandable frame made of nitinol, rather than a balloon [19]. This Echo 2 (Bard, Inc. Warwick, RI) device has fewer steps than the balloon-based frame, and accomplishes the same task (Fig. 7.4).

Mesh Fixation

There are two types of mesh fixation. The first is how the surgeon connects the mesh to the tissue in the operating room, and the second is how the body connects the mesh to the tissue as part of the healing process. To date, there has been no consistent data to suggest one fixation method is better than another. Full thickness anchoring sutures that traverse the mesh, and all layers of the abdominal wall except the skin and most subcutaneous tissue are considered the strongest of all surgical applied fixation methods [20, 21]. There are a variety of mechanical anchoring devices on the market, most of which are helical fasteners that resemble a screw. One fastener has a "U" shape with barbs at the tips to hold it in place, and one resembles a suture, encircling the tissue and mesh, with the ends connected similar to a zip tie. The mechanical devices can deliver both permanent and absorbable fasteners, depending on the version. These types of mechanically delivered fasteners are not as strong as full thickness abdominal wall sutures, because they only go through a portion of the abdominal wall muscle and fascia. There has been no proven benefit of one fixation fastener

a

b

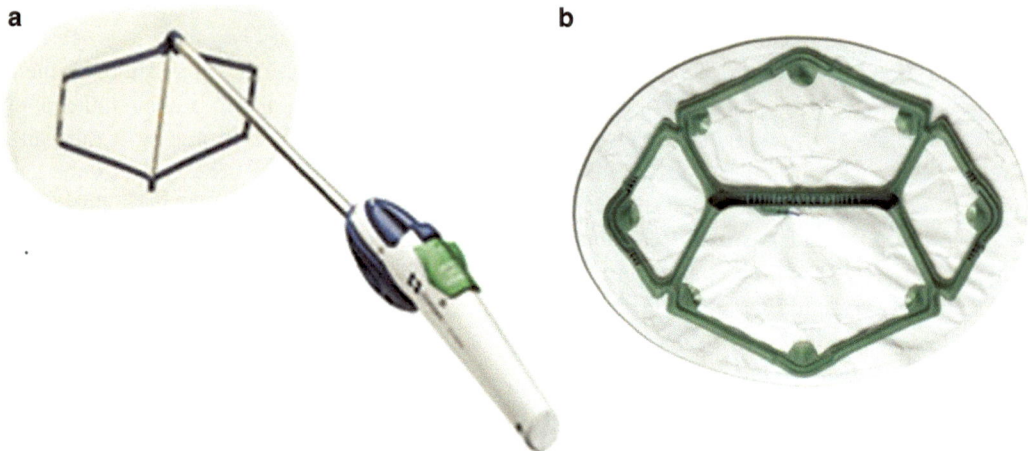

Fig. 7.3 Mesh introduction and positioning systems. (**a**) Medtronic AccuMesh™ device assists with introduction of mesh, mesh spreading with an expandable frame, and positioning using an articulating shaft with 4 degrees of freedom. (**b**) Bard Echo PS™ device utilizes a separate introduction device, and assists with unraveling and placement of the mesh over the defect with a balloon frame, inflated via a central catheter pulled out through the center of the defect

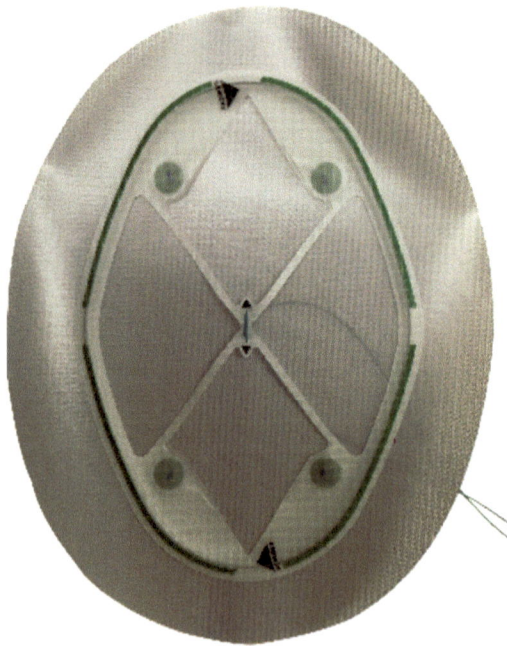

Fig. 7.4 Bard Echo 2™ device utilizes an accessory introduction device, and assists with unraveling and placement of the mesh over the defect with a nitinol frame. The mesh is pulled up to the abdominal wall through the center of the defect with the attached "hoisting" suture, and is removed after fixed to the abdominal wall by simply pulling the frame through a cannula with a grasper

over another, and new fasteners are continually being introduced to the market in an attempt to continuously improve this aspect of laparoscopic ventral hernia repair [22]. Examples of these fasteners can be seen in Fig. 7.5. Finally, it has become popular among users of robotically assisted surgical devices to use a variety of suture types to connect the mesh to the abdominal wall, with a variety of suturing patterns and suture depths. Because the technique is manual, and operative circumstances not uniform, it is unknown how strong and predictable this fixation method will ultimately be. Furthermore, suture choice and suture pattern are highly variable among surgeons, making a comparison to existing methods of fixation difficult at best. However, whatever the depth and pattern the sutures are placed, they will largely be placed through a partial thickness of the abdominal wall, and thus less strong compared to full thickness sutures [23, 24].

Hernia mesh fixation is obviously necessary, but not without complications. Full thickness sutures can cause long-term pain requiring trigger point injections and/or suture removal, and helical tacks can cause postoperative bowel perforation, adhesions, and additional hernia defects [25–27].

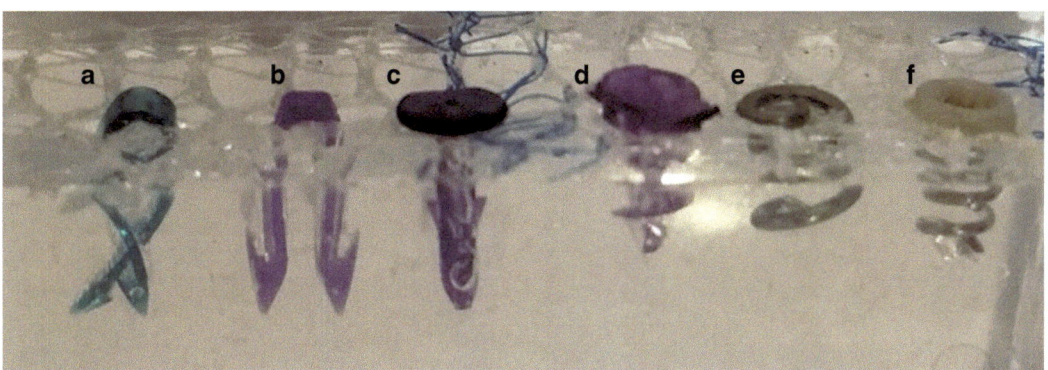

Fig. 7.5 Mesh fixation products. (**a**) Suture-like fixation, permanent (FasTouch™, Via Surgical, Amirim, Israel), (**b**) "U"-shaped fastener, absorbable (Secure Strap™, Ethicon, Cincinnati, OH), (**c**) Barbed nail-type fastener, absorbable (Optifix™, Bard, Warwick, RI) (**d**–**f**) Helical fasteners, ((**d**, **e**) Absorbatack™-absorbable and ProTack™-permanent, Medtronic, Minneapolis, MN; (**f**) CapSure™, Bard, Warwick, RI-permanent)

Long-term pain has not been shown to be clearly related to partial thickness fasteners deployed laparoscopically, or full thickness sutures [28].

In an attempt to avoid the potential postoperative complications from permanent fixation methods, absorbable fixation devices have been developed, and are popular among surgeons. Since the currently available absorbable fasteners take up to a year to absorb, it is unlikely that an absorbable fastener placed through a nerve will allow for nerve regeneration and healing after absorption. Also, the incidence of tack pain is extraordinarily low, given the millions of permanent helical tacks that have been placed, and the rarity of removal with successful pain relief. A study from Denmark published in 2015 examined 816 patients after LVHR, and showed no effect on long-term pain with absorbable tacks compared to permanent tacks [29].

Additionally, absorbable fasteners are thought to be less prone to adhesions. However, adhesions to permanent and absorbable screw-type fasteners were found to be equal at 4 weeks postoperatively in a porcine model [30]. Consider however small bowel, which is perfectly biocompatible. Small bowel can adhere to itself, which is most likely due to tissue trauma. It is certainly possible that adhesions to fixation points may be more related to tissue injury related to the profile of the fastener exposed to the bowel, rather than the absorbability or raw material of the fastener.

Furthermore, absorbable fixation alone will rely on tissue integration as the sole method of mesh fixation in the long term. Since the host tissue response is unpredictable, the strength of the long-term fixation will be more variable, and the mesh:defect ratio becomes more important. Indeed, at least one study of 816 patients from Denmark revealed higher recurrence rates when using absorbable, rather than permanent fasteners [29].

The host response to the foreign body also will fixate the mesh to the anterior abdominal wall during the postoperative period. This process however is much less predictable than the surgical fixation placed in the operating room. As collagen is deposited and remodeled throughout the interstices of the mesh, a greater contact surface should increase the overall strength of the tissue incorporation aspect of the mesh fixation. Closing the defect with the mesh flat against the tissue, without buckling, would obtain a greater contact area.

Mesh Coverage

A common concern among surgeons is the optimum amount of "overlap" required to prevent recurrence. The term refers to the distance between the edge of the defect and the edge of the mesh covering the defect. The problem with this concept is that this distance is a linear measurement that is used in the context of a nonlinear environment, and does not take into account mesh fixation technique/location, and tissue ingrowth. Despite this, it has been shown that increasing the overlap is associated with decreased rates of recurrence [31].

A better perspective may be to consider the ratio of the mesh size to the defect size, the type and relative strength of the fixation, and the clinical scenario regarding the patient's weight and fat distribution, activity level, size and location of the hernia defect, and whether or not the defect is closed. Since it is impossible at the current time to measure the relative importance of these factors, and even take precise measurements in the operating room, the surgeon should size the mesh based on all of these factors, and not just consider the number of centimeters between the defect edge and edge of the mesh. By way of example, the forces exerted on a mesh covering a 10 cm circular defect are different than those from a 4 cm defect. If both size defects are covered with a mesh that has a 5 cm overlap with the same fixation techniques, the mesh covering the 10 cm defect will be subject to larger forces at the fixation points, and theoretically have an increased risk of recurrence compared to the 4 cm defect, despite a 5 cm "overlap". Therefore, known risk factors for recurrence such as larger defect size, obesity, and recurrent nature of the hernia should demand a higher mesh:defect ratio in order to mitigate the increased risk of recurrence to the best of our abilities, as shown conceptually in Fig. 7.2 [32].

Exiting the Abdomen

At the conclusion of the operation, there is often a sigh of relief, a natural human tendency after a period of intense concentration. While not related to the hernia repair itself, it is important to run through a brief checklist prior to exiting the abdomen (Table 7.2). First, look for any ongoing bleeding. This will necessitate an intentional look around the peritoneal cavity, particularly in dependent areas that have been out of the field of

Table 7.2 Checklist prior to exiting the abdomen after LVHR

Task	Rationale
Inspect peritoneal cavity for ongoing bleeding-dependent areas (particularly areas out of the field of view), areas under a large clot	Avoid postoperative hemorrhage
Inspect bowel (particularly areas involved in adhesiolysis)	Avoid missed enterotomy
Inspect port sites after cannula removal	Avoid postoperative hemorrhage and assess need for fascial closure
Inspect mesh while evacuating pneumoperitoneum	Avoid peritoneal contents slipping between mesh and abdominal wall

The order and diligence of the final inspection will vary according to clinical scenario. It is generally recommended to dictate this final inspection, or reason why it was done, in the operative report

view. Areas covered in clot that seem to be thick may need to have at least some of the clot evacuated in order to inspect the underlying area for active bleeding. The next area of inspection should be of the GI tract, particularly areas involved in the adhesiolysis. The intensity of the inspection will be dependent on the surgeon's judgment and intimate knowledge of the operation. Additionally, one should laparoscopically inspect all the port sites after the cannula is removed to inspect for bleeding that may have been tamponaded by the cannula, and need for fascial closure [10]. Finally, the mesh may be inspected as the pneumoperitoneum is evacuated, in an attempt to make sure no intraperitoneal contents slip between the mesh and the abdominal wall. While the order and diligence of the final inspection will vary according to clinical scenario, it is generally a good idea to dictate this into the operative report.

Conclusion

The choice of a laparoscopic approach to ventral hernia repair should come from an algorithmic approach that puts the patient's goals and specific clinical situation at the top of the list in terms of importance. *The choice to proceed with LVHR should not be made simply on the basis of the desire to use a specific surgical device.* Once the choice is made, adhesiolysis should be accomplished with fundamental laparoscopic techniques, including the use of proper ergonomics, sparing/careful use of an energy device, and inspection of the GI tract after adhesiolysis is completed. Careful assessment of the hernia should include operative exposure and inspection of the defect and surrounding abdominal wall in order to look for occult hernias, and allow placement of an appropriate size mesh flat against the abdominal wall. Midline hernias for example, may have a punched out, circular defect of 3 cm, but may be associated with a surrounding elliptical area between the rectus muscles of 5 cm transverse × 8 cm vertical. The abdominal wall deficit should be considered to be the elliptical area between the rectus muscles, not just the punched out defect through which abdominal contents can herniate. Closure of the defect will increase the surface area the mesh is in contact with, and reduce seroma rates, but has not been shown to improve long-term outcomes such as recurrence. Rather than using the linear measurement of "cm of overlap" to select mesh size, consider the mesh:defect ratio, with a tendency to use higher ratios for cases with higher risk for recurrence, such as larger defects, obese patients, and recurrent hernias. The amount and type of fixation will depend on the size of the defect, and whether or not the defect was closed. Stronger and increased amount of fixation should be used for larger defects that are bridged, compared to smaller defects that are closed.

References

1. LeBlanc KA, Booth WV. Laparoscopic repair of incisional abdominal hernias using expanded polytetrafluoroethylene: preliminary findings. Surg Laparosc Endosc. 1993;3:39–41.
2. Earle D, Seymour N, Fellinger E, Perez A. Laparoscopic versus open incisional hernia repair: a single-institution analysis of hospital resource utilization for 884 consecutive cases. Surg Endosc. 2006;20(1):71–5.
3. Arita NA, Nguyen MT, Nguyen DH, Berger RL, Lew DF, Suliburk JT, al e. Laparoscopic repair reduces incidence of surgical site infections for all ventral hernias. Surg Endosc. 2015;29(7):1769–80. https://doi.org/10.1007/s00464-014-3859-1.
4. Earle D. Open versus laparoscopic incisional/ventral hernia repair in the Medicare population. Oral presentation. American Hernia Society annual meeting, Orlando, Florida, March 2013.
5. Earle D. Hospital based outcomes of open versus laparoscopic ventral hernia repair. Oral presentation. American Hernia Society annual meeting, Orlando, Florida, March 2013.
6. Ahmad G, Gent D, Henderson D, O'Flynn H, Phillips K, Watson A. Laparoscopic entry techniques. Cochrane Database Syst Rev. 2015;31:8. https://doi.org/10.1002/14651858.CD006583.pub4.
7. Earle D, Roth JS, Saber A, Haggerty S, Bradley JF 3rd, Fanelli R, al e. SAGES guidelines for laparoscopic ventral hernia repair. Surg Endosc. 2016;30(8):3163–83.
8. LeBlanc KA. The critical technical aspects of laparoscopic repair of ventral and incisional hernias. Am Surg. 2001;67(8):809–12.
9. Morales-Conde S. A new classification for seroma after laparoscopic ventral hernia repair. Hernia. 2012;16(3):261–7. https://doi.org/10.1007/s10029-012-0911-8.
10. Peters JH, Fried GM, Swanstrom LL, Soper NJ, Sillin LF, Schirmer B, al e. Development and validation of a comprehensive program of education and assessment of the basic fundamentals of laparoscopic surgery. Surgery. 2004;135(1):21–7.
11. SB J, MG M, LS F, TN R, LM B, Schwaitzberg SD, et al. Fundamental use of surgical energy (FUSE): an essential educational program for operating room safety. Perm J. 2017;21:16–050. https://doi.org/10.7812/TPP/16-050.
12. Lambrecht JR, Vaktskjold A, Trondsen E, et al. Laparoscopic ventral hernia repair: outcomes in primary versus incisional hernias: no effect of defect closure. Hernia. 2015;19:479.
13. Chelala E, Baraké H, Estievenart J, Dessily M, Charara F, Allé JL. Long-term outcomes of 1326 laparoscopic incisional and ventral hernia repair with the routine suturing concept: a single institution experience. Hernia. 2016;20(1):101–10.
14. Tandon A, Pathak S, Lyons NJ, Nunes QM, Daniels IR, Smart NJ. Meta-analysis of closure of the fascial defect during laparoscopic incisional and ventral herniarepair. Br J Surg. 2016;103(12):1598–607. https://doi.org/10.1002/bjs.10268.
15. Perriello B. J&J's Ethicon recalls Physiomesh flexible composite hernia mesh. http://www.massdevice.com/jjs-ethicon-recalls-physiomesh-flexible-composite-hernia-mesh/. Accessed 10 Oct 2017.
16. Earle D, Mark LA. Prosthetic material in inguinal hernia repair: how do I choose? Surg Clin N Am. 2008;88(1):179–201.

17. Zuvela M, Galun D, Djurić-Stefanović A, Palibrk I, Petrović M, Milićević M. Central rupture and bulging of low-weight polypropylene mesh following recurrent incisional sublay hernioplasty. Hernia. 2014;18(1):135–40. https://doi.org/10.1007/s10029-013-1197-1.
18. Saber AA. Simple technique for mesh placement during laparoscopic ventral hernia repair. Surg Endosc. 2004;18(1):162–4.
19. Ashar B. 510(k) Substantial Equivalence Letter. https://www.accessdata.fda.gov/cdrh_docs/pdf14/K143743.pdf. Accessed 21 Sept 2017.
20. Joels CS, Matthews BD, Kercher KW, Austin C, Norton HJ, Williams TC, et al. Evaluation of adhesion formation, mesh fixation strength, and hydroxyproline content after intraabdominal placement of polytetrafluoroethylene mesh secured using titanium spiral tacks, nitinol anchors, and polypropylene suture or polyglactin 910 suture. Surg Endosc. 2005;19(6):780–5.
21. Reynvoet E, Deschepper E, Rogiers X, Troisi R, Berrevoet F. Laparoscopic ventral hernia repair: is there an optimal mesh fixation technique? A systematic review. Langenbeck's Arch Surg. 2014;399(1):55–63.
22. Berler DJ, Cook T, LeBlanc K, Jacob BP. Next generation mesh fixation technology for hernia repair. Surg Technol Int. 2016;XXIX:109–17.
23. Lyons C, Joseph R, Salas N, Reardon PR, Bass BL, Dunkin BJ. Mesh fixation with a barbed anchor suture results in significantly less strangulation of the abdominal wall. Surg Endosc. 2012;26(5):1254–7. https://doi.org/10.1007/s00464-011-2014-5.
24. Nguyen D, Szomstein S, Ordonez A, Dip F, Rajan M, Lo Menzo E, et al. Unidirectional barbed sutures as a novel technique for laparoscopic ventral hernia repair. Surg Endosc. 2016;30(2):764–9. https://doi.org/10.1007/s00464-015-4275-x.
25. Reynvoet E, Berrevoet F. Pros and cons of tacking in laparoscopic hernia repair. Surg Technol Int. 2014;25:136–40.
26. LeBlanc KA. Tack hernia: a new entity. JSLS. 2003;7(4):383–7.
27. Muysoms FE, Cathenis KK, Claeys DA. "Suture hernia": identification of a new type of hernia presenting as a recurrence after laparoscopic ventral hernia repair. Hernia. 2007;11(2):199–201.
28. Brill JB, Turner PL. Long-term outcomes with transfascial sutures versus tacks in laparoscopic ventral hernia repair: a review. Am Surg. 2011;77(4):458–65.
29. Christoffersen MW, Brandt E, Helgstrand F, Westen M, Rosenberg J, al KH e. Recurrence rate after absorbable tack fixation of mesh in laparoscopic incisional hernia repair. Br J Surg. 2015;102(5):541–7. https://doi.org/10.1002/bjs.9750.
30. Byrd JF, Agee N, Swan RZ, Lau KN, Heath JJ, Mckillop IH, et al. Evaluation of absorbable and permanent mesh fixation devices: adhesion formation and mechanical strength. Hernia. 2011;15(5):553–8. https://doi.org/10.1007/s10029-011-0826-9.
31. LeBlanc K. Proper mesh overlap is a key determinant in hernia recurrence following laparoscopic ventral and incisional hernia repair. Hernia. 2016;20(1):85–99. https://doi.org/10.1007/s10029-015-1399-9.
32. Hauters P, Desmet J, Gherardi D, Dewaele S, Poilvache H, Malvaux P. Assessment of predictive factors for recurrence in laparoscopic ventral hernia repair using a bridging technique. Surg Endosc. 2017;31(9):3656–63.

Intraoperative Considerations for Robotic Repair

8

Ryan M. Juza, Jerome R. Lyn-Sue, and Eric M. Pauli

Introduction

Much like laparoscopic *hernioplasty*, the keys to performing a successful robotic hernia repair lie as much in the attention to ancillary details of the procedure as they do in performing the actual operative steps. Seemingly mundane details like room setup, patient positioning, port placement, and instrumentation all ultimately facilitate the successful completion of the robotic-assisted case. In this chapter we will discuss intraoperative considerations for robotic hernia repair including a review of the technical aspects of the procedures and will provide details and helpful tips for managing difficulties unique to robotic-assisted hernia repair. As of the writing of this chapter, the da Vinci system is the only device available in the United States for hernia repair and our discussion will focus entirely on this system.

Operating Room Setup

Successful robotic *hernioplasty* surgery is dependent on appropriate room setup prior to initiating the operation. Given the considerable amount of

space taken up by the entire da Vinci robotic system (the Patient Cart (PC), the Vision Cart (VC), and the Surgeon Console (SC)), optimization of operating room space takes on a much greater role than a standard laparoscopic operation. These components may not always be easily repositioned around the operative table once the patient has been anesthetized and a sterile field established. Careful planning must therefore go into arranging the components prior to the patient entering the room. Such problems are obviously magnified by smaller operating rooms designed prior to any consideration of the possibility of robotic surgery, and operative procedures that may require bilateral docking during the conduct of the case.

Placing the VC and the PC on the same side of the patient allows the surgical technologist/scrub nurse and instrument table to be on the opposite side of the operative table, thereby facilitating instrument exchanges. We prefer to make this the side where the patient enters and leaves the operating room because it is much easier to move the scrub table than the PC and VC (Fig. 8.1). Keeping the PC and the VC on the same side of the patient allows consistency and standardization for the majority of robotic procedures. This allows improved familiarity and efficiency, especially when dealing with rotating surgical residents, anesthesia providers, and OR nursing/technologist teams.

R. M. Juza · J. R. Lyn-Sue · E. M. Pauli (✉)
Division of Minimally Invasive and Bariatric Surgery, Department of Surgery, Penn State Hershey Medical Center, Hershey, PA, USA
e-mail: epauli@pennstatehealth.psu.edu

© Springer International Publishing AG, part of Springer Nature 2018
K. A. LeBlanc (ed.), *Laparoscopic and Robotic Incisional Hernia Repair*,
https://doi.org/10.1007/978-3-319-90737-6_8

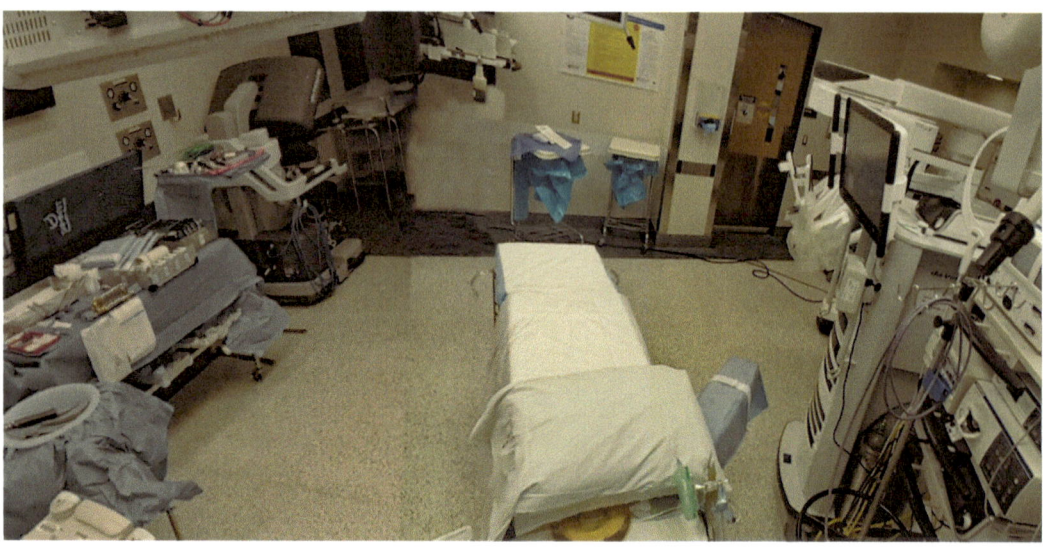

Fig. 8.1 Operating room setup: Patient Cart and Vision Cart on the patient's right, opposite the location of room entry, the Surgeon Console and the scrub table

The bedside assistant is usually positioned on the side opposite the PC to allow greater mobility of the assistant and to facilitate instrument exchanges. An assistant port can be placed to allow the insertion of laparoscopic instruments to provide counter traction during dissection. Bariatric length instruments can be used by the assistant to avoid collisions between the assistant and the robotic arms. This is especially useful in situations where the assistant and PC must be on the same side.

The SC is less position dependent than the VC or the PC and requires only being within reach of the connection cable to communicate with the system. Because of this, we prefer to position the SC away from the operating table in a spot that does not interfere with the circulating nurse, anesthesia, patient transport in and out of the room, or the need to move the PC in the event of a planned double dock method. We use an identical setup for both Si and Xi platforms (Fig. 8.2).

Performing multi-quadrant surgery with the Si platform requires a second docking position to allow working in a separate quadrant. In these cases we first dock on one side of the patient and complete our dissection. We then undock the robot and move it to the opposite side of the patient to continue our dissection (Fig. 8.3).

Many operating rooms have hardwired equipment such as laparoscopic and endoscopic booms, monitors, and gas supplies that are hardwired in such a way as to be preclusive of the above noted setup. This does not prevent robotic surgery from being performed in these rooms, but the ergonomics of the room need to be taken into consideration. When performing robotic surgery in a new room we find it beneficial to practice room setup with all of the key components prior to the arrival of the patient.

Patient Positioning

Patient positioning at the beginning of the case is of greater concern for robotic compared with standard laparoscopic hernia surgery because specific adjustments (most notably adjustments to the patient's position on the operating room table) cannot be made after the robot is docked. If patient positioning is discovered to be suboptimal after docking, the robot must be undocked and moved away from the OR table to allow patient repositioning, significantly decreasing operating room efficiency. This situation is eliminated by the use of OR tables that integrates with the PC so that the two platforms move in sync (TruSystem™ 7000dV OR Table, Trumpf

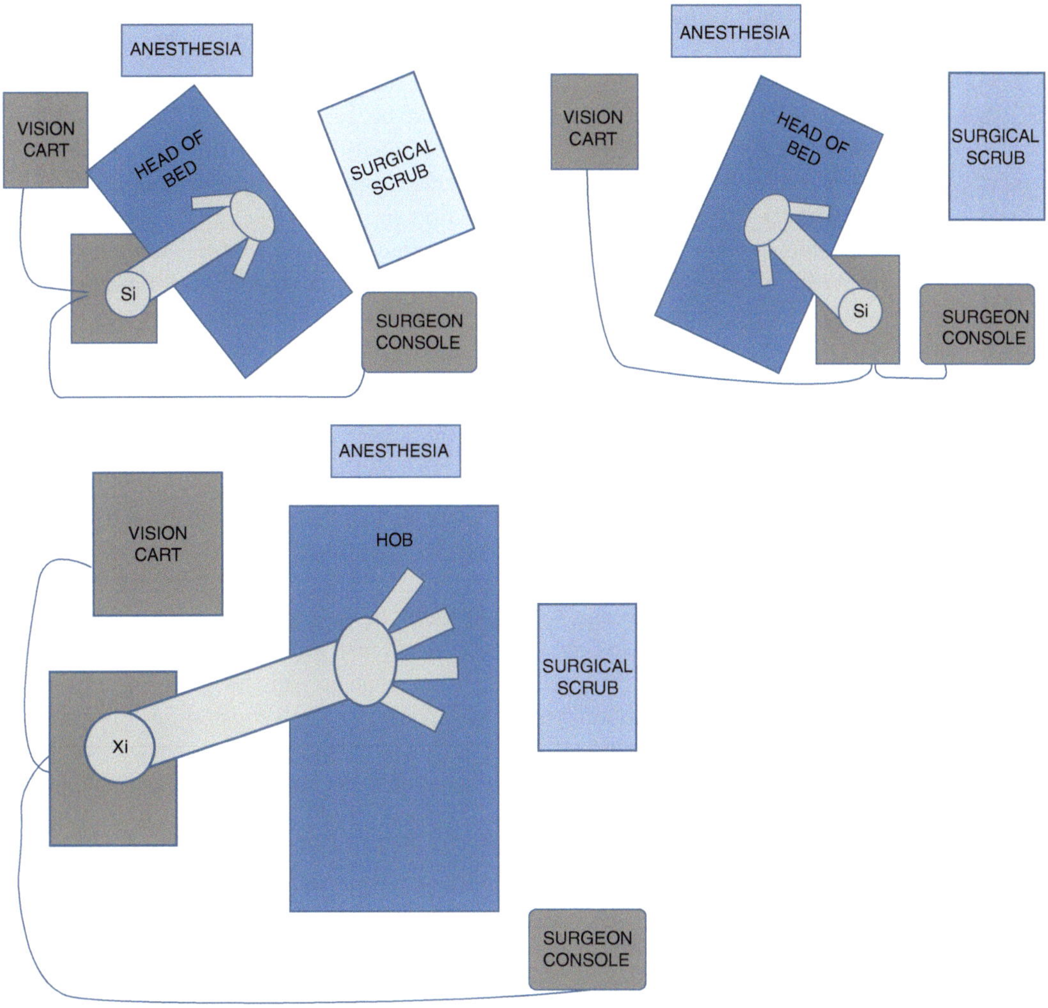

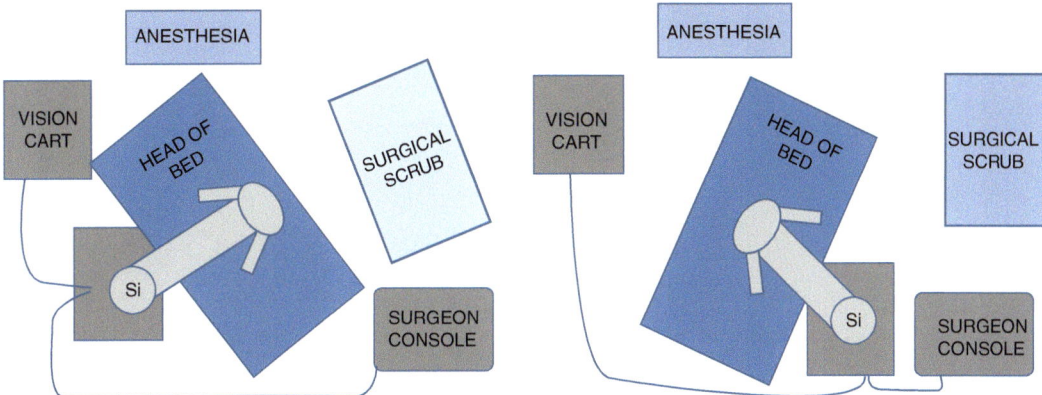

Fig. 8.2 Equipment positioning for Si and Xi cases. In the Xi platform, single position of PC allows secondary docking by rotating the boom 180° eliminating the need for repositioning of the patient cart for double docking

Fig. 8.3 Si room setup to facilitate a double dock for multi-quadrant operations; the bed is repositioned and the PC maneuvered around the foot of the bed. This setup requires minimal repositioning of equipment during the secondary docking procedure

Medical Saalfeld, Germany). Clinical data on the efficacy of the combined use of these systems for hernia repair is limited at this time.

Patients are generally positioned in a supine position with both arms extended and all pressure points padded. We prefer to have the arms extended to allow ports to be placed as lateral as possible on the abdominal wall, thereby increasing the intracorporeal working distance. The operative table is typically elevated above standard operating height to permit easy instrument exchanges by the bedside assistant or scrub nurse/tech without the need to reach below the level of the OR table.

Port Placement and Docking

Once the patient has been secured to the OR table and general anesthesia induced, placement of operating ports can ensue. Port position will vary greatly depending on the location and type of planned hernia repair but can be guided by bony anatomic landmarks and the palpable hernia defect(s) (Fig. 8.4). Accurate port placement is essential to minimize external arm collisions and maximize intracorporeal working space to allow smooth completion of the *hernioplasty*. The camera port is placed approximately 15–20 cm from the hernia in the center of the working field. The instrument ports should be

approximately 8 cm apart from the camera port to allow full range of motion [1]. Prior to docking the robot, final patient position must be obtained because no further position changes can be made once the robot is docked. See *Patient Positioning* for a description of optimal positioning.

Docking the robot with the camera port directly in front of the center column and with the instrument ports equal distance apart from the camera allows for optimal working space while reducing instrument collisions. When extending the camera arm for docking, the optimal position is obtained by aligning the blue arrow at the superior-most pivot within the blue indicator field. This alignment ensures the camera arm is able to move through its full range of motion. After docking the camera port, the instrument ports can be docked. Typically the second and third instrument arms are docked next. When the fourth instrument arm is used, it is typically docked last.

After docking each instrument arm, the arms should be rotated so that the elbows face outward at roughly a 45° angle to prevent collisions. This can be done by clutching the arm at the port and rotating the main pivot outward so that the large number on the arm is facing forward. Finally the port should be "burped" by quickly pressing and releasing the port clutch without tension on the arm. This allows

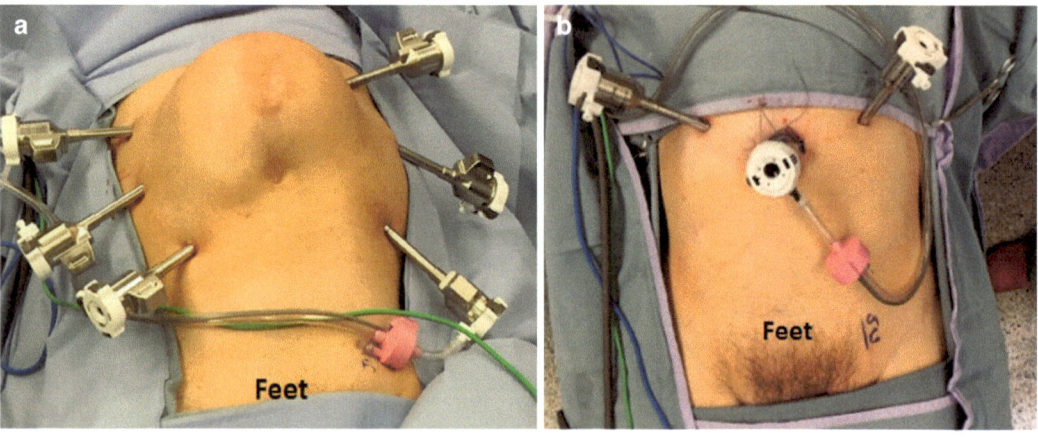

Fig. 8.4 Standard port placement for midline ventral (**a**) and inguinal (**b**) herniorrhaphy

the arm to release to a neutral position that eliminates stress on the abdominal wall and allows the port to move around the fixed pivot point. Additionally, burping the arms upward allows the port to gain more mobility when operating.

The Xi system should be docked in a similar fashion with the instruments in a symmetrical position in relation to the camera port (Fig. 8.5). Because many hernias span a wide stretch of the abdominal wall, obtaining maximum distance between the arms of the PC prior to beginning the operation can reduce the risk that such collisions will occur later in the case as the dissection proceeds through several abdominal wall quadrants. Should arm collisions occur during the operation, the arms can be undocked and the elbows repositioned to a more optimal position. Additionally, bariatric length ports and instruments can be used to increase the distance between working arms and potentially alleviate collisions. After docking the robot we double check for any unwanted contact points on the patient's torso and limbs. If found, we reposition the offending arm and pad the areas as necessary. Throughout the case the bedside assistant remains vigilant for any potential areas of contact.

When working through multiple abdominal quadrants or when operating at multiple insufflation pressures (such as at a reduced pressure to facilitate primary facial closure) ports can shift out of the abdominal cavity. This can result in impaired instrument exchange as well as insufflation of the abdominal wall musculature or subcutaneous spaces, both of which result in delays in the operation. Some surgeons reduce the risk of these events by utilizing balloon tipped trocars through which robot ports are nested.

Nesting

When performing ventral hernia repair, the instruments used are 8 mm in diameter including the camera. We use a 12 mm port to pass sutures and mesh into and out of the peritoneal cavity. To prevent an extra port being used, a robotic 8 mm port is "nested" in the 12 mm port to pass the camera through. The camera is inserted and the arm docked to the robotic port for solid connection. As noted above, nesting within balloon tipped trocars can reduce the likelihood that ports will become dislodged into the abdominal wall and can facilitate the flow of the operation.

Abdominal Wall Thickness

Obesity is a well-known risk factor for the development of hernias and the presence of obesity is a common comorbid condition in patients undergoing robotic *hernioplasty*. The

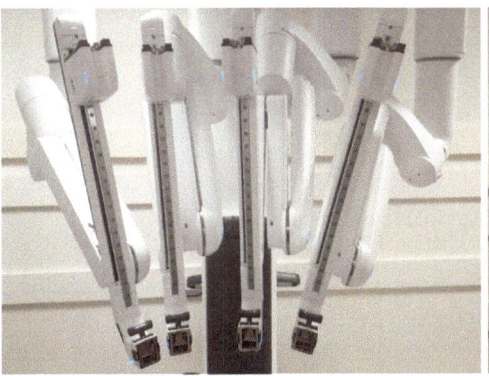
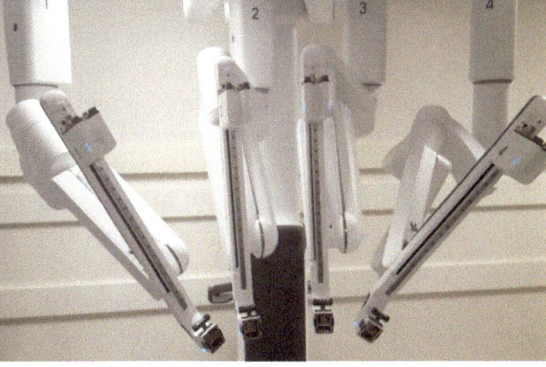

Fig. 8.5 Rotating the arms outward (at approximately 45° angles) creates greater distance at the elbows which reduces the likelihood of collision as the case progresses

use of extra-long ports can help overcome this issue of gaining abdominal access in a thick abdominal wall. In muscular patients as well as patients with thick abdominal walls, the robot has the benefit of offloading the surgeon from the manual forces transmitted through ports to facilitate performing the procedure. This is best accomplished with minimal strain on the abdominal wall if the robotic center of the port coincides with the abdominal wall muscles to minimize excessive torque on the tissues.

There may be instances, however, where the port needs to be advanced or retracted to allow for increased working space. This can also occur when a nested port is retracted in the larger port. When this occurs, the robot senses the extra torque on the instrument and the scale of motion will be affected depending on the settings (1:3 or 1:4). The surgeons console arm will move a greater distance than expected for a prescribed motion in the surgical field if this happens. If this continues, there may be sudden and wide movements in the surgical field, which may cause injury to nearby viscera. The wristed motion and grasping mechanism of the instrument may also be affected adversely.

Instrumentation

The typical instruments we utilize for hernia repair include Prograsp™ grasping forceps, Hot Shears™ and regular or suture cut needle drivers. The regular drivers are used when training residents and fellows to avoid inadvertent suture damage from grasping the suture within the crotch of the driver by inexperienced hands. Alternative instruments include standard grasping forceps in place of Prograsp™, bowel graspers, and hook cautery in place of the Hot Shears™. When an assistant port is used, a bariatric length grasper instrument is typical to provide additional retraction. The bariatric length instrument allows the assistant to stand back from the moving arms to prevent them from being injured.

A 30-degree lens is used for all incisional and inguinal hernias to better visualize the anterior abdominal wall and inguinal region during dissection and suturing, as this permits both a 30-degree up and a 30-degree down view during the conduct of different parts of each procedure. If the surgeon's preference is to perform optical trocar access into the abdomen, then a 0-degree standard laparoscope can be used and then passed off the table after entry.

Inguinal Hernias

For inguinal hernias, we prefer to have the patient in 15–30° Trendelenburg without lateral rotation (Fig. 8.6).

Ventral Hernias

For common midline hernias, we prefer to have the bed flexed around 15° with slight Trendelenburg and the bed tilted away from the ports (Fig. 8.7). This positioning increases the distance between the costal margin and the anterior superior iliac spine and allows for placement of the camera port along mid axillary line with instrument port placement along the anterior axillary line. This position also prevents instrument collisions with the patient's face and thigh closest to the port. Mirror image port placement is utilized on the contralateral side if double docking is required for larger hernias or when performing posterior component separation via transversus abdominis release (Fig. 8.4a).

Atypical Hernias

For hernias in nontraditional locations (e.g., suprapubic or epigastric hernias), port placement for camera and instruments follows standard target organ triangulation with the recommended 8 cm distance between instrument ports and the camera port.

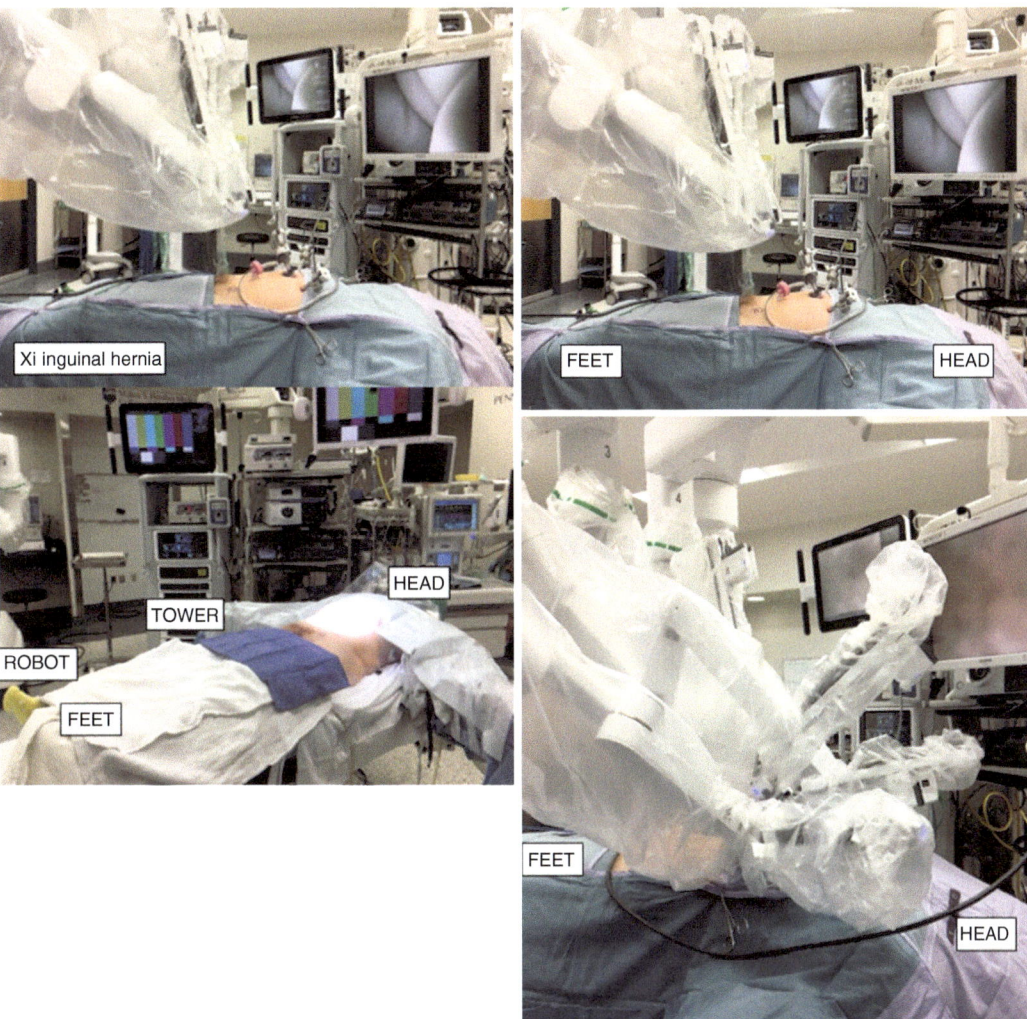

Fig. 8.6 Inguinal hernia docking: the patient is positioned supine in slight Trendelenburg position with no additional table angulation

Abdominal Access

Inguinal Hernia

Abdominal access for inguinal herniorrhaphy is obtained by Hassan cutdown technique in the supraumbilical position. A 12 mm port is placed for the introduction of mesh and suture. During the procedure an 8 mm instrument port is inserted into the 12 mm port (nesting) to function as the robotic camera port.

Ventral Hernia

Abdominal access for ventral hernia is performed via an optical access trocar to the left upper quadrant with a 0° laparoscope. Two addi-

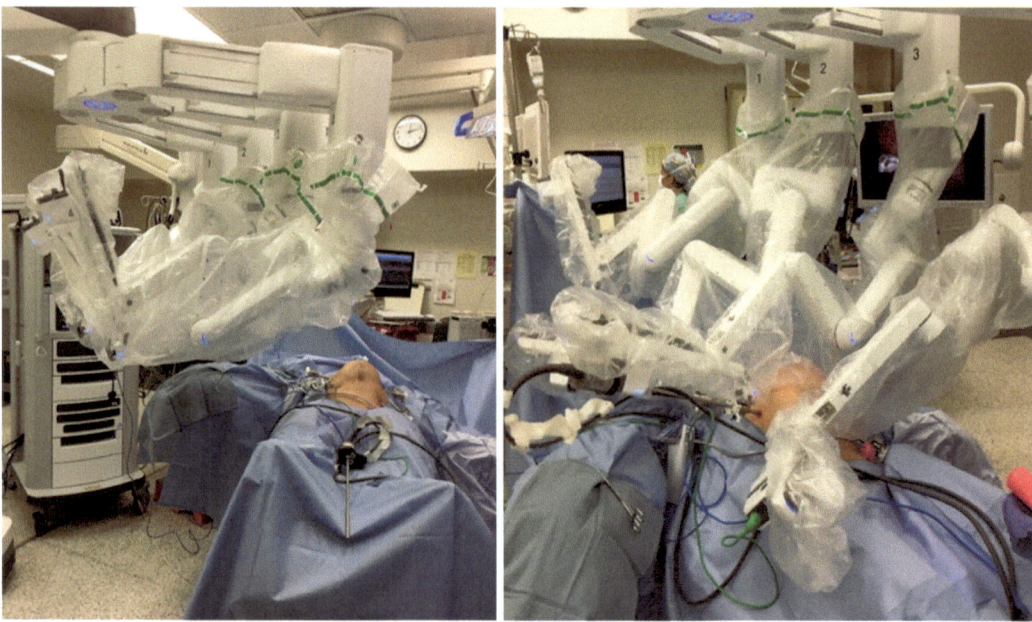

Fig. 8.7 Ventral hernia docking; the patient is supine with a partially break the table, slight Trendelenburg with the working side down

tional ports are placed along the anterior or mid axillary line. One port is a 12 mm disposable port, which allows insertion of the mesh along with necessary sutures with needles and facilitates removal of any specimen (old mesh, hernia contents, hernia sac, etc.). During the procedure an 8 mm instrument port is inserted into the 12 mm port (nesting) to function as the camera port. If there are lateral adhesions preventing necessary port placement, additional contralateral laparoscopic ports may be placed to facilitate laparoscopic lysis of adhesions. After adequate lysis of adhesions is performed, standard robotic port placement can occur and the robot can then be docked.

An additional port may be required for a bedside assistant to perform suctioning, suture exchange, or to provide additional retraction. Prior to placing the assistant port, consideration should be given to the final position of the robot when docked to make it easier for the bedside assistant to function through this port without contorting around the arms of the PC. If necessary (or desired) this port can be placed after

docking to optimize its position for maximum functionality.

Lysis of Adhesions and Reduction of Hernia Content

The robot is an exceptional platform for lysis of adhesions. The 3-D imaging and multiple degrees of freedom allow for fine dissection and easy visualization of tissue planes when working on the anterior abdominal wall. Due to the lack of haptic feedback, care must be taken while grasping bowel during adhesiolysis to prevent traction and avulsion injuries. Direct observation of the tissue in the workspace gives an idea of the degree or traction through "sensory substitution" using visual cues of tissue distortion [2]. If there is difficulty encountered with accessing contents within the hernia sac, the bedside assistant can provide external pressure on the abdominal wall by direct palpation over the hernia. This permits better visualization of the correct dissection plane, optimizes the angles of dissection between the viscera and hernia sac, and can help reduce incarcerated but non-adherent content from the hernia sac.

Common to robot surgery is the use of metal, reusable ports, which are available but less commonly used during standard laparoscopy. This is particularly important when using radiofrequency energy devices as the current can arc to the port causing unwanted burns to the abdominal wall. Additionally, the metal trocars can act as capacitors, storing and then unintentionally discharging current to adjacent structures. Special attention needs to be paid when using radiofrequency energy in robotic surgery to avoid inadvertent (and often unrecognized) thermal injury to the bowel.

Defect Closure

After reduction of the hernia, internal dimensions of the defect can be measured using one of two methods. The intracorporeal method is the easiest and uses the robotic instrument tips as a guide (the width of open grasper measures 2 cm). The instrument tips are transferred end to end to approximate the defect in stepwise fashion. A more accurate method uses an umbilical tape passed into the abdomen and stretched between the length and width of the defect. The assistant then extracts by grabbing the umbilical tape at the edge of the defect and measuring the length extracorporeally. While at the console, the bedside assistant can be instructed to pass a spinal needle to delineate the borders of the hernia in cardinal locations by palpating over the abdomen and watching on the monitor. In this fashion a spinal needle can be passed through the abdominal wall under direct visualization to identify the hernia borders without the surgeon having to step away from the SC. Placing spinal needles can also enhance communication between the surgeon and the bedside team members with regard to mesh size and orientation. The length and width of the defect can be measured in this way and then translated into the required mesh size.

Prior to defect closure, the abdominal insufflation pressure is reduced to 6–8 mmHg pressure to decrease the abdominal circumference and tension. The lowest pressure that provides adequate visualization and working space is used to approximate the native abdominal wall. As noted above, caution must be exercised to recognize when ports are at risk of dislodgement due to desufflation. Closure of the hernia defect is performed using a "barbed suture" to maintain tension during suturing. So-called "barbed sutures" come in unidirectional or bidirectional products which have small "barbs" cut into the suture to grasp the tissue and prevent the monofilament from sliding against tension.

The defect closure is initiated just beyond the apex of the hernia. Sutures are placed 2–3 loops at a time and then tensioned. Placing 2–3 loops at a time makes the suture more manageable and reduces inadvertent knots and a tangled suture. A double-armed suture is used to allow the hernia defect to be closed in two layers. During defect closure, the suture can break if there is too much tension applied to close the hernia. The sutures should be tightened one loop at a time with counter traction on the tissue. If the hernia defect is too wide and defect closure cannot be accomplished by simple suturing, placement of figure-of-eight sutures by an external suture passer assists with offloading the tension and improves the likelihood of defect closure. The bedside assistant provides upward tension on these sutures to partly close the defect while the surgeon continues closure with the barbed suture around the temporary percutaneous figure-of-eight stitch.

Inadvertent breakage of the suture can occur as a result of excessive tension being applied to the stitch or as a result of nicks in the monofilament suture from excessive handling with the robotic instruments. The use of the barbed suture allows the suture line to remain intact even if breakage occurs. The repair can be continued at the break point by tying the broken tip to a new suture or by beginning a new suture line at a location proximal to the break point. A second layer is used for added security as needed.

Instrument Issues

Occasionally instruments will fail to mate with the robotic arm properly. The robot arm indicator light turning yellow and alarm sounding will alert the personnel to this occurrence. In this event, the instrument should be completely removed and then reinserted. If that does not work, check the sterile arm drape and make sure the plastic connector has appropriate connection to the arm. Removing and reseating the sterile drape can alleviate this problem. The instrument can then be reinserted. Sometimes the instrument will malfunction after insertion even if the indicator light does not alert. If the instrument fails to open, close, or articulate properly, one or more of the actuator dials is not making contact with the instrument. The instrument should be removed and the actuator dials on the instrument and sterile drape interrogated for proper contact.

During the procedure, whether it is during adhesiolysis, defect closure, component separation, or mesh fixation, there may be times where the instruments are in a suboptimal working position. This occurs the closer the surgeon is working to the respective port. When this occurs, the bedside assistant can clutch the instrument and port simultaneously away from the working area to allow for more dexterity of the affected instrument. Care has to be taken to ensure that the port tip remains intra-abdominal (the use of nested balloon tip ports also reduces the likelihood of this event). This maneuver may have to be performed on multiple occasions during the procedure.

Desufflation and Port Loss

Desufflation of the abdominal cavity to facilitate defect closure can cause the tips of the cannulae and/or instruments to be in an intramuscular position. This occurs because the relative stability of the robotic arms and the lack of a negative thread design on the cannulae (i.e., smooth outer diameter cannula shaft) permit the abdominal wall to slide off of the ports. Prior to desufflation,

the ports and instruments should be advanced under direct vision to compensate for this anticipated event.

In the event of port loss, there can be difficulty during instrument exchanges and the bedside assistant will report resistance when attempting to advance instruments into the abdominal cavity. If this occurs, the instrument should not be advanced because of the possibility of injury to the abdominal wall structures or to intra-abdominal contents. In the latter instance, the port is actually still intra-abdominal and the resistance being reported is coming from instrument interaction with abdominal viscera. The surgeon should guide the camera to the affected port to ensure correct positioning. Sometimes this is not possible without undocking the camera and/or instrument port.

If an instrument port is partially out of position with a few muscle fibers covering the tip, the introducer can be placed to clear these fibers allowing the bedside assistant to advance the port into the peritoneal cavity. This maneuver can be performed for the camera port also in the event preperitoneal fat/muscle fibers or adhesive strands cause continued smudging of the lens system.

During repair of the hernia defect, multiple instrument exchanges as well as passage of sutures may occur. In the case of moving the port and instrument tip away from the working area to facilitate increased degrees of instrument freedom, from the bedside view the ports may seem out of position. One way to confirm that the ports are still intraperitoneal is to open the vent. If there is a hiss of venting pneumoperitoneum, this suggests the port is in an adequate position. If minimal or no gas returns then the port may be partially or completely obscured in the abdominal wall. This requires repositioning of the port by the assistant.

Mesh can be placed into the abdominal cavity through the 12 mm camera port by removing the nested 8 mm trocar and rolling the mesh around a standard laparoscopic atraumatic grasper before inserting. Care should be taken when passing the mesh as the abdomen can rapidly desufflate when the mesh is inserted. Prior to inserting we aim the port into a large free space and aim up to avoid injuring underlying organs. Additionally it is preferred to manually place the camera in a working port to facilitate placing the mesh under direct visualization.

Mesh Sizing, Delivery, Fixation

The size, delivery, fixation, and coverage (if preperitoneal or retromuscular) of mesh during robotic-assisted hernia repair do not differ substantially from traditional laparoscopic repair but will be reviewed here for completeness sake.

Inguinal Hernia

After creating a peritoneal flap, reducing the hernia and sac, the myopectineal orifice is completely exposed. Mesh size and weight are determined by patient characteristics and surgeon preference. We find that anatomically contoured mesh is generally easier to position intraabdominally with reduced shift of mesh when closing. Undersized mesh is easy to position but may provide inadequate coverage and increased recurrence rates. Oversized mesh may be difficult to position, to completely cover with the peritoneal flap and may buckle during closure creating gaps for inferior recurrence. Performing a wide dissection of the entire myopectineal orifice permits a large piece of mesh to be placed without any of these concerns. Following introduction, the mesh can be secured to the pectineal (Cooper's) ligament and anterior abdominal wall with suture or a laparoscopic tacker. Finally the peritoneal flap can be suture closed (or tacked) over the mesh.

Ventral Hernia

For ventral hernias, the mesh should have 4–6 cm overlap beyond the edges of the defect. The mesh can be indexed externally by drawing lines to mark the correct orientation, or a mesh positioning system can be utilized. Localizing sutures placed at the superior- and inferiormost edges can assist with correct positioning intraabdominally and to hold the mesh to the anterior abdominal wall until it can be sutured in place. The mesh is then inserted into the abdomen. Localizing sutures are grasped using a transfascial suture passer and tied externally by the bedside assistant at the superior and inferior edges of the defect. The mesh should be correctly oriented at this point and ready for final suturing. The mesh is fixed to the abdominal wall by suturing the edges to the abdominal musculature circumferentially using a barbed suture. The sutures are first placed along the side closest to the camera port. Placing sutures then tightening the loops after three throws reduces the risk of the suture being tangled and increases efficiency. When suturing has progressed to the contralateral side, the mesh can be stretched with the second working arm to allow for adequate coverage and overlap without sagging. In the event that intracorporeal suturing is ineffective or not progressing appropriately, a standard laparoscopic tacker can be used to secure the mesh circumferentially. Ultimately the goal is to have a wellsecured mesh, regardless of the modality used.

No Peritoneal Flap or Poor Flap

Patients who have thin peritoneum or have had prior preperitoneal dissection create a challenge when raising peritoneal flaps for mesh coverage. Small holes or linear tears in the peritoneum can be sutured closed with a running suture. Large defects that cannot be closed primarily, or cases where there is insufficient peritoneum for coverage, should have a coated mesh used to prevent intra-abdominal adhesions.

Operative Complications

Multiple studies have been published demonstrating equivalent operative complication rates when comparing the laparoscopic and robotic surgery [3, 4]. Injury during abdominal access, misapplied radiofrequency energy, and bowel injury rates are the same between the two modalities [5]. Therefore when experiencing a complication during robotic-assisted hernia repair, the same principles of management apply as to an injury created laparoscopically. There are some types of complications unique to robotic surgery that warrant specific consideration.

Guided Instrument Exchanges

In robotic surgery the instrument exchanges are typically blind, relying on the stored memory of the robotic arm. Injury can occur when viscera, fat, or other structures shift into the path of the instrument following its removal. This can happen through the release of tension from the extracted instrument but can also occur when motion of a second instrument pushes structures into the anticipated path of the instrument being replaced. As the instrument is reinserted, the structure can be inadvertently pierced or injured out of view of the camera. This demonstrates the importance of good communication with the bedside assistant and carefully reinserting instruments, noting any unanticipated force on the instrument as it is being inserted. We prefer to engage the instrument and then slide it back into position with one-finger pressure. If excessive force is required, the camera should be used to watch the instrument come in. This may require the camera port to be clutched and manually controlled to watch the instrument. The key here is to recognize that an injury may have occurred to prevent an enterotomy or other organ damage from being missed.

Arm Collisions

Collisions between arms and torqueing may also occur without the surgeons notice due to the loss of haptic feedback. When one instrument cantilevers over another, the applied forces may cause unrecognized injury to adjacent structures or cause the instruments to fly off each other as they shift position. The easiest way to recognize this situation is to note when one or both instrument moves spontaneously or lacks 1:1 motion. The bedside assist may be able to hear, see, or feel such collisions and should report concern for collisions to the surgeon.

Avulsion Injuries

This can occur due to the lack of haptic feedback. When grasping tissue, applied force can be judged through "sensory substitution" using visual cues based on the amount of tissue distortion [6]. Sensory substitution does not take the place of tactile feedback however and inadvertent avulsion injuries can occur. These should be managed in the same was as laparoscopic surgical avulsion injuries. Traction of the robot arm outside of the field of view can also result in avulsion that might not occur laparoscopically due to the surgeon perceiving forces on the instruments that are not being seen within the operative field.

Bleeding

If uncontrolled bleeding is encountered, the outer working arm can be used to tamponade the bleeding while preparing to convert. This is accomplished by directly clamping or compressing the bleeding vessel with a grasper before the surgeon removes his head from the console. The robot can then be undocked except for the arm holding pressure. A laparotomy incision can be made and the abdomen entered. Once the site of bleeding is encountered and ready to be controlled directly, the robotic arm can be removed and the PC moved away from the table to permit complete access. Other methods of emergent abdominal access have been described in the literature and include subcostal or hockey stick incisions to gain access [6]. Such situations should be uncommon in hernia repair but it is incumbent upon the operating surgeon to understand options for the management of such emergent situations.

Contact Injuries

Because the robot platform sits above the patient, the translated motion of the external arms may inadvertently contact the patient's body causing injury. Additionally, when ports are torqued they can dig into the patient and create a pressure sore over the course of a long case. This is particularly true if the CO_2 gas port is turned toward the patient. Such injuries can be avoided by ensuring proper patient positioning and carefully examination of all the ports and arms after docking. Any areas of concern should be repositioned or padded with sterile towels to prevent inadvertent injury. The bedside assistant is crucial to monitoring for these contact points and should be thoroughly educated prior to assisting with robotic surgical procedures.

Case reports of other rare complications (such as diaphragm rupture and hemiparesis) have been documented but are not directly attributable to the robotic platform itself [7, 8].

Conclusion

Robotic surgery has seen many advances as the technology matures. The most recent generation of platforms is particularly useful for ventral and inguinal herniorrhaphy. The details of both basic and more intricate aspects of robotic-assisted hernia surgery influence the flow of the operation, the mental workload of the procedure and likely the final outcome of the procedure. By understanding the operative considerations outlined in this chapter and by being prepared to address difficult intraoperative situations, the trained surgeon should be able to reduce their learning curve to performing safe and efficient robotic-assisted hernia repair.

References

1. Gonzalez A, Escobar E, Romero R, Walker G, Mejias J, Gallas M, Dickens E, Johnson CJ, Rabaza J, Kudsi OY. Robotic-assisted ventral hernia repair: a multicenter evaluation of clinical outcomes. Surg Endosc. 2017;31(3):1342–9.
2. Bethea BT, Okamura AM, Kitagawa M, Fitton TP, Cattaneo SM, Gott VL, Baumgartner WA, Yuh DD. Application of haptic feedback to robotic surgery. J Laparoendosc Adv Surg Tech A. 2004;14(3):191–5.
3. Chen YJ, Huynh D, Nguyen S, Chin E, Divino C, Zhang L. Outcomes of robot-assisted versus laparoscopic repair of small-sized ventral hernias. Surg Endosc. 2017;31(3):1275–9.
4. D'Annibale A, Orsini C, Morpurgo E, Sovernigo G. Robotic surgery: considerations after 250 procedures. Chir Ital. 2006;58(1):5–14.
5. Sotelo RJ, Haese A, Machuca V, Medina L, Nuñez L, Santinelli F, Hernandez A, Kural AR, Mottrie A, Giedelman C, Mirandolino M, Palmer K, Abaza R, Ghavamian R, Shalhav A, Moinzadeh A, Patel V, Stifelman M, Tuerk I, Canes D. Safer surgery by learning from complications: a focus on robotic prostate surgery. Eur Urol. 2016;69(2):334–44.
6. Jones KB Jr. When and how to "open" in laparoscopic or robotic surgery. Obes Surg. 2016;26(4):891–5.
7. Naeem T, Kumar S, Fareed K, Jah A, Hindmarsh A, Shah N, Sujendran V. Spontaneous diaphragmatic rupture following robotic prostatectomy. Ann R Coll Surg Engl. 2017;99(2):e44–6.
8. Kurdija J, Jakobsson JG. Transient left-sided paralysis following robotic-assisted laparoscopic uteropexy. Case Rep Anesthesiol. 2015;2015:150715. https://doi.org/10.1155/2015/150715. Epub 2015 May 26.

Zachary Sanford, Shyam S. Jayaraman,
H. Reza Zahiri, and Igor Belyansky

Introduction

The last two decades have proven to be a significant period of evolution in the field of abdominal wall reconstruction (AWR). A variety of "components separation" (CS) techniques have been described and shown to be useful in addressing complex abdominal cases associated with large defects and loss of abdominal domain. Originally reported by Ramirez et al. in 1990 as a rectus abdominis advancement flap with primary tissue closure in the midline, the technique described surgical division of contributions by the external oblique muscle to the linea semilunaris and division of the posterior rectus sheath [1, 2]. The external oblique muscle release is also referred to as anterior component separation.

A disadvantage of traditional open anterior CS is aggressive subcutaneous flap elevation to expose the external oblique muscles. This results in compromise of periumbilical perforators and is associated with an increase in wound morbidity. Accordingly, the motivation arose to achieve perforator sparing anterior CS, thus decreasing the wound morbidity associated with large subcutaneous flaps. Lowe et al. have described the separation of anterior components through a minimally invasive technique dividing the external oblique after the creation of a space by an endoscopic balloon dissector [3]. To follow, several authors have described various minimally invasive approaches to CS with the goal of gaining direct access to the lateral abdominal wall without large skin flaps and minimizing subcutaneous dead space while preserving the rectus abdominis perforator vessels [4–7].

The minimally invasive anterior CS is still associated with possible need for an open laparotomy approach as well as placement of mesh in the intra-abdominal cavity that requires an expensive barrier coated mesh as well as penetrating fixation to secure it in place [1, 3, 4]. Consequently, some of the potential issues associated with intraperitoneal mesh placement (IPOM) are visceral adhesions that in 13% of cases can be clinically significant in future surgeries [8]. In addition, penetrating fixation that is required in IPOM placement has been previously described to be associated with presence of chronic pain [9, 10].

More recently, the transversus abdominis muscle release (TAR) technique has been described by Novitsky et al. focusing on division of the posterior rectus sheath, posterior lamella of the internal oblique and transversus abdominis muscle as an alternative myocutaneous advancement flap [11]. This unique approach enables the repair of a variety of complex and atypical defect locations while

Z. Sanford · S. S. Jayaraman · H. Reza Zahiri
I. Belyansky (✉)
Department of Surgery, Anne Arundel Medical
Center, Annapolis, MD, USA
e-mail: ibelyansky@aahs.org

in one step performing myocutaneous advancement in addition to developing the retromuscular space for a large mesh placement without the disruption of subcutaneous perforators. The retromuscular space developed can extend from one midaxillary line to the other and from the subxiphoid space down to the space of Retzius, bordered posteriorly by an autologous posterior layer that serves as a barrier separating the intra-abdominal viscera from mesh material, of which we prefer to use a non-coated polypropylene macroporous medium weight mesh. Having the ability to sandwich the mesh between two layers also enabled us to safely move away from use of penetrating fixation, improving quality of life (QOL) outcomes without increasing recurrence rates [10, 12].

Open posterior CS was demonstrated to have fewer wound morbidities and risk of mesh exposure to the extracorporeal environment than anterior CS [11]. Unfortunately, wound morbidity in open TAR still ranges from 17 to 29% and the open nature of this intervention is associated with an average length of hospital stay of 6 days [13]. Our current practice is heavily influenced by the following principles:

- Paradigm shift towards defect closure
- Eliminating penetrating mesh fixation without compromising the hernia repair
- Using uncoated mesh and placing it outside of the abdominal cavity
- Minimally Invasive Surgical (MIS) approach when possible

Combining the benefits of a minimally invasive approach with the TAR procedure, a laparoscopic approach to posterior component separation (eTEP) has been described by our group in 2015 [5]. This approach underwent several modifications and initial multicenter experiences, with eTEP access for retromuscular repair recently reported and published [14]. In this chapter we will describe the principles and steps to the eTEP access for Rives Stoppa retrorectus repair and discuss the decisions necessary as to when to perform selective TAR.

Preoperative Planning and Considerations

All prospective MIS AWR candidates undergo standard history, physical exam, and basic laboratory testing to ensure they are appropriately selected for major surgery, with emphasis placed on screening for relative and absolute contraindications to the eTEP approach for incisional and ventral herniae (Table 9.1). Attention to defect size, past or current wound infections, stoma, ostomies, redundant skin, and contour abnormalities are critical in establishing suitable patient selection and the proper operative approach for hernioplasty. It is imperative that past medical and surgical records be accurate and thoroughly reviewed for prior interventions and to interrogate for the presence of potentially aberrant anatomy or mesh fixation devices in the case of patients presenting with recurrent hernia disease. An up-to-date computed tomography study of the abdomen and pelvis is recommended for effective preoperative planning per SAGES guidelines [15]. This assists preoperative planning through assessment of the size of hernia defect, extent of loss of domain, and the components of the abdominal wall available for reconstruction. Very thick oblique muscles can reduce compliance of the abdominal wall and compromise efforts to reapproximate the edges of the defect back together [5]. In addition, age-appropriate cancer screening is conducted including a screening colonoscopy for patients over the age of 50 and an updated Pap smear ± HPV cotesting in women over 21 years of age.

Table 9.1 Absolute and relative contraindications to eTEP approach

Relative	Absolute
Previous incision extending from xiphoid process to the pubic bone	Active mesh infection
Loss of domain	Presence of fistula
Dystrophic or ulcerated skin	
Extensive intra-abdominal adhesions	

On initial encounter all major comorbidities must be addressed by means of a multidisciplinary approach before proceeding to the operating room. Emphasis is placed on assessing cardiopulmonary and endocrine systems as they pose the greatest risk for intraoperative morbidity and mortality. Diabetic patients are to have their HbA1C levels managed below 7.4 with established goals for postoperative glycemic control. Morbidly obese individuals must achieve a target body mass index (BMI) of less than 40 with any patient of a BMI greater than 35 consulted by either a registered dietician or nutritionist to begin a comprehensive weight loss program. Patients with a positive smoking history must demonstrate cessation for at least 4 weeks prior to surgical intervention and may benefit from consultation with substance abuse counselors. Nicotine levels are confirmed with serum cotinine levels in the preoperative area the day of surgery to proceed only in those testing negative for nicotine derivatives.

It is important to discuss with the patient likely outcomes and possible complications of surgery in order to establish a reasonable series of expectations postoperatively. Despite the minimally invasive nature of these procedures, patients may still experience significant amounts of pain requiring inpatient management. Possible complications including seroma, hematoma, deep or superficial abscesses, bowel injury, and their respective management options must be presented. In the event of complex revisional procedures, the possibility for conversion to open surgery is typically higher and warrants additional discussion. Additionally, patients with active infection should be treated with properly selected antimicrobial therapy with resolution of the infection before surgery. Preoperative antibiotics should be properly selected and dosed according to hospital protocol [15, 16]. We recommend routine administration of subcutaneous heparin for DVT prophylaxis in our patient population, beginning prior to the induction of anesthesia and administered throughout the typical duration of the procedure [17, 18]. A VTE

surgical risk model such as the Caprini score method can be used to tailor VTE prophylaxis to the specific patient. Sequential compression devices (SCD) or foot pumps should be used when available.

Operating Room Setup and Patient Positioning

Patients are positioned supine with both arms tucked to their sides. After induction of anesthesia, Foley catheter is routinely placed. The operating room table is flexed with the legs extend down at a minimum of 30° to afford the surgeon and assistant greater instrument range of motion (Fig. 9.1). Failure to sufficiently flex the operating table will result in surgeon's hand collision with the patient's body while dissecting and suturing the defects.

eTEP Access

The enhanced-view totally extraperitoneal (eTEP) access approach was previously described for laparoscopic inguinal hernia repair by Dr. Jorge Daes [19]. This approach introduced the notion that the extraperitoneal space is limitless once the confluence of arcuate line and semilunar line are taken down. We have adopted this

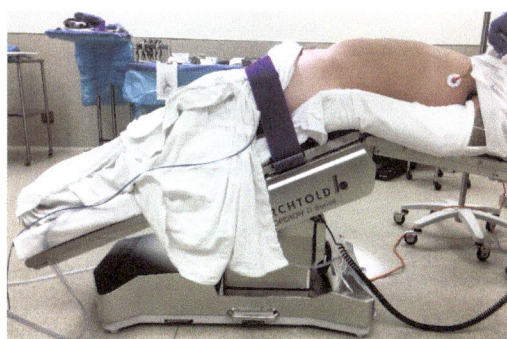

Fig. 9.1 Positioning of the patient for laparoscopic CS. Patient is in Trendelenburg position with hips extended. Bed flexion is best avoided

technique for repair of ventral and incisional herniae [4, 14, 19]. The eTEP access approach relies
on dissection in the naturally occurring retromuscular spaces. Typically, dissection is initiated in
one of the retrorectus spaces and then crosses
over to the contralateral side, thus joining the two
spaces into one large operative region. The key
advantages of this approach are:

- The rapid creation of an extraperitoneal
  domain.
- The technique may enable an entirely extraperitoneal approach.
- If the intra-abdominal cavity is entered, safe
  adhesiolysis can be performed.
- Improved tolerance of pneumoperitoneum.
- Dynamic port setup that can be adjusted based
  on the location of the defect.

Prior to incision, we suggest appreciating and
marking out relevant anatomy at skin level. This
includes the xiphoid process, bilateral subcostal
margins, symphysis pubis, linea alba, and semilunar lines. Preoperative CT scan and physical
exam are used to facilitate the marking of these
landmarks. Positioning of the surgeon, monitor,
and trocars is dependent on the location of the
hernia defect and decision where to crossover.
Monitors are placed at the head of the bed with
trocar sites on the lower abdomen when addressing an upper midline hernia defect and inverted in
instances of lower midline hernia defects.

Upper Midline Defect

When dealing with upper midline defects we prefer to perform the crossover below the level of the
umbilicus, developing preperitoneal and retromuscular spaces that have not been previously violated. Figure 9.2 demonstrates the port position for
upper midline defects. The first incision is made
2 cm below a horizontal line drawn through umbilicus just medial to the right linea semilunaris. The
anterior rectus sheath is identified and incised
sharply. Single site balloon dissector is used to
develop the right retrorectus space in cephalad and
caudal directions. It is critical to avoid over-infla-

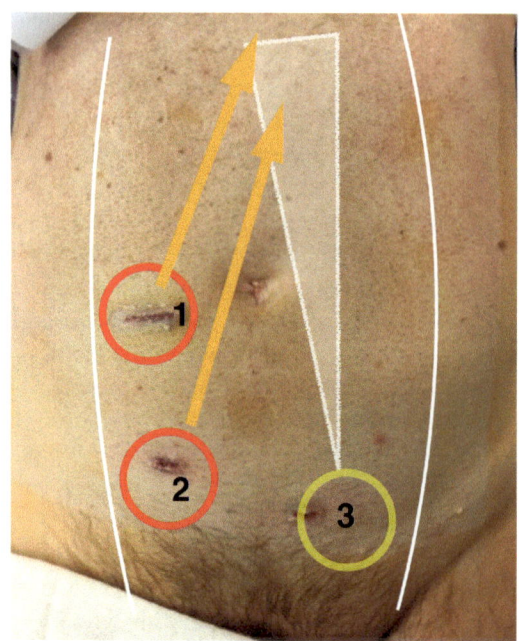

Fig. 9.2 Port positioning for upper midline defects. The
balloon dissector is placed in Port #1. Ports #1 and #2 in
red circles are working ports. Port #3 in yellow is the camera port

tion which may rupture the linea semilunaris and
consequently injure the rectus abdominis muscle.
In addition, special care should be given to appreciating the inferior epigastric vessels that travel
parallel and medial to linea semilunaris in the
vicinity of the #1 port. Once the space of Retzius
is developed, ports #2 and #3 are placed under
direct vision in the lower abdomen. The site of port
#3 can also be used to pass the balloon space-
maker in a cephalad direction to develop the left
retrorectus space. Thus, even before any initiation
of sharp dissection the retromuscular space surrounding the hernia defect is completely dissected
bluntly with the balloon space-maker.

A 30° scope is placed through port #3 after
which we proceed with division of the medial
contributions of the posterior rectus sheath to the
linea alba bilaterally from caudal to cephalad
direction. In the middle we try to preserve the
preperitoneal contributions to the posterior layer
which are made up of the falciform and umbilical
ligaments. In such a fashion the division of posterior rectus sheath and preservation of falciform

Fig. 9.3 View of the retrorectus space. After crossing over and dissection, the retrorectus spaces on both sides are combined into one large retrorectus space. This falciform ligament can be seen below

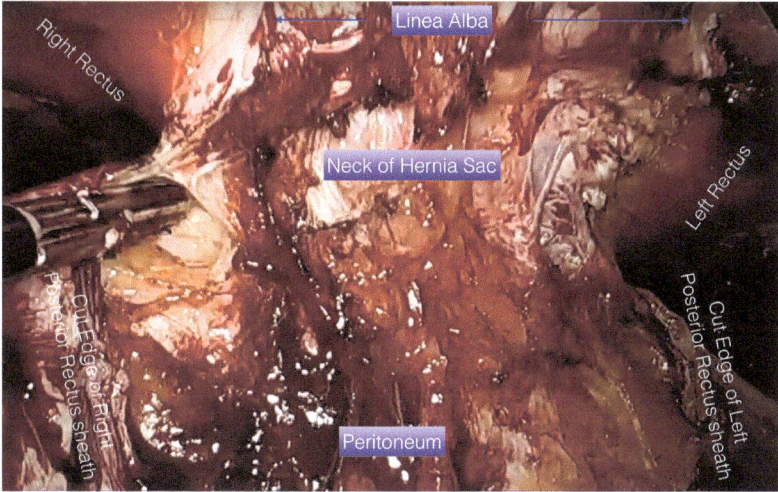

ligament and umbilical ligaments allows us to join the right and the left retrorectus spaces together with midline preperitoneal space (Fig. 9.3).

Following the dissection in these planes we then anticipate to encounter the neck of the hernia sac. In true incisional herniae, the layers surrounding the neck of the sack can be thoroughly fused together and difficult to differentiate. A recent preoperative CT scan, therefore, is an invaluable aid in identification of the hernia and its contents. An attempt may be made in some cases to reduce the entirety of the sac by separating it from its distal attachments, however this is not often attempted. We frequently give consideration to sharply opening the peritoneal layer just proximal to the neck of the sac to reduce visceral contents under direct visualization and perform limited adhesiolysis (Fig. 9.4). Any defects in the posterior layer can be fixed with 3-0 suture. Once the hernia contents are reduced, retromuscular dissection commences with release of the medial aspect of the posterior rectus sheath and concludes just below the level of the xiphoid process.

Lower Midline Defects

For a right-handed surgeon, we found that lower midline defects are easier to address by initiating

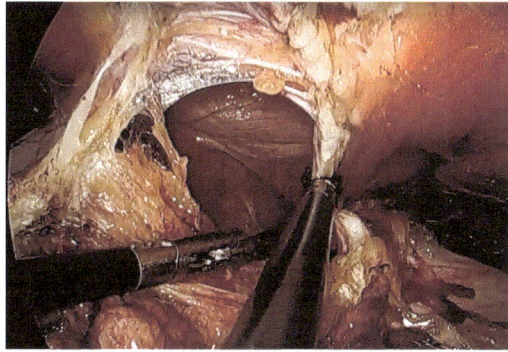

Fig. 9.4 Sharp opening of the peritoneal layer proximal to the neck of the hernia sac, allowing for reduction of visceral contents under direct visualization and limited adhesiolysis

the dissection in the upper portion of left retrorectus space. Figure 9.5 demonstrates the typical port position that we chose to use for this approach. Balloon dissector is used at port position #1 to develop the left retrorectus space, followed by direct visualization for placement of port #2 into the developed space with an optional port #3. Blunt dissection in the left retrorectus space is performed in a caudal direction and the pubis is identified. As the upper midline has not previously been violated above the level of umbilicus, the medial aspect of the left posterior rectus sheath is incised and the preperitoneal space entered just superficial to falciform ligament (Fig. 9.6). The right posterior rectus sheath is

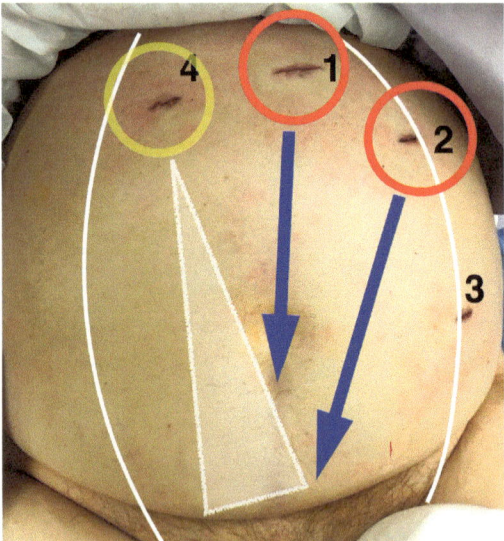

Fig. 9.5 Port placement for a right-handed surgeon addressing a lower midline defects. We initiate the dissection in the upper portion of left retrorectus space. Balloon dissector is used at port position #1 to develop the left retrorectus space, followed by direct visualization for placement of port #2 into the developed space with an optional port #3. Port #4 is used as a camera port

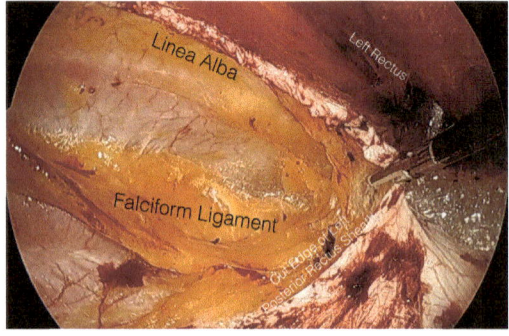

Fig. 9.6 Medial aspect of the left posterior rectus sheath is incised and the preperitoneal space entered just superficial to falciform ligament

identified and its medial aspect incised and released in a cephalad to caudal direction followed by blunt dissection in the right retrorectus space (Fig. 9.7). Port #4 is then placed under direct vision through the upper aspect of right rectus abdominis muscle which is then used as the camera port. The retrorectus dissection is carried out in the caudal direction completing bilateral release of the posterior rectus sheaths.

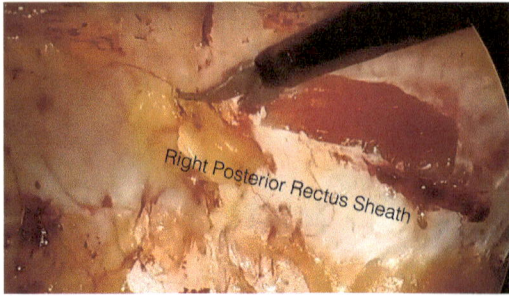

Fig. 9.7 The right posterior rectus sheath is identified and its medial aspect incised then released in a cephalad to caudal direction followed by blunt dissection in the right retrorectus space

When encountering the hernia sac we try to sharply dissect the distal attachments, thus mobilizing it downward. Alternatively, the sac can be sharply entered and laparoscopic adhesiolysis performed as needed.

Transversus Abdominis Release

For more complex defects that require large mesh placement, the transversus abdominis release (TAR) procedure is added [20, 21]. We have found that incorporation of the TAR is beneficial in cases with wide (>10 cm) defects, narrow (<5 cm) retrorectus spaces, or when dealing with a poorly compliant abdominal wall. Any defects in the posterior layer are closed with 2-0 absorbable suture. The abdominal wall defect is primarily closed using 0 barbed suture in running fashion, while pneumoperitoneum is dropped to 8 mmHg.

For defects wider than 10 cm, primary fascial closure can rarely be achieved under physiologic tension unless additional CS in the form of l-TAR is added to the procedure. The edge of the cut posterior rectus sheath (PRS) on one side is retracted medially and a thin, almost transparent layer of connective tissue that covers the transversus fibers is identified as the posterior lamina of the internal oblique muscle and incised with hook electrocautery, thus exposing the transversus abdominis muscle fibers (Fig. 9.8). Care must be taken to stay medial to the perforating nerves and vessels at the linea semilunaris to maintain functional segmental innervation to the rectus

(Fig. 9.9). Hook cautery is used to elevate and transect the exposed transversus fibers, revealing the glistening transversalis fascia underneath. This is continued from cephalad to caudad until the transversalis fascia is seen as a glistening line extending the entire craniocaudal length of the abdominal wall. Blunt dissection is now used to develop the plane just deeper to the transversus muscle fibers and superficial to the transversalis fascia resulting in a retromuscular preperitoneal plane, thereby achieving the TAR (Fig. 9.10). The plane can be extended in the lateral direction as far as the mid axillary line. A unilateral TAR can achieve as much as 7 cm of medial fascial mobilization at the level of the umbilicus. Bilateral TAR can be performed as needed.

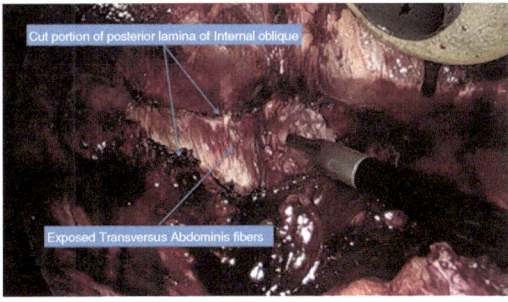

Fig. 9.8 The cut edge of PRS is retracted medially revealing the posterior lamina of the internal oblique muscle, a thin layer of connective tissue covering. Once identified and incised with hook electrocautery the transversus abdominis muscle fibers can be appreciated

Closure

Posterior Layer
The edges of the PRS are sutured together in the midline with 2-0 absorbable or barbed suture starting near the xiphoid process running caudally. Starting at the dome of the bladder the surgeon and assistant switch positions and suture is run cranially, meeting in the middle where the two sutures are tied together.

Anterior Layer
Pneumoperitoneum is dropped to 8–10 mmHg. The defect being closed is at the top of the monitor and is sutured "upside down" with backhanded needle driving. A 0 barbed suture is used for this closure due to technical ease of use afforded in this situation. If a large subcutaneous sac is present, one or more bites of the sac are included in the suture line for plication in order to reduce the likelihood of developing a postoperative seroma (Fig. 9.11). With the previously performed posterior CS, the defect edges should come together in a reasonably tension-free fashion. The defect is closed with V-lock suture, completed with four or five throws run in a backwards fashion.

Mesh Placement
Once both anterior and posterior fascial layers are closed, the mesh is deployed in the

Fig. 9.9 When incising the lateral edge of the PRS sheath to expose the transversus abdominis, care must be taken to prevent injury to the neurovascular bundles near the linea semilunaris

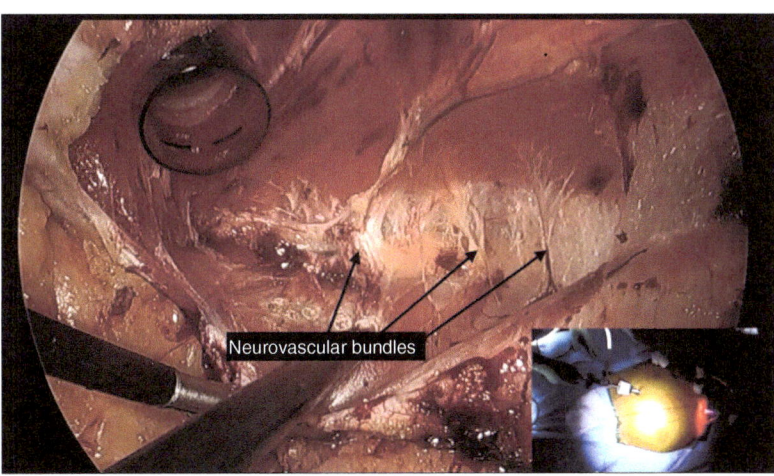

Fig. 9.10 The transversalis fascia is separated from the transversus abdominis by blunt dissection achieving TAR

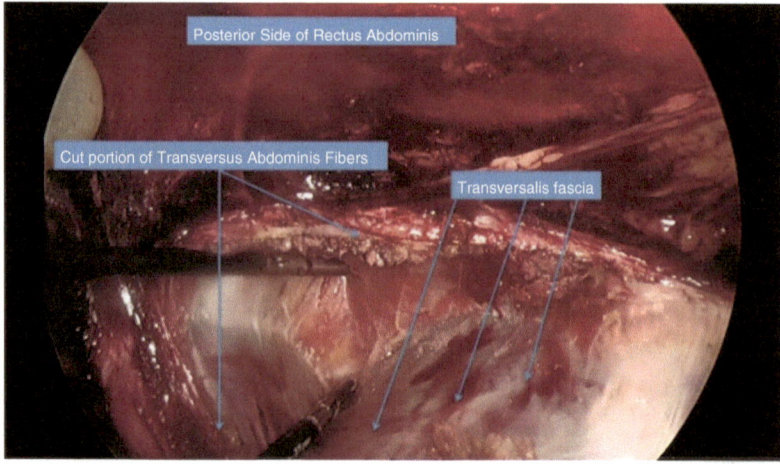

Fig. 9.11 Closure of the anterior layer. A 0 barbed suture is used in a back-handed fashion with an "upside down" view to take bites of the edges of the defect while including the sac (if a large subcutaneous portion is present) in between to reduce the chance of postoperative seroma

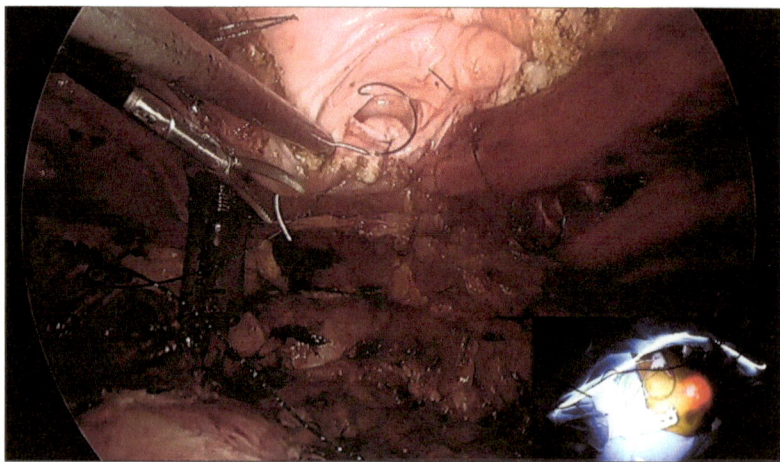

retromuscular sublay position. The developed retromuscular space is measured for appropriate mesh size selection. Our preference is medium weight macroporous polypropylene mesh which is deployed through our 12 mm trocar (Fig. 9.12). There is no need for antiadhesion barriers as there now exists an autologous barrier between the mesh and viscera, a significant advantage of the sublay position. Mesh placement in the retromuscular space has allowed for the discontinuation of aggressive penetrating fixation techniques with transfascial sutures, transitioning first to fibrin glue and, more recently, to complete cessation of mesh fixation as our data illustrates penetrating fixation is associated with higher incidence of chronic pain without the added benefit of low-

ered rates of recurrence. Pneumoperitoneum is released under direct vision, assuring the mesh is lying flat and wrinkle-free between the posterior and anterior layers.

Formerly, we once placed drains just superficial to the mesh in all repair cases. We are now more selective with drain placement and do not utilize it for most patients. To date, we have not observed an increase in wound morbidity as a result.

Transabdominal Approach

Alternatively, traditional laparoscopic transabdominal approach can be used. Standard

Fig. 9.12 Placement of a medium weight macroporous polypropylene mesh deployed through the 12 mm trocar. There is no need for antiadhesion barriers as there now exists an autologous barrier between the mesh and viscera

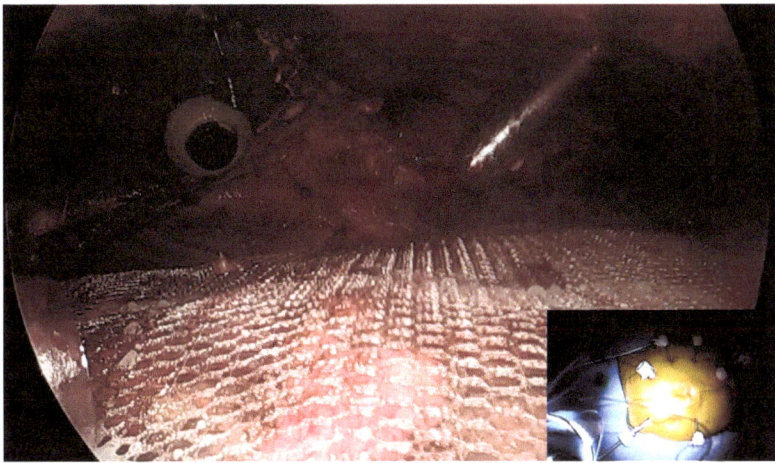

laparoscopic entry to the peritoneal cavity can be achieved and adhesions taken down. The PRS is then incised just lateral to the defect or the linea alba. Dissection can proceed from there as we described in l-TAR originally, prior to our adoption of the eTEP access approach [5].

Postoperative Management

After recovery from anesthesia, patients are transferred from the PACU for admission to the wards or alternatively discharged to home as determined by the complexity of the surgery. Those that underwent an eTEP access Rives Stoppa repair (retrorectus mesh placement) are typically discharged home the same day. Diet is advanced as tolerated and patients are encouraged to ambulate as early and often as possible to prevent postoperative ileus. The average length of stay at our center following TAR via the eTEP access approach is approximately 1–2 days. Prolonged postoperative ileus, although uncommon, is the primary cause for length of hospital stay.

Immediately following surgery, pain is controlled with patient-controlled analgesia (PCA) devices, substituted the following morning to oral analgesics. The minimally invasive approach has allowed us to significantly reduce dependence on PCA and associated large volumes of narcotics for postoperative analgesia.

Patients are provided incentive spirometry (IS) to assist in their pulmonary toilet and instructed to use these devices ten times per hour while awake to minimize any respiratory complications from splinting. Sequential compression devices (SCD) are placed and subcutaneous unfractionated or low molecular weight heparin is used for DVT prophylaxis until the patient is ambulating. Abdominal binders are offered to all patients for their psychological benefit and are advantageous in promoting early ambulation [22, 23]. Drain(s), when used, are left in place until their output is <30 cc per day.

Patients are discharged from the hospital once they are sufficiently ambulating, tolerate oral intake, have a return of bowel function, and tolerate pain control without the need for intravenous medications. Typically, patients are seen 4 weeks following surgery for their first postoperative clinic visit; however, visits are scheduled sooner if they are discharged with a drain in place.

Future Directions

Controversies abound in the ventral hernia literature regarding the best anatomical approach, ideal mesh material, and the best plane for prosthetic placement. Better definiton of indications, contraindications and complication rates for each approach and further refinement of techniques are avenues for future research that will continue to improve care for these complex patients with major hernia disease.

On the subject of minimally invasive surgical techniques, robotics deserves special mention. Increasing case volumes and ergonomic challenges of laparoscopic surgery pose significant physical strain on surgeons, potentially leading to chronic pain and earlier or more frequent burn out for experienced surgeons [24]. Robotic surgery allows for an increased degree of freedom with more elegant technical maneuvering while offering improved ergonomics and comfort to the operating surgeon. Nevertheless, many questions remain unanswered on the subject of robotic-assisted surgery, including its impact on operative and postoperative costs [25]. Data on comparative outcomes for ventral hernia repair is scarce, with less than a handful of studies currently in the literature. This topic is better addressed in a different chapter of this text.

Prospective large-scale trials are ideal for providing the best quality evidence to compare and contrast different approaches hernia repair. MIS CS is but one field within hernia repair that is still in relative infancy and is as yet not widely practiced. The eTEP access approach to laparoscopic CS may perhaps lend itself to rapid learning and technical adoption [14]. Although the preliminary data are encouraging, more studies are necessary, particularly on long-term outcomes as it joins the armamentarium of the hernia surgeon.

References

1. Ramirez OM, Ruas E, Dellon AL. "Components separation" method for closure of abdominal-wall defects: an anatomic and clinical study. Plast Reconstr Surg. 1990;86(3):519–26.
2. Criss CN, Petro CC, Krpata DM, et al. Functional abdominal wall reconstruction improves core physiology and quality-of-life. Surgery. 2014;156(1):176–82.
3. Lowe JB, Garza JR, Bowman JL, Rohrich RJ, Strodel WE. Endoscopically assisted "components separation" for closure of abdominal wall defects. Plast Reconstr Surg. 2000;105(2):720–9; quiz 730.
4. Butler CE, Campbell KT. Minimally invasive component separation with inlay bioprosthetic mesh (MICSIB) for complex abdominal wall reconstruction. Plast Reconstr Surg. 2011;128(3):698–709.
5. Belyansky I, Zahiri HR, Park A. Laparoscopic transversus abdominis release, a novel minimally invasive approach to complex abdominal wall reconstruction. Surg Innov. 2016;23(2):134–41.
6. Maas SM, de Vries RS, van Goor H, de Jong D, Bleichrodt RP. Endoscopically assisted "components separation technique" for the repair of complicated ventral hernias. J Am Coll Surg. 2002;194(3):388–90.
7. Mommers EH, Wegdam JA, Nienhuijs SW, de Vries Reilingh TS. How to perform the endoscopically assisted components separation technique (ECST) for large ventral hernia repair. Hernia. 2016;20(3):441–7.
8. Chelala E, Barake H, Estievenart J, Dessily M, Charara F, Alle JL. Long-term outcomes of 1326 laparoscopic incisional and ventral hernia repair with the routine suturing concept: a single institution experience. Hernia. 2016;20(1):101–10.
9. Carbonell AM, Harold KL, Mahmutovic AJ, et al. Local injection for the treatment of suture site pain after laparoscopic ventral hernia repair. Am Surg. 2003;69(8):688–91; discussion 691–2.
10. Colavita PD, Tsirline VB, Belyansky I, et al. Prospective, long-term comparison of quality of life in laparoscopic versus open ventral hernia repair. Ann Surg. 2012;256(5):714–22; discussion 722–3.
11. Krpata DM, Blatnik JA, Novitsky YW, Rosen MJ. Posterior and open anterior components separations: a comparative analysis. Am J Surg. 2012;203(3):318–22; discussion 322.
12. Weltz ASSA, Zahiri RZ, Schoeneborn A, Park A, Belyansky I. Operative outcomes after open abdominal wall reconstruction with retromuscular mesh fixation using fibrin glue versus transfascial sutures. Am Surg. 2017;83(9):937–42.
13. Martin-Del-Campo LA, Weltz AS, Belyansky I, Novitsky YW. Comparative analysis of perioperative outcomes of robotic versus open transversus abdominis release. Surg Endosc. 2018;32(2):840–5.
14. Belyansky IDJ, Radu VG, Balasu-bramanian R, Zahiri HR, Weltz AS, Sibia US, Park A, Novitsky Y. A novel approach using the enhanced-view totally extraperitoneal (eTEP) technique for laparoscopic retromuscular hernia repair. Surg Endosc. 2018;32(3):1525–32.
15. Earle D, Roth JS, Saber A, et al. SAGES guidelines for laparoscopic ventral hernia repair. Surg Endosc. 2016;30(8):3163–83.
16. Sanchez-Manuel FJ, Lozano-Garcia J, Seco-Gil JL. Antibiotic prophylaxis for hernia repair. Cochrane Database Syst Rev. 2012;2012(2):CD003769.
17. Hull RD, Brant RF, Pineo GF, Stein PD, Raskob GE, Valentine KA. Preoperative vs postoperative initiation of low-molecular-weight heparin prophylaxis against venous thromboembolism in patients undergoing elective hip replacement. Arch Intern Med. 1999;159(2):137–41.
18. Venturi ML, Davison SP, Caprini JA. Prevention of venous thromboembolism in the plastic surgery patient: current guidelines and recommendations. Aesthet Surg J. 2009;29(5):421–8.

19. Daes J. The enhanced view-totally extraperitoneal technique for repair of inguinal hernia. Surg Endosc. Apr 2012;26(4):1187–9.
20. Ghali S, Turza KC, Baumann DP, Butler CE. Minimally invasive component separation results in fewer wound-healing complications than open component separation for large ventral hernia repairs. J Am Coll Surg. 2012;214(6):981–9.
21. Tandon A, Pathak S, Lyons NJ, Nunes QM, Daniels IR, Smart NJ. Meta-analysis of closure of the fascial defect during laparoscopic incisional and ventral hernia repair. Br J Surg. 2016;103(12):1598–607.
22. Christoffersen MW, Olsen BH, Rosenberg J, Bisgaard T. Randomized clinical trial on the post-operative use of an abdominal binder after laparoscopic umbilical and epigastric hernia repair. Hernia. 2015;19(1):147–53.
23. Rothman JP, Gunnarsson U, Bisgaard T. Abdominal binders may reduce pain and improve physical function after major abdominal surgery—a systematic review. Dan Med J. 2014;61(11):A4941.
24. Park A, Lee G, Seagull FJ, Meenaghan N, Dexter D. Patients benefit while surgeons suffer: an impending epidemic. J Am Coll Surg. 2010;210(3):306–13.
25. Higgins RM, Frelich MJ, Bosler ME, Gould JC. Cost analysis of robotic versus laparoscopic general surgery procedures. Surg Endosc. 2017;31(1):185–92.

Robotic Component Separation

Clayton C. Petro and Yuri W. Novitsky

Historical Context: The Evolution of Component Separation Techniques

For large ventral hernias, primary fascial closure and recreation of the linea alba can be difficult to achieve without undue tension. Component separation techniques involve strategic division of fascial and muscular layers of the abdominal wall that relieve such tension and thereby allow for an increased abdominal domain. In the 1980s, Jean Rives and René Stoppa described division of the posterior rectus sheath in their series of large incisional hernias. This retrorectus dissection provides both medial fascial advancement and allows for placement of a prosthetic reinforcement in the retrorectus space [1]. However, when bilateral release of the posterior rectus sheathes is insufficient to gain adequate medial advancement, further myofascial release is necessary. In 1990, Oscar Ramirez described division of the external oblique fascia from its insertion on the internal oblique aponeurosis in a cadaver study, coining the term "component separation." Importantly, he first quantified the

medial advancement gained by a bilateral posterior rectus sheath release (Rives-Stoppa technique) as 6, 10, and 6 cm in the upper, middle, and lower thirds of the abdominal wall, respectively. Adjunctive bilateral division of the external oblique myofascial layer allowed for additional advancement, crudely measured to be 10, 20, and 6 cm [2]. This approach would become one of the most common ways to achieve sufficient facial medialization for large ventral incisional hernias, and today some still consider the term "component separation" to specifically regard division of the external oblique myofascial layer.

While Ramirez's technique grew in popularity, limitations were noted. Access to the external oblique aponeuroses' insertion on the internal oblique typically requires significant undermining of skin and subcutaneous tissue anterior to the rectus fascia. These soft tissue flaps, reliant on blood supply from anterior perforators of the epigastric vessels, can be at risk of devascularization and subsequent wound morbidity has been reported from 26 to 63% [3, 4]. Such wound morbidity could prove to be more significant if a prosthetic enforcement is placed in the onlay position—anterior to the fascia and just beneath the soft tissue flaps—leaving the prosthetic directly exposed to and involved with any superficial surgical site morbidity. In order to minimize soft tissue mobilization and devascularization, modifications to Ramirez's external oblique release were developed. The periumbilical "perfo-

C. C. Petro
Department of Surgery, Cleveland Clinic, Cleveland, OH, USA

Y. W. Novitsky (✉)
Department of Surgery, Columbia University Medical Center, New York, NY, USA
e-mail: yn2339@cumc.columbia.edu

© Springer International Publishing AG, part of Springer Nature 2018
K. A. LeBlanc (ed.), *Laparoscopic and Robotic Incisional Hernia Repair*,
https://doi.org/10.1007/978-3-319-90737-6_10

rator sparing" technique preserves some of the anterior epigastric perforating vessels to the skin flaps. Saulis and colleagues retrospectively reported a dramatic reduction in wound morbidity (2%) when compared to the traditional technique (20%) at their institution [5]. Completely obviating the need for soft tissue flaps, Lowe et al. described division of the external oblique muscle through either a paramedian incision or an intramuscular tunnel in the avascular plane between the external and internal oblique muscles utilizing a balloon dissection and laparoscopic equipment [6]. A recent meta-analysis of 3055 patients confirmed a decrease in wound morbidity from 35 to 21% utilizing the endoscopic approach when compared to the traditional open technique [7].

Still, limitations to external oblique component separation and variations persist. There are scenarios when periumbilical perforator sparing techniques may not be possible: (1) large ventral hernias with loss of domain where the skin and soft tissue may tether fascial medialization or (2) previous mesh onlay. Large recurrences after a previous external oblique component separation also proved to be another challenging group of patients. Most notably, regardless of the specific approach, no external oblique division technique has an ideal space for prosthetic reinforcement. As previously mentioned, onlay prosthetics are susceptible to superficial wound morbidity. Perforating sparing techniques are a catch-22 in that they limit the space in which to place the prosthetic while a larger subcutaneous pocket for wider overlap paradoxically potentiates superficial soft tissues devascularization. A mesh underlay leaves the abdominal viscera exposed to a prosthetic akin to laparoscopic repairs. Despite the use of coated or barrier meshes, long-term sequelae of intraperitoneal mesh include longer re-operative times, secondary mesh infection, and increased incidence of an unplanned bowel resection or enterotomy in the 25% of these patients who will require a future abdominal operation [8, 9]. The Rives-Stoppa retrorectus space is limited laterally by the linea semilunaris above the arcuate line. Finally, the absence of an ideal space for wide prosthetic overlap is most vexing when managing subxyphoid, suprapubic, and non-midline defects adjacent to

boney prominences. These limitations of external oblique release inspired the conception of other component separation techniques that have gained wide popularity in the last decade.

In 2008, Carbonell et al. described a novel progression to the Rives-Stoppa retrorectus dissection that allows for wide prosthetic overlap lateral to the semilunar line [10]. After release of the medial posterior rectus sheath and lateral retrorectus dissection, the lateral posterior rectus sheath—consisting solely of fibers from the posterior lamina of the internal oblique—can be divided to expose the underlying transversus abdominis muscle. This allows the plane between the internal oblique and transversus abdominis muscles to be accessed and matured laterally. A subtle but critical anatomical point that allows for this dissection is that the transversus abdominis muscle and its associated aponeurosis inserts onto the posterior rectus sheath more medially than indicated by some anatomical texts. Completely detaching the posterior rectus sheath medially and laterally was termed a "posterior component separation" (PCS), and Ramirez's external oblique release somewhat retroactively became known as an "anterior component separation" (ACS). While Carbonell's PCS and intramuscular dissection addressed the issue of providing a space for wide lateral prosthetic reinforcement by laterally extending the Rives-Stoppa retromuscular plane, limitations persist. As opposed to an ACS, PCS does not divide any of the lateral abdominal wall muscles opposing medial tension. Also, laterally perforating neurovascular bundles traveling in the intramuscular plane between the internal oblique and transversus abdominis muscles are sacrificed during this lateral dissection. While the clinical significance of subsequent rectus muscle denervation is unknown, division of these nerves and vessels seems to counter one of the theoretical aims of recreating the linea alba—improving core abdominal function by restoring the rectus muscles to the midline and giving lateral abdominal muscles a stable insertion point.

Subsequently in 2009, Novitsky reported a distinct adjunct to the Rives-Stoppa retrorectus dissection, now known as a posterior component separation with transversus abdominis muscle release (TAR). In this technique, the posterior rectus sheath is again divided medially and the retrorectus space is matured laterally in a Rives-Stoppa fashion. At the lateral extent of the retrorectus dissection, just medial to laterally perforating neurovascular bundles, the posterior lamina of the internal oblique is divided to expose the underlying transversus abdominis muscle. This step is similar to the Carbonell's PCS, with the conscious effort to preserve lateral neurovascular bundles by dividing the posterior rectus sheath medial to these perforators that pierce the posterior lamina of the internal oblique to enter the retrorectus space. Once the transversus abdominis muscle is exposed, it can be separated from the underlying peritoneum and divided to access the retromuscular space between the transversus abdominis muscle and peritoneum. Maturing the retromuscular plane can be done laterally all the way to the psoas muscle. This retromuscular dissection serves two critical purposes. One, it creates a large peritoneal sac contiguous with the posterior rectus sheath that can be used to completely isolate the viscera and allow for "giant prosthetic reinforcement of the visceral sac" originally utilized by Rives and Stoppa in the descriptions of large inguinoscrotal hernia repairs [11]. Specifically, a TAR allows for wide prosthetic reinforcement of the visceral sac *above* the arcuate line. The second reason to develop this plane is that in our own cadaver studies, retromuscular dissection was the critical step that allowed for anterior facial medialization (akin to Ramirez's ACS cadaver study) to allow for repair of large (~20 cm) defects [12]. The retromuscular plane also can be matured superiorly to the preperitoneal space beneath the xyphoid and cephalad to the central tendon of the diaphragm. Inferiorly, below the arcuate line, the preperitoneal plane is matured below the pubis into the space of Retzius to expose the Cooper's ligaments bilaterally. Given the wide retromuscular plane of dissection, subxyphoid, suprapubic, and off-midline hernias can also be addressed. To review, TAR allows for numerous advantages in regard to large ventral incisional hernia repair:

- Myofascial release—Division and separation of the transversus abdominus muscle allowing for considerable rectus coplex medialization without the need for any soft tissue flaps and the associated wound morbidity encountered during ACS.
  - Division of a muscle—transversus abdominis—whose vector of force directly opposes fascial medialization.
  - Can be utilized when a previous ACS has been done [13].
- A lateral extension of the Rives-Stoppa retrorectus dissection that creates a cephalad extension of the visceral sac above the arcuate line for giant prosthetic reinforcement.
  - Further allows for management of off-midline, subxyphoid, and suprapubic herniations adjacent to boney prominences.
  - The wider retromuscular space allows prosthetic placement in a plane with bilaminar fascial coverage to potentiate ingrowth, while also providing an environment isolated from the viscera and superficial wound morbidity.
  - Knowledge of favorable mesh characteristics in regard to preventing chronic mesh infection when placed in a contaminated scenarios (wound class II–III), coupled with a favorable space for prosthetic placement makes repairs in contaminated fields less of a surgical faux pas [14, 15].
- Preservation of laterally perforating neurovascular bundles that supply the rectus muscles. To support the importance of preserving this innervation, we have demonstrated that restoration of the linea alba improves rectus abdominis function after TAR [16].
  - Restoration of the midline via TAR also allows for reversal of atrophy and compensatory hypertrophy of the external and especially synergistic internal oblique muscles demonstrated on CT imaging [17].

As major proponents of this technique, we also understand the importance of introspection and critical review. Some skeptics highlight the importance of the transversus abdominis muscle as an internal girdle whose circumferential tension stabilizes the lumbosacrum. Potential associations between transversus abdominis dysfunction and low back pain as well as spinal instability are theoretical causes for concern given complete transection during a TAR [18]. To date, no such deleterious effects have been reported, and subsequent reversal of atrophy of the external and internal oblique muscles may provide a mechanism of compensation.

Complimentary Limitations of Modern Techniques Inspire Ingenuity

While no technique is ideal for all scenarios, the TAR appears to be an incredibly useful operation for the armamentarium of the general surgeon, as attributed by its growing popularity during the past decade. Still, our largest series of 428 TARs repaired with synthetic mesh generated a wound morbidity rate of 18.7%, including a 9.1% rate of surgical site infection. The large operations generated a median hospital stay of 6 days, with associated morbidity including a 6.8% rate of urinary tract infections and 6.3% rate of venous thromboembolic events [19]. So while the TAR operation is versatile and effective—offering a recurrence rate of 3.7%—it relegates the patient to the consequences of a large laparotomy. Adaptation of a less invasive approach, offering the same benefits of open repair, would seem to be the next logical step.

Meanwhile, undergoing its own evolution in parallel since 1993, laparoscopic ventral hernia repair (LVHR) has been adopted by general surgeons to address 20–27% of ventral hernias [20, 21]. However, unlike open retromuscular repairs, these techniques have traditionally culminated in the placement of an intraperitoneal prosthetic directly exposed to the underlying viscera at the expense of the aforementioned sequelae. Defects bridged by a prosthetic in the absence of fascial approximation leave a dead space for seroma formation, fail to recreate the anatomy of a functional abdominal wall, and are subject to mesh eventration or "pseudo-recurrence" [22, 23]. Conversely when primary fascial closure precedes intraperitoneal onlay mesh, it is done so in the absence of any fascial release to mitigate tension. Finally, despite demonstrating improvements in length of hospital stay, time to recovery, wound morbidity, and recurrence, LVHR is notoriously painful, suppressing some of the benefits anticipated with a less invasive approach [24–27].

Given the outlined benefits of an open TAR technique for large ventral hernias at the expense of a large laparotomy, and the inverse technical sacrifices made during LVHR to reap the benefits of a minimally invasive approach, one can conceptually appreciate everything a minimally invasive TAR would accomplish. Conveniently, as advanced minimally invasive techniques to address ventral hernias were being conceptualized, so too was robotic technology. The da Vinci robot (Intuitive Surgical, Sunnyvale, CA, USA) touts several advantages over traditional laparoscopy including six degrees of motion, three-dimensional images, superior ergonomics, and tremor-less precision during intracorporeal suturing [28]. Approved by the Food and Drug Administration in 2000, it was first used for ventral hernia repair in 2002 by Ballantyne [29]. The robot was initially utilized to mimic traditional laparoscopic repairs with intraperitoneal mesh placement or preperitoneal mesh placement in the absence of any myofascial release [30, 31]. Not until 2012 did Abdallah et al. describe a robotic retrorectus dissection akin to a Rives-Stoppa technique in series of small herniations associated with rectus diastasis [32]. While a review article in 2015 and two recently published hernia textbooks offer early descriptions of the evolving robotic TAR (rTAR) technique [21, 33, 34], a manuscript offering outcomes of the robotic retromuscular dissection was only recently published by Warren et al. less than a year from the time this chapter is being written [35]. As experience and technical considerations for rTAR are evolving, herein we will aim to describe our approach to this fairly challenging robotic repair.

Patient Selection

Early considerations of attempting a rTAR were obviously met with skepticism. Because of the complexity of recurrent ventral incisional hernia-tions addressed with an open TAR, minimally invasive attempts were understandably difficult for most surgeons to envision. Patient selection is obviously going to be critical. As permutations of robotic hernia repairs are evolving, so are the inclusion criteria. Conservatively, to optimize the technical feasibility and safety of the technique, rTAR candidates ideally have:

- Midline defects of 8–15 cm without loss of domain.
  - Smaller defects may be amendable to intra-peritoneal, preperitoneal, or an isolated ret-rorectus repair done either open, laparoscopically, or robotically.
  - Larger defects may create too much ten-sion at the time of fascial closure, depend-ing on abdominal wall compliance.
- Limited redundant soft tissue and no chronic skin infections/ulcerations that would typi-cally be removed during open repairs.
- No large amounts of previous mesh or concern for chronic mesh infection that would also typically be excised during an open repair.
- Ability for safe laparoscopic access, port placement, and subsequent lysis of adhesions to free the viscera from the anterior abdominal wall.
- No or limited history of obstructive symptoms that would compel the surgeon to lyse inter-loop adhesions. This is a relative contraindication.

As comfort with the robotic technique evolves, inclusion and exclusion criteria will as well. Optimal patients should be identified for early attempts, and candid conversations should be had regarding the risk of technical unfeasibility. If laparoscopic access cannot be achieved, the patient and surgeon should agree preoperatively on whether to abort the procedure or convert to an open repair, and the informed consent form should reflect this. Not only should the surgeon be well trained in the robotics platform, but he/she should be comfortable with the open tech-nique, if necessary. Furthermore, a thorough understanding of abdominal wall anatomy and subtle points appreciated during the open TAR technique aid in the robotic dissection.

While a complete discussion of our patient-driven medical optimization goals for complex ventral hernia patients are beyond the scope of this chapter, some details are worth mentioning. We expect that patients will take an active and conscientious role in losing weight before sur-gery and we often refer patients for medically monitored weight loss through a protein sparing modified fast regimen for extreme cases refrac-tory to traditional weight loss attempts. Diabetics are expected to optimize their hemoglobin A1c to below 7.5, and preoperative levels >9 will prompt endocrinology consultation and case cancella-tion. Smokers are expected to quit for a minimum of 4 weeks before their operation and appropriate preoperative blood testing can be done to confirm patient sincerity when indicated. Our center for perioperative medicine coordinates universal decolonization of methicillin-resistant staph aureus (MRSA) before surgery and MRSA-positive patients receive perioperative antibiotic prophylaxis that includes coverage of MRSA (typically vancomycin). Finally, preoperative nutritional optimization with arginine and omega-3 fatty acid supplements is provided and encouraged for all patients starting 5 days before surgery. These have traditionally been our expec-tations before an open TAR. If the surgeon decides to proceed with robotic repair in an un-optimized patient, these factors should play a role in the decision to convert to open if a minimally invasive approach is not technically feasible. For example, the patient may be counseled that if laparoscopic peritoneal access cannot be gained, that an open repair will be deferred until the patient loses more weight.

rTAR Operative Details

- Patients are placed in a supine position and arms are tucked so that the arm boards are not an obstacle during movement of the robot patient-side cart (Fig. 10.1).
- We utilize a double-dock technique when performing a rTAR, meaning that the retromuscular dissection on each side of the abdominal wall is achieved with the robot docked on the contralateral side. The da Vinci Xi has the ability to rotate its boom 180° so that bilateral docking can be achieved without moving the patient or the patient-side cart. Earlier models of the da Vinci (ex. Si) require movement of the robot to the other side of the patient, or rotating the patient 180° for the contralateral dissection depending on the setup of the operating room. When necessary, this transition should be discussed and negotiated with the anesthesia team and operating room staff before the operation. At our institution, we rotate the foot of the operating table away from where the patient-side cart will approach the bed, and the da Vinci Xi boom obviates the need to move the bed or side cart when docking on the contralateral side.
- The abdomen should be widely prepped and draped in the event that open conversion is necessary.
- We prefer to gain intra-abdominal access using a 5 mm optical trocar and 0° laparoscope away from previous incisions. Typically, this is done just beneath the costal margin just lateral to the mid-clavicular line. Either side is feasible but we prefer the left when possible.
- Pneumoperitoneum to 15 mmHg of carbon dioxide is achieved.
- The next 8 mm trocar is then placed 1–2 finger breadths medial and cephalad to the anterior superior iliac spine. The long bariatric trocars are helpful here to minimize collisions with hips and thighs during upper abdominal dissection.
- The subcostal port is upsized to the 8-m robotic trocar and the 3rd port is placed in between the first 2 at approximately anterior axillary line (Fig. 10.2).
- At this point, initial adhesiolysis can be done using traditional laparoscopic equipment and may have already been necessary to make room for lateral port placement. During adhesiolysis, a conscious effort should be made to preserve the peritoneum that will eventually provide a barrier to the retromuscular prosthetic. Alternatively, docking of the robot could be done to aid adhesiolysis, understanding that the benefits of improved visualization and ergonomics are at the cost of losing haptic feedback. Loss of haptic feedback and a contained visual field are important considerations and require utmost care to minimize risks of visceral injuries. There should be a low threshold to perform a standard laparoscopic lysis of adhesions until an adequate working space for the robot has been achieved. Finally, if the adhesions are considered treacherous or one encounters a "frozen" abdomen

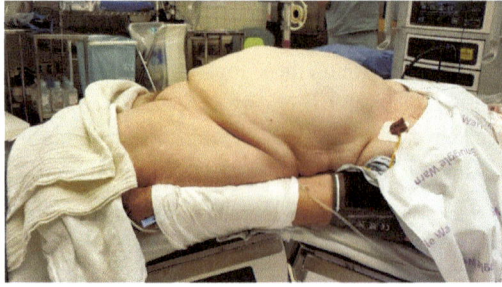

Fig. 10.1 Patient positioning. The table is flexed to lower the thighs to minimize external collisions. The arms are tucked

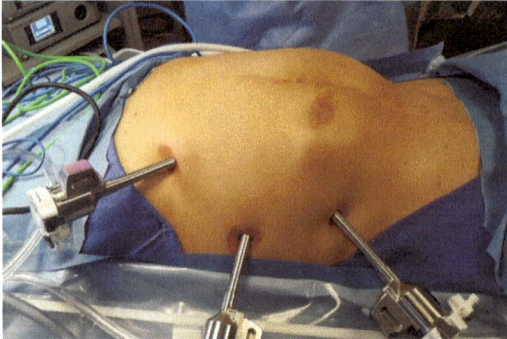

Fig. 10.2 Our typical trocar strategy

where preservation of the visceral sac seems unlikely, a minimally invasive approach should be abandoned.

- The robot is docked by bringing the patient-side cart toward the operating room table at 90° to the torso with the center column aligned with the patient's hip. Arms 1/2/3 or 2/3/4 can be docked to the ports, as only 3 of 4 are typically utilized.

- For right-handed surgeons, a dV Fenestrated bipolar (or Prograsp) is placed in the left-handed port and the dV monopolar scissors is placed in the right-handed port. A standard angled camera is placed through the middle port.

- Once the visceral adhesions are cleared from the hernia sac and the anterior abdominal wall, the posterior sheath is incised with the monopolar scissors just lateral to the edge of the hernia sac to expose the rectus muscle (Fig. 10.3). This posterior rectus sheath division can be extended superiorly, following the belly of the rectus muscle.

- The avascular retrorectus plane is then matured laterally to the linea semilunaris and superiorly/inferiorly at least 5–8 cm beyond the defect. The pneumoperitoneum allows for uniform retraction to aid this dissection. Although for smaller hernias, this retrorectus only Rives-Stoppa dissection may be sufficient for closure of the anterior fascia, exces-

sive tension on the posterior closure and limited space for mesh placement limit utilization of this approach in our practice.

- The lateral extent of the retrorectus dissection reveals the perforating neurovascular bundles that are identified and preserved, similarly to the open technique. Identification and preservation of those bundles is not only important to maintaining innervation of the rectus muscles, but also serves to identify the semilunar line.

- In the upper third of the abdomen, where the belly of the transversus abdominis muscle is most prominent medially to the semilunar line, the lateral posterior rectus sheath (consisting solely of fibers from the posterior lamina of the internal oblique aponeurosis) is incised just medial to the neurovascular perforators to expose the underlying transversus abdominis muscle (Fig. 10.4).
  - Using the neurovascular perforators as a landmark will typically prevent intramuscular dissection or potentially catastrophic division of the semilunar line.

- The transversus abdominis muscle can then be separated from the underlying transversalis fascia and maturation of the pretransversalis plane laterally as far as the psoas muscle allows from wide release of the posterior and anterior components as they become more dissociated. An ideal superior retromuscular

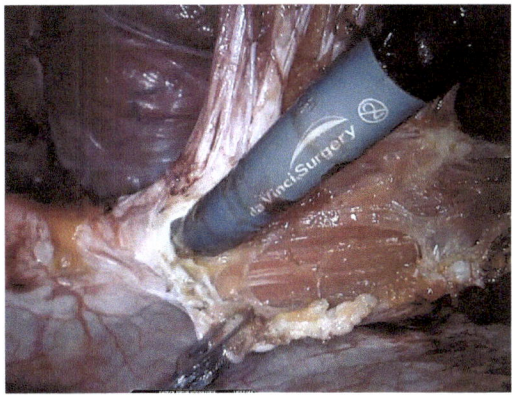

Fig. 10.3 Initial incision of the medial aspect of the posterior rectus sheath. It is important that the fibers of the rectus muscle are seen

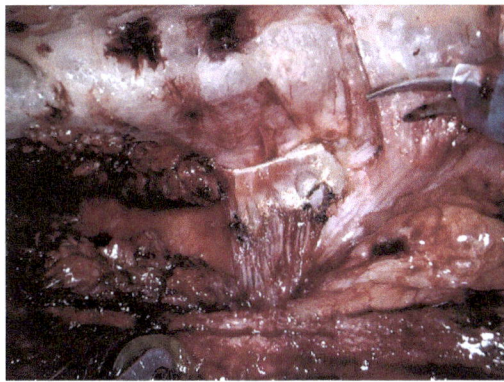

Fig. 10.4 Incision of the transversus abdominis muscle just medial to the semilunar line and neurovascular bundles. Care must be taken not to divide the underlying transversalis fascia and peritoneum

dissection leaves the transversus abdominis naked, with an intact visceral sac consisting of transversalis fascia and peritoneum. While dissection in the preperitoneal plane is also possible, we avoid it due to significant risks of tearing thin peritoneum, especially in the subcostal areas.

- The lateral division of the posterior rectus sheath and transversus abdominis release can be initiated inferiorly, but the medial transversus abdominis becomes aponeurotic at the mid-abdomen. Starting the development of the pretransversalis plane superiorly will aid the inferior retromuscular dissection in our opinion.
- Eventually, the inferior TAR dissection will culminate in division of the arcuate line just medial to its junction with the semilunar line and the posterior rectus sheath with its contiguous peritoneum/transversalis fascia is completely disconnected from the anterior fascia and muscles of the lateral abdominal wall. The initiated superior and lateral retromuscular dissections will become contiguous with the inferior preperitoneal plane (space of Retzius) utilized for laparoscopic inguinal hernias where Cooper's ligaments can be visualized. The inferior transversalis fascia fibers below the arcuate line are swept up to the abdominal wall so as not to injure the inferior epigastric vessels.
  - Overall, our preferred plane of the retromuscular dissection is pretransversalis in the upper abdomen and preperitoneal in the lower abdomen with the transition between the two layers at approximately the level of the umbilicus.
- Once the unilateral TAR dissection is complete, any defects in the posterior layers need to be closed. We utilize either interrupted figure of 8's 2-0 Vicryl sutures or running 3-0 barbed absorbable sutures.
- Next, three robotic ports are placed on the contralateral side to perform a mirror-image dissection. These ports will enter the retromuscular space directly without piercing the underlying peritoneum. Conversely, when the contralateral TAR is complete, port site

defects in the posterior sheath will need to be closed, along with any other posterior sheath tears. Once again, we typically use interrupted 2-0 Vicryl or running 3-0 barbed absorbable sutures.
- Superiorly, if extension into the subcostal and/ or subxyphoid space is necessary for prosthetic overlap, there are a few anatomical considerations of which to be aware. A superior and lateral dissection in the preperitoneal space *below* the costal margin, exposing the muscle fibers of the diaphragm, confirms development of the correct retromuscular plane after a TAR.

When completed, bilateral posterior component separations with a TAR should allow for primary fascial closure with acceptable tension, as well as a sufficient retromuscular space to accommodate large prosthetic overlap in all directions.

- First, the medialized posterior rectus sheathes are closed using a running 2-0 V-loc suture with the dV SutureCut needle driver in the dominant hand (Fig. 10.5). If too much tension is encountered, this could be a sign of incomplete retroperitoneal dissection.
- Similarly, closure of the anterior fascial sheath is accomplished using several running nonabsorbable #1 V-loc suture (Fig. 10.6). Every 3–4 throws, a bite of the soft tissue or hernia

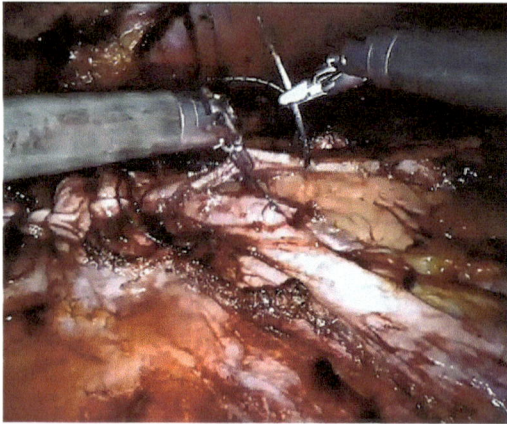

Fig. 10.5 Restoration of the visceral sac via closure of the posterior layers using a running 2-0 absorbable V-lock suture

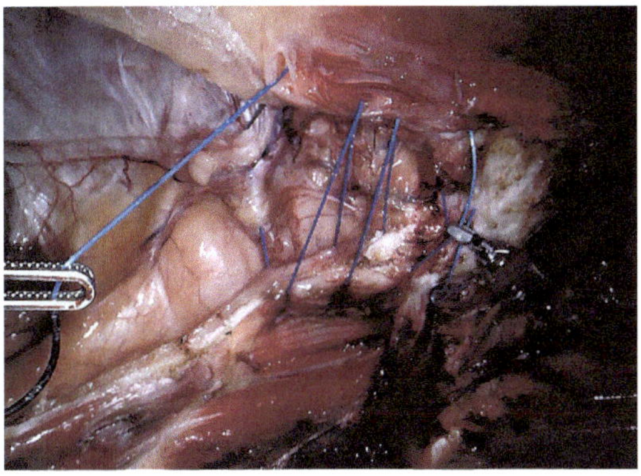

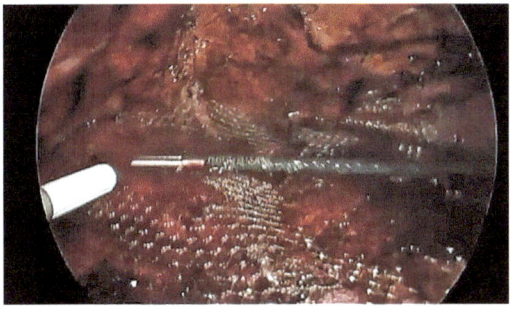

Fig. 10.6 Restoration of the linea alba with approximation of the medialized anterior rectus sheaths using #1 nonabsorbable barbed suture

Fig. 10.7 Laparoscopic placement of a sublay mesh with optional fixation with fibrin glue

sac is incorporated to minimize the dead space for seroma formation. The sutures are pre-placed at a regular pneumoperitoneum, but tightened when the pressure is decreased to 4–5 mmHg.

- Next, the retromuscular pocket is measured with a ruler to size the prosthetic to subsequently achieve a giant prosthetic reinforcement of the visceral sac.
- The robot is undocked and a piece of appropriately sized midweight uncoated macroporous polypropylene (*SoftMesh*, Bard, Murray Hill, NJ, USA) is placed on top of the visceral sac. While fibrin glue, absorbable tacks or transfascial suture fixation have all been tried, and we typically add no additional mesh fixation (Fig. 10.7).
- No port sites need to be closed since the mesh underlays them.

Postoperative Care

We tend to use a multimodal pain control regimen outlined in our previous descriptions of our enhanced recovery pathway [36, 37]. Diet advancement and transition to enteral medications is typically accelerated in comparison to open repairs, and is mostly dictated by the extent of adhesiolysis and duration of the operation. Over the course of 12 months our operative times decreased from greater than 6 h to 2.5–4 h, much like the early experience reported by Carbonell [21]. As our operative times have improved, patients with a minimal adhesiolysis are given clear liquids on the day of surgery and are advanced as tolerated to a regular diet the next day. If they are tolerating a regular diet, ambulating in the halls, and their pain is controlled on enteral pain medication, they are typically ready for discharge the next day.

Outcomes

Presented at the SAGES 2016 annual meeting, Warren et al. reported a retrospective comparison of 103 LVHRs and 53 robotic ventral repairs (rVHR) at their institution between 2013 and 2015 [35]. Techniques were not standardized, and rVHR included preperitoneal (26%), intraperitoneal (4%), retrorectus (27%), and rTAR (43%) mesh placement. The benefits of abdominal wall reconstruction by fascial closure (rVHR 96.2 vs. LVHR 50.5%; $p < 0.001$) and extraperitoneal mesh placement (96.2 vs. 9.7%; $p < 0.001$) were achieved in almost all robotic approaches. Longer operative times (245 vs. 122 min, $p < 0.001$) and more frequent postoperative seroma formation (47.2 vs. 16.5%, $p < 0.001$) for rVHR are countered with equivalent rates of surgical site infection (3.8 vs. 1%, $p = 0.592$) and a shorter median length of stay (1 vs. 2 days, $p = 0.004$). While the improvement in length of stay is consistent with our anecdotal experience, no difference was shown in narcotic requirement to suggest the robotic approach was less painful. Notably, LVHR patients in this study were also statistically older (60.2 vs. 52.9 years; $p = 0.001$) and selection bias no doubt favored the rVHR group. The anomalous 9% rate of bowel injury in the LVHR group and four open conversions speaks to the complexity of the LVHR group and also likely played a role in prolonging that cohort's median length of stay. While one could attribute the lower incidence of bowel injury and open conversion to improved visualization and ergonomics offered by the robotic technique, this may be a dangerous assumption and can more likely be explained by a less complex robotic cohort. Loss of haptic feedback, fixed camera angles, and instrument exchanges by novice assistants can be dangerous properties of the robotic approach early in the learning curve, especially during visceral adhesiolysis.

The largest retrospective review of robotic ventral hernia repair to date was recently published by Carbonell et al. using data extracted from the Americas Hernia Society Quality Collaborative (AHSQC) database [38]. Their aim was to compare hospital length of stay for 111 robotic retromuscular repairs (rRMR)—including 85% rTAR and 15% robotic retrorectus dissections—with a propensity score matched group of patients who underwent open retromuscular repair (83% TAR, 17% retrorectus) using logistical regression to match patient variables, medical comorbidities, and hernia characteristics. They found a median length of stay of 2 days for rRMR compared to 3 days for open equivalents ($p < 0.001$) with no difference in readmission rates or surgical site infection. Increased seroma formation was again associated with the robotic approach (25% vs. 4%) and could be related to less frequent use of drains placed after robotic dissections (21% vs. 70%). While the propensity score matching algorithm appears to account for most variables impacting hospital length of stay, the authors admit they were not able to account for surgeon or institutional characteristics. Surgeons pioneering the robotic approach may be more likely to employ enhanced recovery pathways and feel comfortable with accelerated discharge.

Limitations and Vitality of the Robotic Technique

Conservatively, rVHR is feasible for a select group of patients. Whether or not the technique has value in terms of reduced cost or improved patient outcomes will be the subject of intense scrutiny in our value-conscious healthcare landscape. The upfront cost a hospital system invests on the purchase of a robot as well as its maintenance, and the disposable cost of multiuse instruments immediately puts the platform at a disadvantage, not to mention the added expense of barbed suture and increased operative times for rVHR. Not surprisingly, the focus of early reports on rVHR reduction in hospital stay can be a major step in justifying the sincere debt. Furthermore, operative times have dropped dramatically as experience accrues, and extraperitoneal placement of uncoated polypropylene prosthetic reinforcement obviates the need for their more expensive barrier mesh counterparts used in most laparoscopic repairs. Future analysis of resources utilized for pain control and time to return to work could also favor the robotic approach.

Most intriguingly, robotic retrorectus and rTAR are unique to general surgery in that they cannot be routinely reproduced in a minimally invasive approach without use of the robot. Most comparisons in the colorectal, foregut, and thoracic literature compare a laparoscopic technique to a robotic replication of that technique. While safety and feasibility can typically be demonstrated, a clinical benefit has not been demonstrated for most procedures, making it difficult to justify the increased cost of the robotic platform. A notable exception has been the evolution of robotic prostatectomy that touts equivalent cancer outcomes to open repair through a minimally invasive technique that is easy to learn and teach [39]. Comparatively, laparoscopic prostatectomy is notoriously challenging and difficult to learn. Retrospective analyses comparing open and robotic prostatectomy confirm a shorter hospital stay and return to normal activity with the robotic approach to justify the increased cost. Interestingly, robotic prostatectomy has been widely accepted into clinical practice despite the absence of any randomized controlled trials.

In this chapter, we have outlined in detail the benefits of an open retrorectus dissection supplemented with the TAR release in comparison to alternative open and laparoscopic techniques. For the right patient, a rTAR can achieve the benefits of the open TAR technique through a minimally invasive approach, simultaneously avoiding limitations of each traditional operation. Importantly, the cost of the robotic approach appears to be offset by savings in decreased hospital stay. The quality of the operation, as substantiated by patient outcomes, could further legitimize its value and vitality. Robotic prostatectomy has already set a precedent for wide adoption of a robotic technique driven by improved patient outcomes despite increased cost. As we move forward, we need to be critical of how we define and study outcomes in our hernia patients, being cognizant that both patients and surgeons can be susceptible to marketing bias.

References

1. Stoppa RE. The treatment of complicated groin and incisional hernias. World J Surg. 1989;13(5):545–54.
2. Ramirez OM, Ruas E, Dellon AL. "Components separation" method for closure of abdominal-wall defects: an anatomic and clinical study. Plast Reconstr Surg. 1990;86(3):519–26.
3. Girotto JA, Chiaramonte M, Menon NG, Singh N, Silverman R, Tufaro AP, et al. Recalcitrant abdominal wall hernias: long-term superiority of autologous tissue repair. Plast Reconstr Surg. 2003;112(1):106–14.
4. Gonzalez R, Rehnke RD, Ramaswamy A, Smith CD, Clarke JM, Ramshaw BJ. Components separation technique and laparoscopic approach: a review of two evolving strategies for ventral hernia repair. Am Surg. 2005 Jul;71(7):598–605.
5. Saulis AS, Dumanian GA. Periumbilical rectus abdominis perforator preservation significantly reduces superficial wound complications in "separation of parts" hernia repairs. Plast Reconstr Surg. 2002 Jun;109(7):2275–80.
6. Lowe JB, Garza JR, Bowman JL, Rohrich RJ, Strodel WE. Endoscopically assisted "components separation" for closure of abdominal wall defects. Plast Reconstr Surg. 2000;105(2):720–9.
7. Switzer NJ, Dykstra MA, Gill RS, Lim S, Lester E, de Gara C, et al. Endoscopic versus open component separation: systematic review and meta-analysis. Surg Endosc. 2015;29(4):787–95.
8. Snyder CW, Graham LA, Gray SH, Vick CC, Hawn MT. Effect of mesh type and position on subsequent abdominal operations after incisional hernia repair. J Am Coll Surg. 2011;212(4):496–502.
9. Patel PP, Love MW, Ewing JA, Warren JA, Cobb WS, Carbonell AM. Risks of subsequent abdominal operations after laparoscopic ventral hernia repair. Surg Endosc. 2017;31(2):823–8.
10. Carbonell AM, Cobb WS, Chen SM. Posterior components separation during retromuscular hernia repair. Hernia. 2008;12(4):359–62.
11. Stoppa RE, Rives JL, Warlaumont CR, Palot JP, Verhaeghe PJ, Delattre JF. The use of Dacron in the repair of hernias of the groin. Surg Clin North Am. 1984;64(2):269–85.
12. Majumder A, Miller HJ, Sandoval V, Fayezizadeh M, Wen Y, Novitsky YW. Objective assessment of myofascial medialization after posterior component separation via transversus abdominis muscle Releas. J Am Coll Surg. 2016;223(4):S57.
13. Pauli EM, Wang J, Petro CC, Juza RM, Novitsky YW, Rosen MJ. Posterior component separation with transversus abdominis release successfully addresses recurrent ventral hernias following anterior component separation. Hernia. 2015 Apr;19(2):285–91.
14. Blatnik JA, Krpata DM, Jacobs MR, Gao Y, Novitsky YW, Rosen MJ. In vivo analysis of the morphologic characteristics of synthetic mesh to resist MRSA adherence. J Gastrointest Surg. 2012;16(11):2139–44.
15. Carbonell AM, Criss CN, Cobb WS, Novitsky YW, Rosen MJ. Outcomes of synthetic mesh in contaminated ventral hernia repairs. J Am Coll Surg. 2013;217(6):991–8.
16. Criss CN, Petro CC, Krpata DM, Seafler CM, Lai N, Fiutem J, et al. Functional abdominal wall reconstruction improves core physiology and quality-of-life. Surgery. 2014;156(1):176–82.
17. De Silva GS, Krpata DM, Hicks CW, Criss CN, Gao Y, Rosen MJ, et al. Comparative radiographic analysis of changes in the abdominal wall musculature morphology after open posterior component separation or bridging laparoscopic ventral hernia repair. J Am Coll Surg. 2014;218(3):353–7.
18. Willard FH, Vleeming A, Schuenke MD, Danneels L, Schleip R. The thoracolumbar fascia: anatomy, function and clinical considerations. J Anat. 2012;221(6):507–36.
19. Novitsky YW, Fayezizadeh M, Majumder A, Neupane R, Elliott HL, Orenstein SB. Outcomes of posterior component separation with transversus abdominis muscle release and synthetic mesh sublay reinforcement. Ann Surg. 2016;264(2):226–32.
20. LeBlanc KA, Booth WV. Laparoscopic repair of incisional abdominal hernias using expanded polytetrafluoroethylene: preliminary findings. Surg Laparosc Endosc. 1993;3(1):39–41.
21. Vorst AL, Kaoutzanis C, Carbonell AM, Franz MG. Evolution and advances in laparoscopic ventral

and incisional hernia repair. World J Gastrointest Surg. 2015;7(11):293–305.

22. Carter SA, Hicks SC, Brahmbhatt R, Liang MK. Recurrence and pseudorecurrence after laparoscopic ventral hernia repair: predictors and patient-focused outcomes. Am Surg. 2014 Feb;80(2):138–48.

23. Orenstein SB, Dumeer JL, Monteagudo J, Poi MJ, Novitsky YW. Outcomes of laparoscopic ventral hernia repair with routine defect closure using "shoelacing" technique. Surg Endosc. 2011;25(5):1452–7.

24. Heniford BT, Park A, Ramshaw BJ, Voeller G. Laparoscopic ventral and incisional hernia repair in 407 patients. J Am Coll Surg. 2000;190(6):645–50.

25. Carbonell AM, Harold KL, Mahmutovic AJ, Hassan R, Matthews BD, Kercher KW, et al. Local injection for the treatment of suture site pain after laparoscopic ventral hernia repair. Am Surg. 2003;69(8):688–91.

26. Ramshaw BJ, Esartia P, Schwab J, Mason EM, Wilson RA, Duncan TD, et al. Comparison of laparoscopic and open ventral herniorrhaphy. Am Surg. 1999;65(9):827–31.

27. Itani KM, Hur K, Kim LT, Anthony T, Berger DH, Reda D, et al. Comparison of laparoscopic and open repair with mesh for the treatment of ventral incisional hernia: a randomized trial. Arch Surg. 2010;145(4):322–8.

28. Schluender S, Conrad J, Divino CM, Gurland B. Robot-assisted laparoscopic repair of ventral hernia with intracorporeal suturing. Surg Endosc. 2003;17(9):1391–5.

29. Ballantyne GH. Robotic surgery, telerobotic surgery, telepresence, and telementoring. Review of early clinical results. Surg Endosc. 2002;16(10):1389–402.

30. Allison N, Tieu K, Snyder B, Pigazzi A, Wilson E. Technical feasibility of robot-assisted ventral hernia repair. World J Surg. 2012;36(2):447–52.

31. Sugiyama G, Chivukula S, Chung PJ, Alfonso A. Robot-assisted transabdominal preperitoneal ventral hernia repair. JSLS. 2015;19(4):1–3.

32. Abdalla RZ, Garcia RB, RIDD C, CRPD L, Abdalla BMZ. Procedimento de Rives/Stoppa modificado robô-assistido para correção de hérnias ventrais da linha média. ABCD arq bras cir dig. 2012;25(2):129–32.

33. Ballacer C, Parra E. Robotic ventral hernia repair. In: Novitsky YW, editor. Hernia surgery: current principles. Cham: Springer; 2016.

34. Hope WW, Cobb WS, Adrales GL, editors. Textbook of hernia. Cham: Springer; 2017.

35. Warren JA, Cobb WS, Ewing JA, Carbonell AM. Standard laparoscopic versus robotic retromuscular ventral hernia repair. Surg Endosc. 2017;31(1):324–32.

36. Belyansky I, Zahiri HR, Park A. Laparoscopic transversus abdominis release, a novel minimally invasive approach to complex abdominal wall reconstruction. Surg Innov. 2016;23(2):134–41.

37. Majumder A, Fayezizadeh M, Neupane R, Elliott HL, Novitsky YW. Benefits of multimodal enhanced recovery pathway in patients undergoing open ventral hernia repair. J Am Coll Surg. 2016;222(6):1106–15.

38. Carbonell AM, Warren JA, Prabhu AS, Ballecer CD, Janczyk RJ, Herrera J. et al. Reducing length of stay using a robotic-assisted approach for retromuscular ventral hernia repair: a comparative analysis from the Americas Hernia Society Quality Collaborative: Ann Surg; 2017. p. 27.

39. Estey EP. Robotic prostatectomy: the new standard of care or a marketing success? Can Urol Assoc J. 2009;3(6):488–90.

Omar Yusef Kudsi and James Avruch

Introduction

Lumbar hernias are a rare clinical entity involving herniation of the intra-abdominal or retroperitoneal contents through congenital or acquired weaknesses in the posterolateral abdominal wall. First reported in 1731 on autopsy, they were formally credited to the French surgeon and anatomist Jean Louis Petit, who described a strangulated hernia emerging from the inferior lumbar triangle in 1783 [1]. In the modern era lumbar hernia is usually the result of prior urologic or aortic surgical intervention, although congenital and traumatic herniation is still described. Lumbar herniation is a possible etiology of both acute incarceration and strangulation of abdominal/retroperitoneal viscera as well as chronic lower back and flank pain.

The first lumbar hernia repair was described by Ravaton [2] in 1750, acutely incarcerated in a pregnant woman. The existence of the superior lumbar triangle was posited independently by Grynfellt and Lesshaft in 1870. S. Charles Kasdon described in the New England Journal of Medicine in 1954 [3] the case of an obese 67-year-old woman with a chief complaint of pain in the region of the left buttock radiating medially to the tip of the spine. In this era before the advent of computed tomography, the woman was admitted to four different hospitals over the course of 14 months and underwent state-of-the-art workup, including X-rays, intravenous pyelogram, sigmoidoscopy, and barium enema. Eventual operative exploration of the left lumbar area under general anesthesia revealed, after section of the subcuticular fascia, "a lobulated fat mass, 6-8 cm in diameter, and moderately well circumscribed, [was] protruding through a [3 cm] defect in the posterior sheath of the lumbodorsal fascia." This fat pad was connected via a well-defined stalk to the retroperitoneal fat overlying the sacrospinalis muscle. The stalk was transected and transfixed, and the lumbodorsal fascial defect was closed using interrupted fine silk suture. After a period of convalescence the patient's chronic and disabling back pain was cured. The author urged readers to consider lumbar herniation in the differential diagnosis of back pain, as "its removal was a simple procedure, and gave complete relief of symptoms." In 1970 Orcutt [1] described the case of a man who had felt a "tender knot" develop in his side after straining to lift some heavy implements. Examination revealed a tender, soft mass in the posterior axillary line immediately underneath the 12th rib which was easily reducible. He underwent flank exploration with high ligation of

O. Y. Kudsi (✉)
Department of Surgery, Good Samaritan Medical Center, Tufts University School of Medicine, Brockton, MA, USA

J. Avruch
Department of General Surgery, St. Elizabeth Medical Center, Boston, MA, USA

© Springer International Publishing AG, part of Springer Nature 2018
K. A. LeBlanc (ed.), *Laparoscopic and Robotic Incisional Hernia Repair*,
https://doi.org/10.1007/978-3-319-90737-6_11

a mass of herniated fat emerging from a defect under the 12th rib with complete resolution of symptoms.

Epidemiology

There have been approximately 300 cases described in the literature [2]. Because this is a seldom-reported entity, the true incidence of this type of hernia is unknown. They occur more commonly in males with a peak incidence between 60 and 70 years of age [4], typically presenting as a reducible bulge, asymptomatic or painful, in the suprailiac area and accentuated with Valsalva maneuver. They represent 2% or less of all abdominal wall hernias [5]. In a series of 109 cases published by Virgilio in 1925 it was found that hernia through the space of Grynfellt was more common than that through Petit's triangle. Hafner et al. [6] in their 1962 paper reviewing lumbar hernia and presenting two cases of Petit defect hernias reviewed the records of Henry Ford Hospital in Detroit and found only nine lumbar hernias (Grynfeltt, Petit, and diffuse) in the registration records of one million new patients. An extrapolation of this statistic suggests that a general surgeon will see at most one of this type of hernia in a career. The true incidence, however, is likely much higher than this. Hundreds of elective surgical procedures which can cause acquired secondary lumbar hernias are being performed yearly [7]. Traumatic lumbar hernia is a recognized entity, and likely underreported. It behooves the laparoscopic and robotic surgeon to be familiar with the relevant surgical anatomy and repair techniques for these uncommon hernias.

Etiology/Pathogenesis

The etiology of lumbar hernia is either congenital or acquired (Table 11.1). Twenty percent of reported lumbar herniae are congenital and 80% are acquired. Regardless of etiology, the natural history of the lumbar hernia is an increase in size along with back pain, and a certain number of

Table 11.1 Classification of lumbar hernias

I. Congenital
II. Acquired
a. Primary (spontaneous)
b. Secondary (posttraumatic, postinfectious, postsurgical)

reducible lumbar hernias will become incarcerated and/or strangulated; rates of up to 18–25% have been reported [8, 9] along with cases of large and small bowel obstruction [10, 11]. Thus the general consensus among authors is that these hernias should be surgically repaired once recognized.

Congenital lumbar herniation has been described in the pediatric surgical literature in association with other hereditary anomalies, most commonly the lumbocostovertebral syndrome, neuroblastoma, meningomyelocele, and caudal regression syndrome [12]. It can also be associated with congenital aplasia of the lumbodorsal musculature, which results in bilateral hernias. To date 54 cases have been reported in the literature [13]; reported repairs of these hernias are primary or with prosthetic mesh; there have been no reported laparoscopic repairs in these patients who usually present before the age of 2 years.

Acquired lumbar hernia is further broken down into primary (spontaneous) herniation and secondary herniation. Fifty-five percent of the reported lumbar herniae in the literature are spontaneous herniation through the anatomical weak points in the lumbodorsal fascia. Herniation through the upper (Grynfeltt) triangle is more common than herniation through the lower (Petit) triangle [14]; this is likely due to the presence of the fascial orifice for the 12th intercostal neurovascular bundle. Spontaneous lumbar hernia is caused by increased intra-abdominal pressure such as in morbid obesity, strenuous physical activity, or chronic cough. Patients will describe the sensation of spontaneous herniation when it occurs, as in the case described previously. Predisposing factors in spontaneous hernia are those which cause anatomical alterations in the lumbodorsal fascia and thinning of the overlying musculature and suprafascial fat pad, such as extreme thinness, chronic debilitating illness, and increased age [15].

Secondary lumbar hernia is due to previous insult to the lumbodorsal fascia, usually in the form of previous surgical incision or trocar placement, prior infection associated with the area, or trauma both blunt and penetrating. The urologist and prolific scholar Herman L. Kretschmer reported a series of 11 lumbar hernias containing the kidney in 1951 [16]. Incisional lumbar hernias complicate 7% of retroperitoneal approaches [17]. While more old-fashioned types of procedures such as open nephrectomy and the retroperitoneal approach to aortic aneurysm repair are known common causes of lumbar hernia, they have now been described after laparoscopic extraperitoneal nephrectomy [18] and latissimus dorsi myocutaneous flap for breast reconstruction [19]. Lumbar herniation after iliac crest bone graft harvest was described as early as 1945, a procedure still commonly performed by orthopedic surgeons. In terms of infection, suppurative conditions of the flank including renal and perirenal abscess and infected retroperitoneal hematoma can predispose to future lumbar herniation.

Lumbar hernia can be due to blunt or penetrating trauma. In their review of 66 cases of traumatic lumbar hernia, Burt et al. [20] found that the majority of traumatic lumbar hernias (70%) were from the inferior (Petit) lumbar triangle; this is in contrast to congenital and other acquired hernias, which have a propensity for the superior (Grynfeltt) lumbar triangle. Seventy-one percent were due to motor vehicle collision. On impact in a motor vehicle collision, the force of deceleration is transmitted to the occupant via the seatbelt, and the lap belt portion can slip over the top of the iliac crests, a so-called "submarining" of the lap belt. This force can cause tearing of musculofascial structures in combination with a sudden massive increase in intra-abdominal pressure which can cause herniation through the lumbodorsal fascia. The diagnosis of traumatic lumbar hernia can be delayed, and in their series the diagnosis was delayed in 27% of hernias for months or years; patients may present with suprailiac bulging and a history of a remote trauma. Traumatic lumbar hernia need not be repaired at the time of initial diagnosis, especially if there are serious associated intra-abdominal and orthopedic injuries. These hernias can be safely followed and referral can be made for elective repair [21].

Computed tomography is the study of choice for patients who are referred with symptomatic flank bulges. CT provides a detailed delineation of the muscular and fascial layers of the posterolateral abdominal wall and any defects that may be present (Fig. 11.1). Lumbar hernia can contain all manner of extraperitoneal, retroperitoneal, and intraperitoneal contents. A normal CT of the lumbar region in a symptomatic patient is sufficient to completely exclude the diagnosis of lumbar hernia as a cause of pain; this is especially important in post-incisional patients, as in the absence of hernia the pain is likely intercostal neuralgia and appropriate therapy can be instituted [17].

Anatomy

The surgical lumbar region (Fig. 11.2) is defined as the area inferior to the lower edge of the 12th rib, superior to the iliac crest, lateral to the erector spinae muscle, and medial to the external oblique [14]. In this location, the lumbar wall is comprised of, from deep to superficial, the following anatomic layers: (1) extraperitoneal tissue/fat; (2) transversalis fascia; (3) deep muscular layer which consists of quadratus lumborum muscle and the psoas; (4) middle muscular layer consisting of erector spinae, internal oblique, and serratus posterior inferior muscles; (5) the thoracolumbar fascia, which is the fused fascial layer of all the muscles of the lumbar area; (6) superficial muscular layer which consists of the latissimus dorsi muscle laterally and the external oblique muscle medially; (7) superficial lumbar fascia; and (8) the skin [15] (Fig. 11.3). The two potential hernia defects within this space are the superior (Grynfeltt) lumbar triangle and the inferior (Petit) lumbar triangle. Grynfeltt was the first to note, in 1866, that the aponeurotic fibers of the transversalis fascia part to permit passage of the

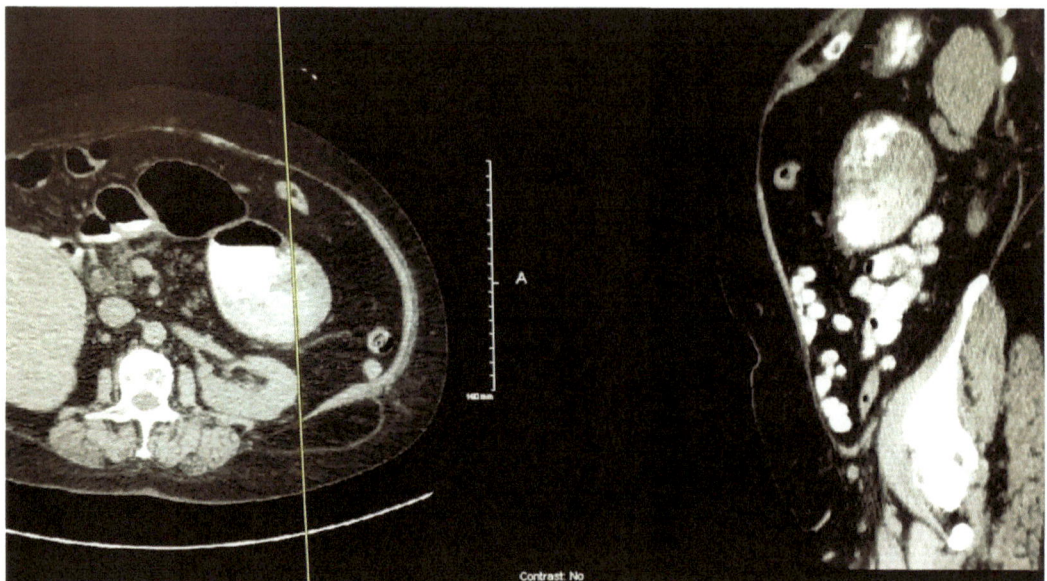

Fig. 11.1 Typical CT appearance of left-sided lumbar hernia containing preperitoneal fat

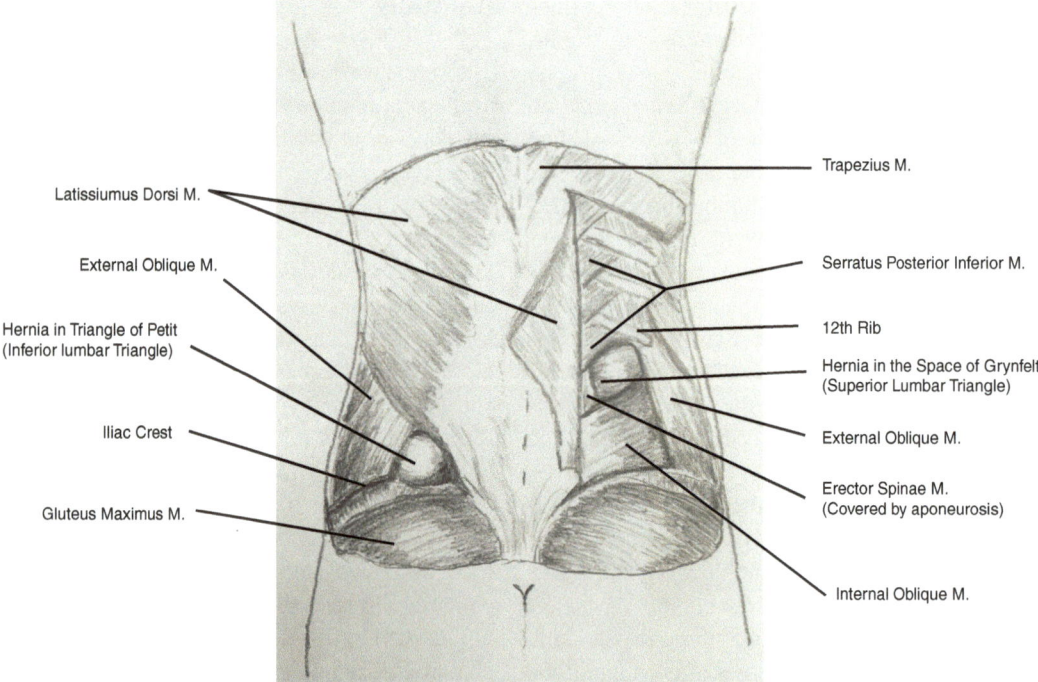

Fig. 11.2 Lumbar region anatomy showing hernia spaces

Fig. 11.3 Cross-sectional view of lumbar region

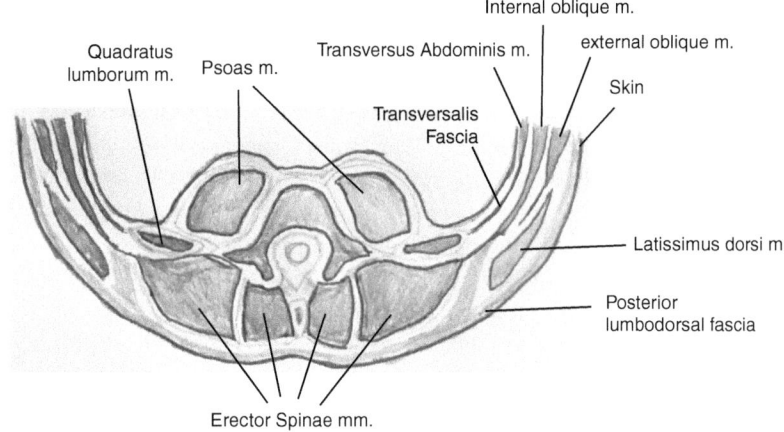

Quadratus lumborum m.

Psoas m.

Transversus Abdominis m.

Internal oblique m.

external oblique m.

Skin

Transversalis Fascia

Latissimus dorsi m.

Posterior lumbodorsal fascia

Erector Spinae mm.

Fig. 11.4 Intracorporeal view showing course of nerves through the lumbar region

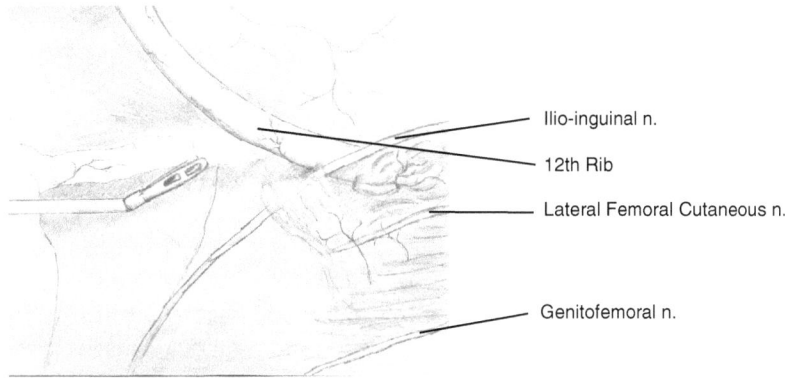

Ilio-inguinal n.

12th Rib

Lateral Femoral Cutaneous n.

Genitofemoral n.

12th intercostal neurovascular bundle inferior to the 12th rib and above the origin of the internal oblique, and that this orifice, located within a natural weak point in the lumbodorsal fascia, was a potential spot of herniation [22]. The superior defect is deeper and larger than the inferior. It is bound by the posterior border of the internal oblique muscle anteriorly, the anterior border of the sacrospinalis muscle posteriorly, and has the 12th rib and the serratus posterior inferior muscle as its base, the external oblique and the latissimus dorsi muscles as its roof, and the aponeurosis of the transversus abdominis as its floor [19]. Cadaveric studies have found that it is anatomically present in more than 90% [22], with its morphology dependent on the development of the surrounding muscles and the position and

length of the 12 rib. Short, round-chested people will have a larger superior triangle due to the more horizontal position of the 12th rib [5]. The inferior triangle of Petit is smaller and more superficial, and is more consistently triangular. It is bounded by the iliac crest inferiorly, the latissimus dorsi medially, and the external oblique laterally, with the internal oblique muscle as its floor.

In terms of surgical anatomic considerations, when performing a laparoscopic repair of the lumbar hernia, the mesh is laid in the retroperitoneal space. When the triangles are viewed from the retroperitoneal perspective, the paths of the sensory nerves arising from the lumbar nerve roots must be kept in mind to avoid tacks or sutures in these locations (Fig. 11.4).

Laparoscopic/Robotic Repair of Lumbar Hernias

There is no consensus on the optimal repair technique of the flank hernia [14, 23]. Techniques for open repair of these hernias used to be extremely varied, however these techniques of primary repair involving rotational muscle flaps or grafts have fallen out of favor [5]. In the modern era open repairs invariably utilize extensive preperitoneal dissection and placement of mesh, except in the pediatric population, where primary repair is favored.

The lumbar hernia can be quite challenging to repair due to the regional anatomy. Dissection and proper overlap of the mesh is limited by the presence of bone (the 12th rib superiorly and iliac crest inferiorly) [24]. The edges of the fascial defect can be difficult to define due to the location, there can be a lack of adequate surrounding fascia, and if the hernia is incisional or posttraumatic there can be thinning and atrophy of the surrounding muscles due to neuropraxia [9]. Primary lumbar hernias (Petit and Grynfeltt hernias) are small and emerge through a well-defined fascial defect, generally without attenuation of the surrounding tissues, and rarely contain visceral contents. Repair of spontaneous lumbar hernias is therefore easier and can be approached with whatever technique the surgeon is most comfortable—open, laparoscopic preperitoneal, and laparoscopic transabdominal all appear to work equally well [9]. For incisional (the majority) and posttraumatic lumbar hernias, recent evidence supports the use of laparoscopy for repair in defects less than 15 cm. The first report of a minimally invasive approach to lumbar hernia was first published in 1996 by Burick and Parascandola [25], and since then there have been multiple reports of the success of the laparoscopic approach [26]. In their retrospective study of laparoscopic versus open lumbar hernia repair, Moreno-Egea et al. [9] compiled 20 additional reports of laparoscopic lumbar hernia repair. In their series of 55 patients (35 laparoscopic versus 20 open repairs) they found mean operative time, length of stay, analgesic consumption, and pain at 1 month were significantly less with laparoscopic repair. Rate of hernia recurrence was 15% in the open repair group versus only 2.9% in the minimally invasive group. Recurrence was related primarily to the size of the hernia. Their conclusion was that laparoscopic repair of hernias with defects 15 cm or less was certainly safe and efficacious, and offered clear benefits over open surgery.

Operative Technique

Minimal invasive lumbar hernia repair can be performed via different approaches. We describe a technique for robotic-assisted transabdominal laparoscopic repair of a left-sided lumbar hernia.

Patient Positioning

The patient is placed in supine position for induction of general endotracheal anesthesia. The patient is then repositioned into the lateral decubitus on a bean-bag. For excellent exposure the operating room table is flexed in order to stretch the lumbar space. It is important to cushion all bony prominences to avoid any harm to the patient.

Trocar Placement

Laparoscopic access to abdominal cavity is performed by Veress needle technique in left subcostal space (Fig. 11.5). After insufflation of the abdominal cavity to 15 mmHg, we place an 8.5 mm reusable port at the same site of Veress needle and explore abdominal cavity to ensure no adhesions that will prohibit the placement of the remaining reusable trocars. A 30-degree scope is used to facilitate the directed visualization. Two additional 8.5 mm trocars are placed in a "C" shape at least 8 cm away from each other (this is necessary with the use of the Intuitive Si robot). The primary consideration in trocar placement is that trocars must be sufficiently distant from the working site, including both the fascial defect and the desired 3–5 cm overlap of the mesh. Robotic scissors, needle driver, and bipolar grasper are the instruments of choice for the authors.

Fig. 11.5 Lateral positioning and Veress needle access

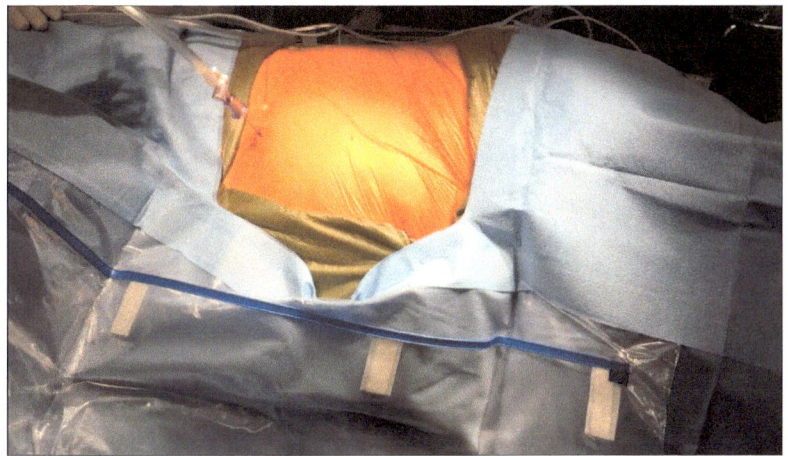

Fig. 11.6 Docking the robotic arms

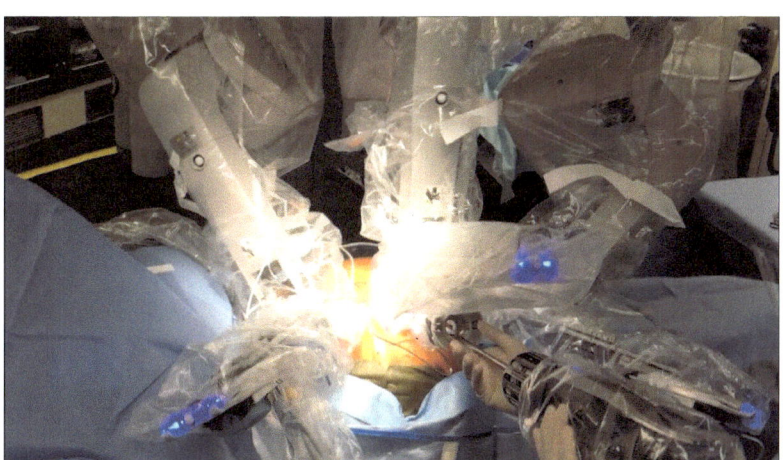

Docking the Robot

The robot is brought in from the flank. Fine adjustment should be made to bring the robotic arms in line with the dissection. Sufficiently distant trocar placement is essential prior to docking to limit the collision of the robotic arms (Fig. 11.6). It is important to ensure that all arms are bumped up to ensure both that there is no tension on abdominal wall and that the range of movement for each arm is sufficient. Proper port placement and docking of the robot entails a learning curve, ensuring proper port placement and arm docking will limit extra time needed for troubleshooting during the case.

Identification of the Lumbar Hernia

The peritoneum of the left paracolic gutter is incised from the 10th rib to the iliac crest. Peritoneum and retroperitoneal tissues are dissected at least 5 cm away from the hernia defect to ensure proper mesh coverage. Reduction of all hernia contents is performed to demonstrate the dimensions of the hernia defect (Fig. 11.7).

Defect Closure

The hernia defect is closed primarily using a 12- or 18-in. length number 0 Stratafix absorbable suture on a CT-1 needle (Ethicon, NJ). Barbed sutures facilitate closure but other types can be

Fig. 11.7 Identification of the hernia defect

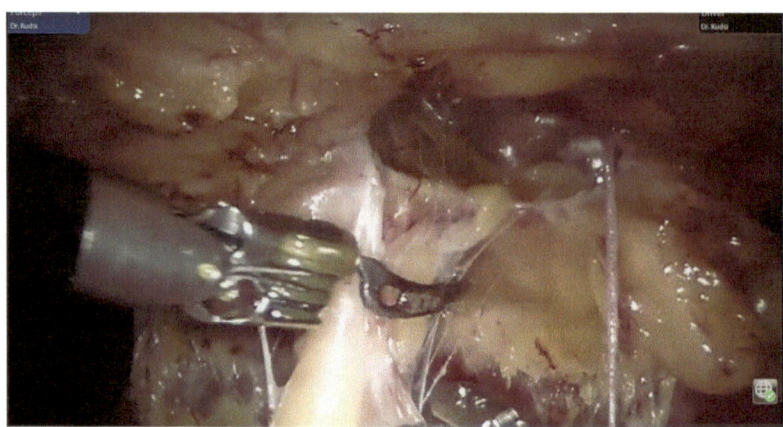

Fig. 11.8 Closure of the hernia defect

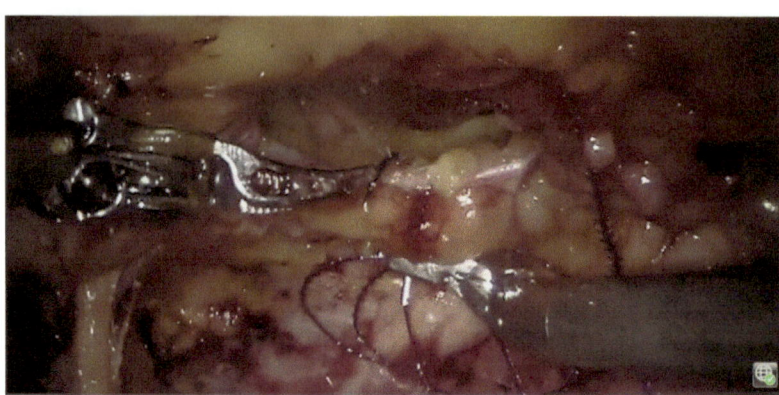

used according to the surgeon's preference (Fig. 11.8). Decreasing the pneumoperitoneum to 6 mmHg and utilizing the shoelace concept by taking all fascial bites and then tightening each one separately to decrease defect size will facilitate fascial closure in larger defects.

Mesh Placement and Fixation

It is important to size the mesh based on the defect prior to closure of the defect. Mesh should be sized with 3–5 cm overlap in mind. The authors prefer self-fixating polyester mesh but non-barrier coated synthetic polypropylene mesh is a suitable alternative. The mesh is fixed either via interrupted absorbable sutures at four corners, or in the case of self-fixating mesh, there is no need for suturing or tacking (Fig. 11.9). Techniques involving suturing the mesh or the use of absorbable tack fixation of the mesh being careful to respect the path of the nerves that arise from the anterior rami of the T12/L1 nerve roots

that splay out over the psoas muscle (ilioinguinal, iliohypogastric, and genitofemoral) have been described [27]. In practice, however, the course of these nerves can be difficult to identify. The benefit of using self-fixating mesh is to avoid the possibility of grabbing any nerves while fixing the mesh in the lumbar space (Fig. 11.10). Biosynthetic glue has been described as a method for mesh fixation as well.

Peritoneum Closure

The peritoneum of the left paracolic gutter is then closed using absorbable 3-0 sutures (Fig. 11.11). The authors prefer number 9-in. length 3 V-lock 180 wound closure device (Medtronic Inc. Minneapolis, MN) on GS-21 needle. Suturing the peritoneal pocket closed is a delicate step. It is crucial to assess the peritoneal flap at the end and close any tears in the pocket that are larger than 1 cm with interrupted absorbable sutures.

Fig. 11.9 Self-fixating mesh placement with sufficient overlap

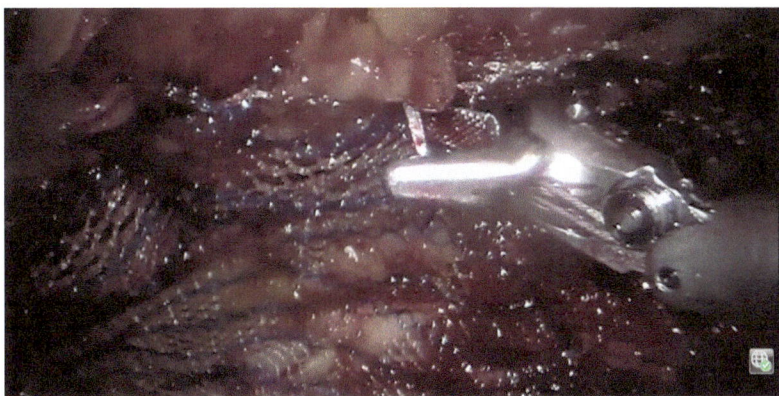

Fig. 11.10 Mesh placement

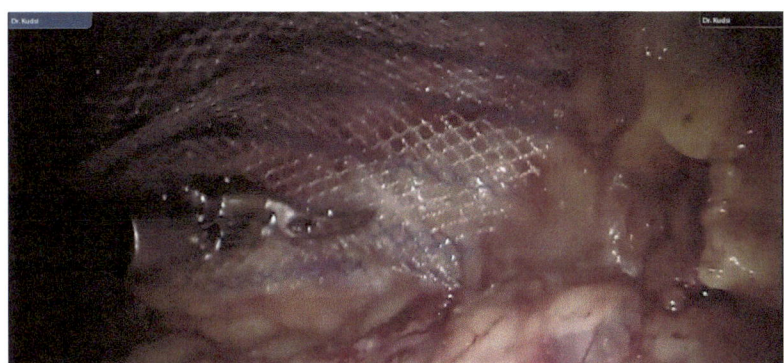

Fig. 11.11 Closure of the peritoneum

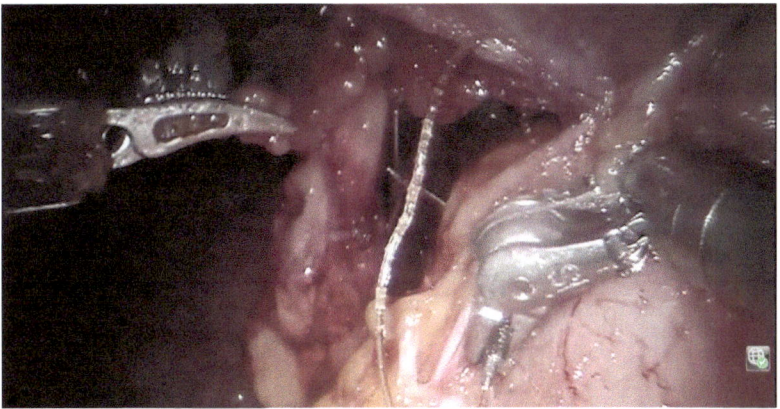

Postoperative Care

In our experience robotic-assisted lumbar hernia repair is performed in the ambulatory setting. The patient is given an abdominal binder to wear during the recovery period. Patients followed up in the office within 30 days and were asked to follow up at 1 year for assessment.

Conclusion

Lumbar hernia, although rare, can be a significant cause of chronic lumbar pain, cosmetic deformity, and potential morbidity from incarceration and strangulation of retroperitoneal and intra-abdominal contents, and all patients diagnosed with lumbar hernia should be referred for elective repair. The recognition and incidence of these hernias will continue to increase, and knowledge of repair of these hernias is essential to the practice of hernia specialists. The minimally invasive approach lends itself well to repair of circumscribed lumbar hernia defects. Adequate mesh overlap is essential, and repair of these rare hernias can be technically challenging. The increased freedom of laparoscopic articulation provided by robotic technology and the opportunity for these patients to be treated in the ambulatory setting makes this the ideal surgical modality.

References

1. Orcutt T. Hernia of the superior lumbar triangle. Ann Surg. 1971;173(2):294–7.
2. Suarez S, Hernandez JD. Laparoscopic repair of a lumbar hernia: report of a case and extensive review of the literature. Surg Endosc. 2013;27:3421–9.
3. Bonner CD, Kasdon SC. Herniation of fat through the lumbodorsal fascia as a cause of low-back pain. N Engl J Med. 1954;251(27):1102–4.
4. Macci V, et al. The triangles of Grynfeltt and Petit and the lumbar tunnel: an anatomo-radiologic study. Hernia. 2017;21:369–76.
5. Armstrong O, et al. Lumbar hernia: anatomic basis and clinical aspects. Surg Radiol Anat. 2008;30:533–7.
6. Hafner CD, Wylie JH, Bush BE. Petit's lumbar hernia: repair with Marlex mesh. Arch Surg. 1963;86:180–6.
7. DeLong MR, Tandon VJ, Rudkin GH, Da Lio AL. Latissimus dorsi flap breast reconstruction—a nationwide inpatient sample review. Ann Plast Surg. 2017;78:S185–8.
8. Cavallaro G, et al. Anatomical and surgical considerations on lumbar hernias. Am Surg. 2009;75(12):1238–41.
9. Moreno-Egea A, Alcaraz AC, Cuervo MC. Surgical options in lumbar hernia: laparoscopic versus open repair. A long-term prospective study. Surg Innov. 2013;20(4):331–44.
10. Teo KAT, Burns E, Garcea G, Abela JE, McKay CJ. Incarcerated small bowel within a spontaneous lumbar hernia. Hernia. 2010;14:539–41.
11. Hide IG, Pike EE, Uberoi R. Lumbar hernia: a rare cause of large bowel obstruction. Postgrad Med J. 1999;75(882):231–2.
12. Lafer DJ. Neuroblastoma and lumbar hernia: a causal relationship? J Pediatr Surg. 1994;29(7):926–9.
13. Wakhlu A, Wakhlu AK. Congenital lumbar hernia. Pediatr Surg Int. 2000;16:146–8.
14. Moreno-Egea A, Baena EG, Calle MC, Martinez JAT, Albasini JLA. Controversies in the current management of lumbar hernias. Arch Surg. 2007;142:82–8.
15. Stamatiou D, Skandalakis JE, Skandalakis LJ, Mirilas P. Lumbar hernia: surgical anatomy, embryology, and technique of repair. Am Surg. 2009;75(3):202–7.
16. Kretschmer HL. Lumbar hernia of the kidney. J Urol. 1951;65:944.
17. Salameh JR, Salloum EJ. Lumbar incisional hernias: diagnostic and managament dilemma. JSLS. 2004;8:391–4.
18. Gagner M, Milone L, Gumbs A, Turner P. Laparoscopic repair of left lumbar hernia after laparoscopic left nephrectomy. JSLS. 2010;14:405–9.
19. Varban O. Lumbar hernia after breast reconstruction. Int J Surg Case Rep. 2013;4:869–71.
20. Burt B, Afifi HY, Wantz GE, Barie PS. Traumatic lumbar hernia: report of cases and comprehensive review of the literature. J Trauma. 2004;57:1361–70.
21. Bathla L, Davies E, Fitzgibbons RJ, Cemaj S. Timing of traumatic lumbar hernia repair: is delayed repair safe? Report of two cases and review of the literature. Hernia. 2011;15:205–9.
22. Goodman EH, Speese J. Lumbar hernia. Ann Surg. 1916;63(5):548–60.
23. Dakin GF, Kendrick ML. Challenging hernia locations: Flank hernias. In: Jacob BP, Ramshaw B, editors. The sages manual of hernia repair. New York: Springer; 2013. p. 531–40.
24. Moreno-Egea A, et al. Open vs laparoscopic repair of secondary lumbar hernias: a prospective nonrandomized study. Surg Endosc. 2005;19:184–7.
25. Burick AJ, Parascandola SA. Laparoscopic repair of a traumatic lumbar hernia: a case report. J Laparoendosc Surg. 1996;6:259.
26. Arca MJ, et al. Laparoscopic repair of lumbar hernias. J Am Coll Surg. 1998;187:147–52.
27. Claus CMP, Nassif LT, Aguilera YS, Ramos EB, Coelho JCU. Laparoscopic repair of lumbar hernia (Grynfelt): technical description. Arq Bras Cir Dig. 2017;30(1):56–7.

Suggested Reading

Baker ME, et al. Lumbar hernia: diagnosis by CT. Am J Roentgenol. 1987;148:565–7.
Esposito TJ, Fedorak I. Traumatic lumbar hernia: case report and literature review. J Trauma. 1994;37(1):123–6.
Heniford BT, Iannitti DA, Gagner M. Laparoscopic inferior and superior lumbar hernia repair. Arch Surg. 1997;132:1141–4.

J. Tyler Watson and Karl A. LeBlanc

Introduction

The creation of a stoma is necessary to treat many different conditions. The first colostomy was described in medical literature by Littre in 1710, although the first successful colostomy recorded was not until 1793, when one was created on an infant with an imperforate anus. It is well known that stomas create a high-risk environment for herniation, as they require passage of the intestine through the abdominal wall. Goligher felt that some degree of herniation was virtually assured following colostomy formation [1]. There are various complications from stomas that necessitate revision, including poor fit of the appliance, difficult irrigation, or cosmetic deformity related to the ostomy itself. Issues relating solely to herniation are also seen, such as incarceration or strangulation. While the mere presence of a hernia does not mandate repair, these complications may require attention, and patients often present with an extremely large hernia requiring extensive surgery that could have been associated with less risk and, perhaps, a greater chance of long-term success if managed earlier.

Devlin classified parastomal hernias into four subtypes [2]. The *interstitial* type has the hernia sac within the aponeurotic layers of the muscles of the abdominal wall, such as between the transversus abdominus and internal oblique. The *subcutaneous* type has the sac above the muscle but below the skin and is the most common of these types of hernias. The *intrastomal* type involves a loop ostomy in which the herniated intestine slips between these loops. The fourth type is that of the prolapse where the bowel (frequently the small intestine) passes through a circumferential hernia sac that encloses the stoma itself. While this classification is logical anatomically, its clinical applicability is limited. The European Hernia Society has recently based a classification upon the size of the hernia and the presence or absence of an incisional hernia (Table 12.1) [3]. This system may prove to be more clinically relevant but studies are still lacking. Adding "P" to the type of hernia signifies a primary hernia and an "R" is added if it is recurrent.

There is a differing clinicoradiological classification that has been described. In this classification, the contents of the hernia are used to characterize the type of hernia (Table 12.2). This system has not been used extensively and it has yet to be shown that this is clinically relevant in regard to the best method of repair.

J. T. Watson
Our Lady of the Lake Regional Medical Center, Baton Rouge, LA, USA

K. A. LeBlanc (✉)
Surgeons Group of Baton Rouge, Our Lady of the Lake Physician Group, Clinical Professor, Surgery, Louisiana State University Health Sciences Center, Baton Rouge, LA, USA

© Springer International Publishing AG, part of Springer Nature 2018
K. A. LeBlanc (ed.), *Laparoscopic and Robotic Incisional Hernia Repair*,
https://doi.org/10.1007/978-3-319-90737-6_12

Table 12.1 European Hernia Society parastomal hernia classification

Type	Description
I	Hernia defect ≤5 cm without cIH
II	Hernia defect ≤5 cm with cIH
III	Hernia defect >5 cm without cIH
IV	Hernia defect >5 cm with cIH

cIH concomitant incisional hernia

Table 12.2 Moreno-Matias parastomal hernia classification

Type	Description
0	Normal (no herniation)
I	Hernia sac containing stoma loop
II	Hernia sac containing omentum
III	Hernia sac containing intestine other than stoma

Incidence of Parastomal Hernia

The incidence of this condition is difficult to quantify with any certainty due to the lack of a uniform description in the past, but it unquestionably represents a major clinical condition that deserves attention. The incidence of this problem has a wide range in the literature, from 4 to 81%, secondary to a broad variation in length of follow-up used in the studies; however, the generally accepted rate is approximately 50%. There is a variance between the clinical examination rate of 52% versus the CT examination rate of 78% [4–6]. Other studies have shown a much smaller discrepancy between clinical examination and CT scan (44% vs. 47%) [4]. However, this latter series evaluated only patients that underwent surgery for the hernia and is probably not representative of the entire population of parastomal hernia patients.

It has been shown that the type of ostomy influences herniation rates. A recent meta-analysis noted that the rate of herniation with a defunctionalizing loop ileostomy (2.45%) was statistically significantly lower than that of a loop colostomy (6.25%) [7]. These cannot be adequately compared to that of end ostomies as these are generally shorter term and temporary.

There is evidence that the placement of the stoma in the extraperitoneal plane (13%) leads to

statistically fewer hernias than if placed in the transperitoneal plane (41%) during laparoscopic colectomy [8–11]. This has also been shown to be true for open surgery as well. A recent meta-analysis revealed approximately the same reduction in the incidence of herniation with the extraperitoneal colostomy (6.3%) versus the transperitoneal colostomy (17.8%) [8]. This study also found a lower incidence of prolapse with the former approach (1.1% vs. 7.3%).

While not the focus of this chapter, prevention might be the best treatment of these hernias. The use of one of the synthetic absorbable or biologic meshes at the creation of these ostomies may represent the biggest advance in this field. There is a substantial amount of evidence that the use of mesh lowers the rate of parastomal herniation [9–14]. Additionally, several trials have shown that the use of mesh lowers hernia rates from 36% with no mesh to 7% with prophylactic mesh. One trial with reported results after 5 years revealed an occurrence of hernia without mesh of 81 and 13% with mesh placement [15].

Parastomal Hernia Repair Considerations

In general, a type of mesh is used in nearly all of the repairs due to the high rate of recurrence with the primary fascial closure or relocation. The use of a biologic product has been shown to be associated with an extremely high rate of recurrence similar to that of primary repair. In one study the rate of recurrence was nearly 90% with a median time to recurrence at 10 months [16]. The use of a synthetic mesh product seems to be the best approach to the repair of these hernias. This is also influenced by the method of repair. This is further detailed later in this chapter.

Laparoscopic Technique

The laparoscopic approach can be used for all types of primary or recurrent parastomal hernias as classified by the European Hernia Society. The previously endorsed keyhole approach, which allows the intestine to exit through the mesh, should not be considered a viable procedure due to reported recurrence rates as high as 56% [17, 18]. The senior author modified this technique to use two overlapping meshes with favorable results but has since abandoned that method in favor of the onlay (Sugarbaker) repair [19]. The onlay repair is technically easier to perform and decreases the amount of prosthetic material required.

Preoperative preparation includes a first-generation cephalosporin and antithrombotic prophylaxis. A urinary drainage catheter is occasionally inserted into any stoma but is always used for a urostomy. This will aid in identification of the intestinal conduit and also drain the urostomy. The author prefers to close all ostomies except for urostomy hernias with silk suture to prevent extrusion of intestinal contents during the operation. Additionally, the location of the ostomy appliance is marked with a skin-marking pen (to assure no transabdominal sutures are placed in that area) and covered with a sponge. An Ioban drape (3M Company, St. Paul, MN) is applied onto the skin (Fig. 12.1).

The overall procedure is similar to the laparoscopic incisional hernia repair. A noncutting optical trocar is used to enter the abdomen in the upper quadrant opposite the site of the ostomy. This will be followed by three additional trocars. The camera port is usually placed in the upper midline (Fig. 12.2). These are all normally 5 mm trocars but occasionally one of them will be replaced with a 12 mm to ease insertion of the meshes. The presence of additional hernias, which are not uncommon, can alter the final number and location of the trocars. Adhesiolysis will be done with or without the use of an energy source based upon the type of tissue that is adherent to the abdominal wall.

Once the entire area that will be covered by the meshes has been freed of both adhesions and preperitoneal fat, a ruler is inserted into the abdominal cavity. The dimensions of the defect will be measured but it is important to also measure the overlap of 5 cm that will cover the defect. This size has been shown to reduce recurrence rates in incisional hernia repair [20]. It has been the author's preference to repair these hernias with a threefold approach. To accomplish this, two different mesh materials are used. After the measurements have been made, a 5 × 7 cm Bio-A® (W. L. Gore & Associates, Elkhart, DE, USA) that has been shaped for hiatal hernia repair is cut to enlarge the "U"-shaped opening and round the edges (Figs. 12.2 and 12.3). An appropriately sized DualMesh PLUS (W. L. Gore & Associates, Elkhart, DE, USA) is chosen, and three permanent (expanded polytetrafluoroethylene) sutures are placed. Two of these are placed on the portion that will be positioned lateral to the hernia defect 8–10 cm apart to allow the creation of a tube through which the intestine will pass (Fig. 12.4).

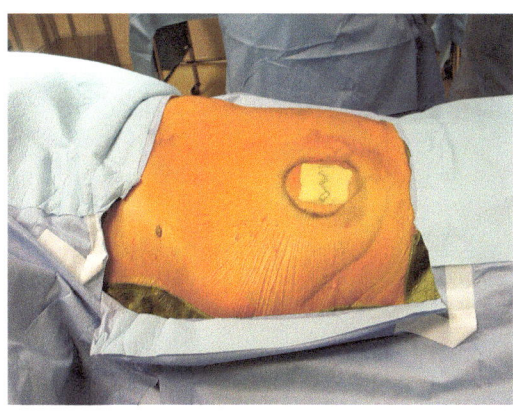

Fig. 12.1 Fully draped ileostomy hernia

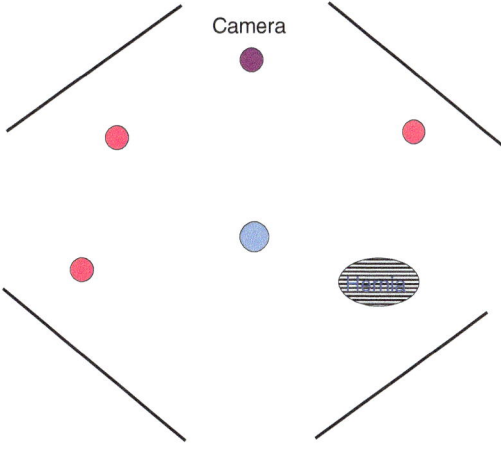

Fig. 12.2 Typical 5 mm trocar positions for laparoscopic paracolostomy hernia repair

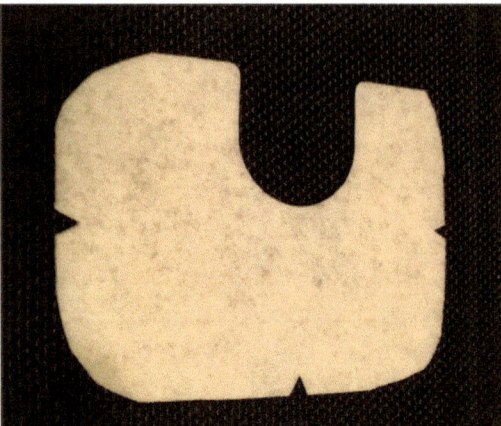

Fig. 12.3 Bio-A cut to size; the notches are placed to aid in positioning

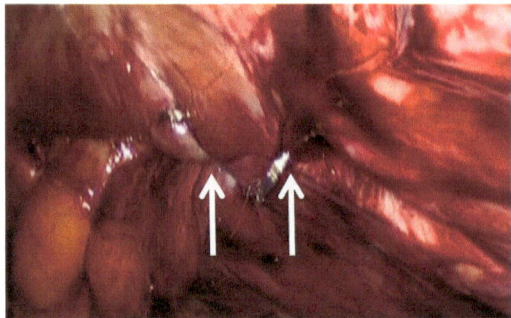

Fig. 12.5 *Arrows* indicate the partially closed defect. The ostomy is to the left

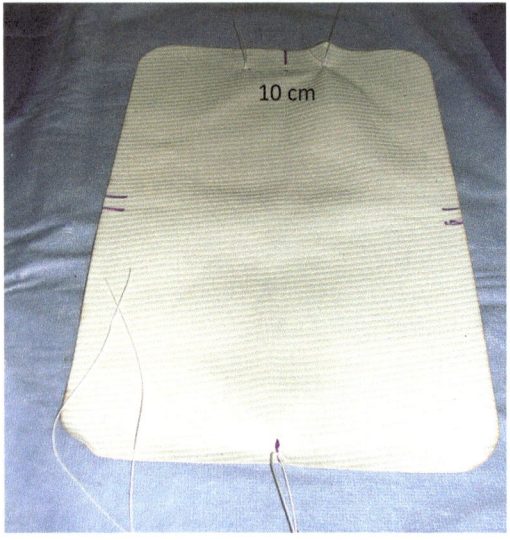

Fig. 12.4 Three sutures are preplaced. The upper sutures are 10 cm apart and will be used to fixate the mesh lateral to the ostomy hernia

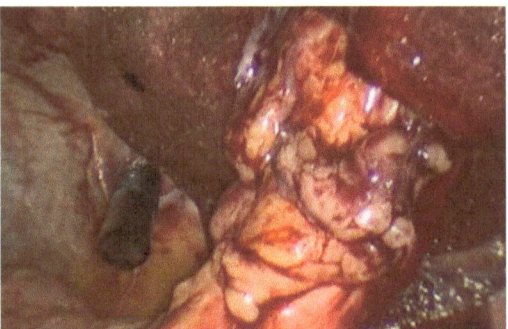

Fig. 12.6 Fixation of the Bio-A with absorbable fasteners

These should be no closer than 8 cm together due to the risk of obstructing the intestine once these are tied into place. If there is a doubt as to the spacing, the larger opening is preferred. The single suture will allow the other side of the mesh to be located accurately and held in place during fixation.

The first step in the repair will be the closure of the defect itself (Fig. 12.5). Any suture can be used, but the author prefers the Ti-Knot device (LSI Solutions, Victor, NY, USA). This serves to allow placement of the absorbable product onto

intact (i.e., closed) fascia, which will facilitate ingrowth. Following this, the Bio-A is brought into the abdominal cavity, positioned to cover the closure and then fixed with an absorbable fixation device (Fig. 12.6). In this figure, a larger Bio-A was chosen due to the size of the fascial closure.

The DualMesh PLUS is then introduced into the abdominal cavity. In most cases, it can be rolled tightly and pulled into the abdomen via a 5 mm trocar site (Fig. 12.7). In this figure, the mesh was brought into the abdominal cavity via a trocar placed next to the repair so that the trocar site would be covered by the onlay mesh. Once positioned correctly, the lower of the two sutures will be pulled through the abdominal wall lateral to the lateralized intestine from a skin incision using a suture-passing device (Fig. 12.8). Through that same incision another pass of the suture-passing device approximately 1 cm lateral of the site of the initial suture will allow the formation of the "tube" through which the intes-

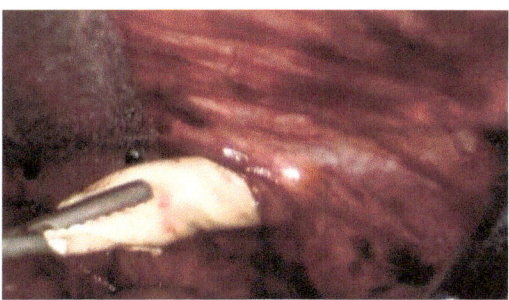

Fig. 12.7 Mesh is pulled into the abdominal cavity via a trocar site

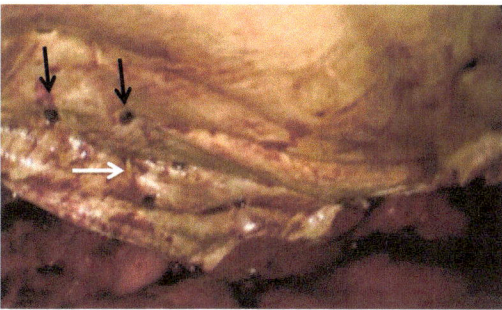

Fig. 12.9 The white arrow indicates a transfascial suture; the black *arrows* indicate "screw-like" absorbable fasteners

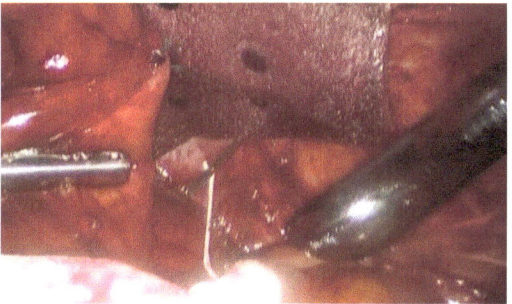

Fig. 12.8 ePTFE suture grasped by a suture passing device to pull it through the abdominal wall adjacent to the bowel

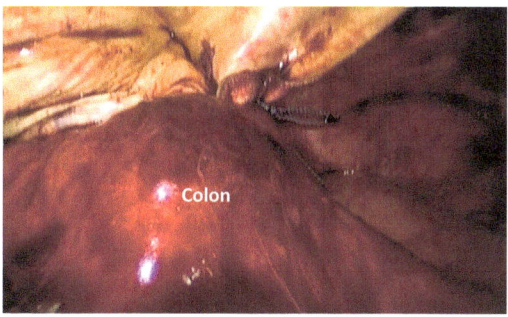

Fig. 12.10 Mesh sutured with permanent suture at the intestinal junction

tine will pass. The location of these sutures is critically important. If they are put too far apart the mesh might be pulled too tightly and act as a bow-string resulting in an obstruction of the intestine or the development of an erosion and/or fistula [21]. The correct lateral placement of the mesh is critical in the prevention of recurrence of the hernia [22].

After assurance that these two sutures are correctly placed, the single suture will be brought through the anterior abdominal wall. It is frequently helpful to move the camera to the lower trocar on the opposite side of the abdomen to place this and the other two sutures. Once the correct position of all three sutures is confirmed, they are tied. The mesh is then pulled tightly in all directions and fixed with an absorbable fixation device, although a permanent one could be used depending upon the preference of the surgeon. These are placed 2–3 cm apart along the periphery and adjacent to the bowel underneath the mesh. Once this

has been done, additional transfascial sutures are placed approximately 5–10 cm apart (Fig. 12.9). The decision of how many additional sutures is based upon the location of the hernia, the prior number of repairs, the presence of prior mesh (although it is best to excise this if possible) and associated comorbidities of the patient.

To prevent the possibility of intestine slipping into the entry point of the intestine under the mesh (and a subsequent recurrent hernia), the intestine is sewn to the mesh with a permanent suture (Fig. 12.10). Once this is complete, the abdomen is deflated, trocars are removed, and the site of all transfascial suture incisions is inspected. In many cases, there will be dimpling due to the fact that the subcutaneous tissue has been caught by the knots of the suture. A hemostat must be used to lift up at these sites to remove the dimpling at that time, as these can be a permanent cosmetic deformity. The skin incisions are closed with an absorbable suture.

Drains are not generally used but will be needed if the contents of the hernia are very large. These patients resume a regular diet the following day and can be discharged from the hospital once there is ostomy function. Awaiting return of ostomy function is necessary to assure that the repair has not compromised the stomal opening. In many cases, however, the patient can be discharged prior to that event.

Results of Laparoscopic Technique

The author has performed the above technique in 18 patients and has had two recurrences with an average follow-up of 30 months. Both of these were recurrent when the operations were performed. One of these patients gained 50 pounds and the intestine slipped into the entry site of the ileostomy. The mesh had not been sutured to the intestine in this patient, and this technique was used on all patients thereafter. The other patient developed a mesh infection of a mesh that was placed prior to the parastomal hernia repair. When that material was removed, the parastomal mesh was removed as well. Unsurprisingly the hernia recurred and has since been repaired robotically with no evidence of failure. Two additional patients had to be returned to the operating room to loosen the lateral transfascial sutures as these were too tight. Consequently, the 8–10 cm gap between these stitches has since been required.

Other studies have reported favorable results with the laparoscopic method. Several have noted that the use of a keyhole is associated with an unacceptably high recurrence rate. Favorable results with a product specifically designed for these hernias but incorporating a keyhole within it were initially reported [23]. This study had only a 4.2% rate of recurrence. Wara and Anderson also reported a low rate of recurrence (3%) but did incur a complication rate of 22 with 4.2% infection rate [6]. Recently, however, Mizrahi et al. reported their experience with this same product. Their recurrence rate was 46.4% [24]. That product is no longer available.

Berger and Bientzle reported on two different methods: the pure Sugarbaker and the keyhole plus Sugarbaker (sandwich method) on 66 patients. The combined recurrence rate was 12%. They later utilized only the sandwich method with polyvinylidene fluoride in 47 patients with a 2% recurrence rate [25, 26]. Others have reported similar results, with a recurrence rate from 4 to 10.5% [27–29]. This methodology is very similar to that described in this chapter except that both of the meshes were permanent and a keyhole was used rather than the shape described herein.

Hansson et al. performed an extensive meta-analysis on the topic of parastomal hernia repair methods (Table 12.3) [30]. They concluded that the primary sutured repair should not be done and that a mesh repair in any location was preferred. It appeared that the sublay (retromuscular) location is the best location for the open repair. They also analyzed the use of the mesh using either Sugarbaker or keyhole in both open and laparoscopic approaches (Table 12.4). They concluded that the laparoscopic keyhole had too high a rate of recurrence to be recommended. The laparoscopic sandwich repair appears to be the optimal technique.

An even more recent meta-analysis regarding only laparoscopic methodology provided similar results [31]. Fifteen articles were eligible for review with a total number of 469 patients. There were favorable outcomes overall but the recurrence rate was much better with the Sugarbaker repair (Table 12.5).

Table 12.3 Meta-analysis of different repairs (numbers are percentages; *IPOM* intraperitoneal onlay mesh)

Repair type	Infection	Other complications	Mortality	Recurrence rate
Suture only	11.8	10.8	3.8	69.4
Open Onlay Mesh	4.5	8.3	0	17.2
Open Sublay Mesh	4.8–8.4	7.1	0–8.4	6.9
Open IPOM	4.4	17.8	0	22.2
Laparoscopic IPOM	6.0	12.7	1.2	14.2

An extensive analysis of evidence-based medicine has found that there is level 3 evidence that the laparoscopic repair of parastomal hernias can be performed safely and level 4 evidence that the recurrence rate after laparoscopic repair is lower than the open approach [32]. Based upon these findings the group concluded that the recommen-dations are as follows: Laparoscopic repair of parastomal hernias should be considered a safe alternative to the open approach (Grade B). Additionally, the laparoscopic repair is a valid alternative option to open repair because the rate of recurrence is lower than the open approach (Grade C).

Table 12.4 Meta-analysis of mesh repairs (numbers are percentages)

Mesh repair type	Recurrence rate
Open Sugarbaker	15.0
Open Keyhole	14.2
Laparoscopic Keyhole	34.6
Laparoscopic Sugarbaker	11.6
Laparoscopic Sandwich (Sugarbaker and Keyhole)	2.1

Table 12.5 Outcomes of laparoscopic parastomal hernia repair

Outcome	Percentage
Postoperative morbidity overall	1.8
Surgical site infection	3.8
Mesh infection	1.7
Obstruction requiring reoperation	1.7
Other complication	16.6
Recurrence rate overall	17.4
Sugarbaker repair	10.2
Keyhole repair	27.9

Robotic Technique

The robotic repair of these hernias is very similar to the laparoscopic method. The position of the trocars is similar to the laparoscopic locations. Four trocars and three robotic arms are generally used. Three trocars are for the robot arms and a fourth one (a 12 mm or 15 mm) is used for introduction of sutures and mesh as well as removal of the needles (Fig. 12.11). These larger trocars will be placed above the rib margin to protect the fascia after the procedure is done. Prior to the introduction of these subcostal trocars, an optical 5 mm trocar is placed first to insufflate the abdomen, inspect the abdomen for adhesions, etc. and placement of the robotic trocars. After these are placed the 5 mm trocar is replaced with a larger one. This also allows for the insufflation of the abdomen prior to placement of the robotic

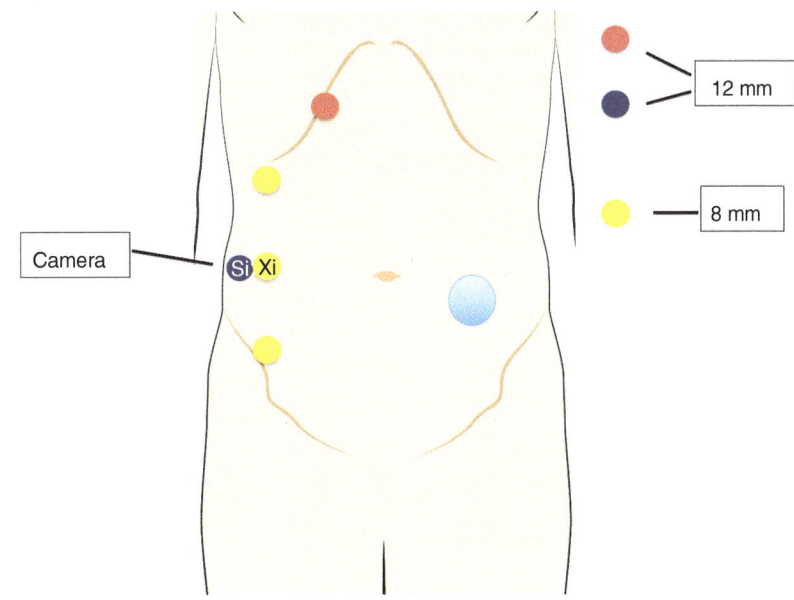

Fig. 12.11 Robotic port placement (the lighter blue circle represents that parastomal hernia)

trocars, which will allow a few more centimeters to place them compared to placement pre-insufflation. Note there are two different locations of the camera trocar for the different robots.

The adhesiolysis and exposure of the intestine and fascial defect are similar to the laparoscopic approach. The author prefers to repair this type of hernia with three different meshes exactly like the laparoscopic repair described above with specific modifications that will be noted below. The size of either mesh is not chosen until the defect and areas to be covered have been assessed and measured. The partial closure of the defect is done with barbed polypropylene sutures rather than the Ti-Knot.

The DualMesh PLUS or the newer Synecor product (W. L. Gore & Associates, Elkhart, DE, USA) is sized to provide at least a 5 cm overlap of the product to the fascial defect. The ultimate choice of size will also be significantly influenced by the presence of an additional incisional hernia (which will occur in at least 25% of cases). The location of any incisional hernia will also dictate not only the size of this mesh but if an additional mesh should be used solely to cover the incisional defect itself. The mesh is then marked on both sides to delineate the center of both axes of the product. At least three absorbable (rather than the permanent used laparoscopically) sutures will be placed into the mesh (Fig. 12.12). These are used for positioning of the mesh only and will be cut after their purpose is served. Two purple polyglactic acid 910 (#0)

sutures are placed one side approximately 10 cm apart as shown on the mesh on the right in the figure. These are sometimes placed closer if the hernia is from an ileostomy or urostomy. Instead of using all three sutures of the same color, it is sometimes helpful for identification inside the abdomen to use a different color, such as a white polyglactic acid 910 (#0) suture for the single one. The mesh on the left in Fig. 12.12 would be used if an associated incisional hernia is also found that will not be covered by the parastomal mesh. It has a centrally located polyglactic acid suture for placement and positioning. The third mesh is the Bio-A that would be used similarly to the laparoscopic repair discussed earlier in this chapter.

Once the dissection of adhesions and the reduction of the hernia contents are complete, the sidewall of the abdomen is inspected to evaluate the amount of adipose tissue that could lie between the mesh and the fascia. It is important that this is dissected away from the tissues so that the mesh is approximated to firm fascia rather than fat to assure rapid and adequate tissue ingrowth. After this is completed, the fascial defect and the area that is to be covered with the DualMesh PLUS or Synecor is measured intracorporeally with a ruler that is inserted into the abdominal cavity through the fourth trocar that was placed earlier. The measurement is done on both the transverse and vertical directions (Fig. 12.13). It is sometimes helpful to measure the exact location of the mesh as it relates to the

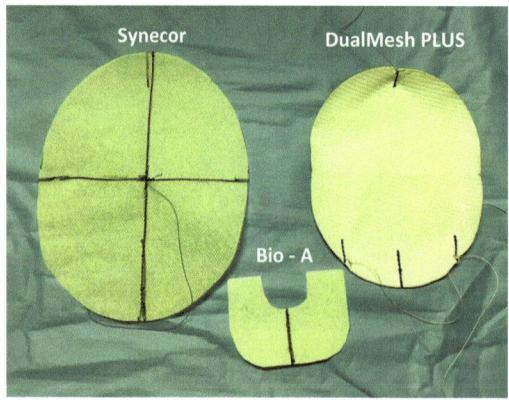

Fig. 12.12 Prosthetic materials that can be used

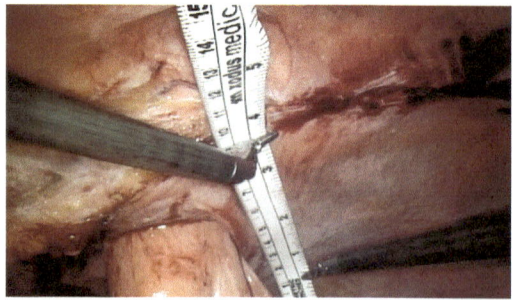

Fig. 12.13 Measurement of the area to be covered by the mesh

fascial defect. This could impact the size selected. Occasionally, as shown in this figure, the fascial defect will be closed prior to measurement to assure the exact location of mesh overlap. Ten centimeters is added in all directions to dictate the size of mesh chosen. In some cases, this may need to be modified, such as if there is an existing mesh present or if there is an associated incisional hernia that will also be repaired with the same prosthetic. It is preferable to remove any preexisting mesh, if possible.

The fascial defect is then re-approximated with barbed sutures (Fig. 12.14). The Bio-A will be introduced and placed onto the abdominal wall. The closure described above will be covered with the material and the side with the cut-out will face the intestine. This will then be secured with an absorbable tacking device similar to the laparoscopic repair (Fig. 12.15). To accomplish this, one of the robotic instruments will be removed and the device placed. It is usually necessary to undock the arm to complete this maneuver.

The second mesh product can now be introduced and positioned. The location of the exact middle of intestine is pinpointed on the lateral abdominal wall and an incision is made there, as is done laparoscopically. The sutures will be pulled tightly to assess mesh position and to note any constriction of the bowel (Fig. 12.16). Due to the location of these sutures on the mesh, this will create a small flap of mesh. This is generally used to suture the mesh to the bowel or mesentery to eliminate the risk of herniation through this potential site.

Next, the white suture is pulled through the wall of the abdomen at the site that confirms that the mesh is centered and positioned properly (Fig. 12.17). The previously placed lines on the mesh are helpful at this time. The mesh is drawn tightly (Fig. 12.18). If it is loose, the suture should be moved to assure that the mesh is snug. The absorbable fixation device may or may not be used to fixate the mesh lateral to the intestine to ease suture fixation. A barbed polypropylene suture (#2) is used to secure one side of the mesh.

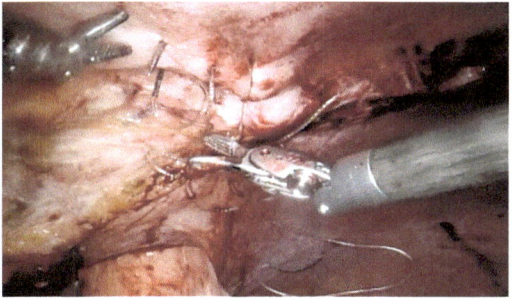

Fig. 12.14 Closure of the fascial defect with barbed permanent suture

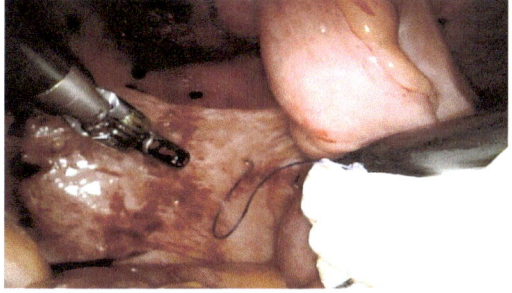

Fig. 12.16 The absorbable sutures are pulled through the lateral abdominal wall to position the mesh

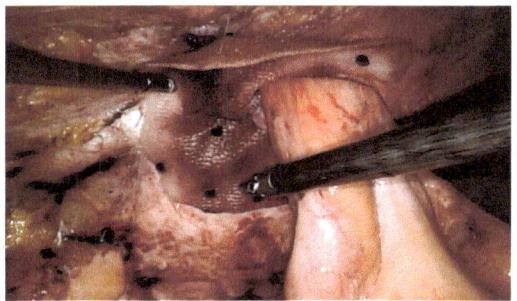

Fig. 12.15 Fixation of the Bio-A with an absorbable fastener

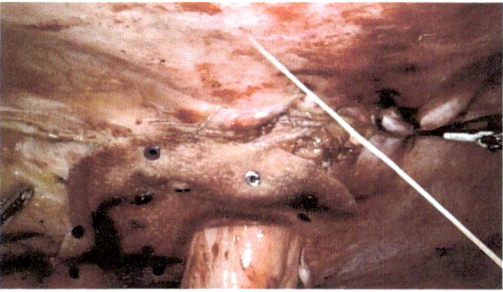

Fig. 12.17 The white absorbable suture is pulled through the abdominal wall to center the mesh

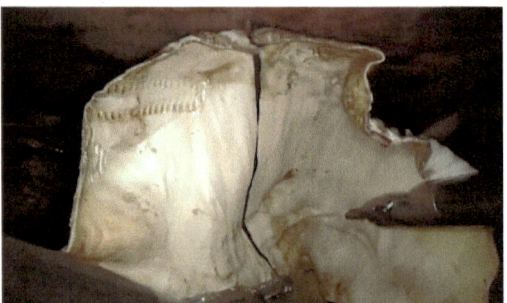

Fig. 12.18 The mesh is pulled tightly against the abdominal wall

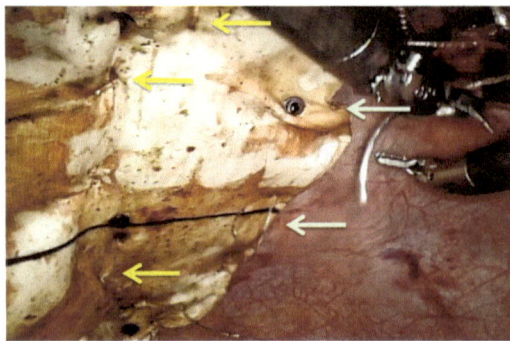

Fig. 12.20 Second row of sutures on the opposite side of the intestine (yellow arrows indicate the inner row of suture near intestine; light blue indicates the outer row of suture)

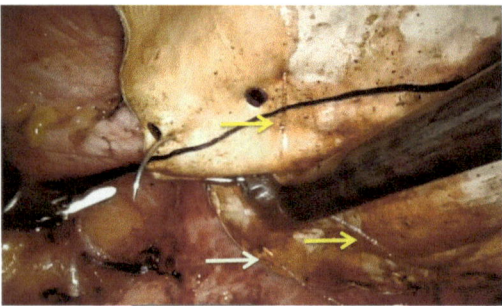

Fig. 12.19 Fascial fixation of one side of the mesh (yellow arrows indicate the inner row of suture near intestine; light blue indicates the outer row of suture)

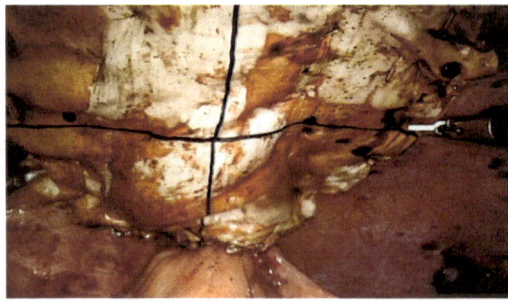

Fig. 12.21 Completed robotic parastomal hernia repair

This is a double-armed suture. One arm will run adjacent to the intestine and the other near the edge of the mesh (Fig. 12.19). A second double-armed and barbed suture will be used to suture on the side opposite the initial one next to the intestine and the other arm on the lateral aspect of the mesh (Fig. 12.20). This will create the tunnel for the intestine to enter, as is typical of the Sugarbaker repair. The final step is to suture the mesh to the intestine with a smaller barbed polydioxone suture similar to the laparoscopic technique. This results in a repair that is reliable (Fig. 12.21).

Postoperative Management

Abdominal binders are generally not used, as this seems to interfere with ostomy function. The nasogastric tube and urinary catheter are removed on postoperative day one. Meals are advanced as appropriate. Patients are usually discharged on the second or third postoperative day.

Most of these hernias will develop a seroma. Generally they are small unless the hernia contents were long standing and of large amount. Patients should be informed of such preoperatively. Unless very symptomatic no treatment is necessary. If needed, aspiration or drainage via interventional radiology could be done.

Results

To date, we have performed 16 parastomal hernias using the robotic assistance. At the time of this writing, the follow-up ranged from 6 to 42 months. One patient early in this experience did have to be returned to the operating room due to an obstruction that was caused by suture that fixed the mesh to the anterior abdominal wall. The mesh was slit and re-sutured to the intestine. There have been no other adverse events or recurrences during this time frame. It now has become our preferred method of repair.

Conclusion

The laparoscopic repair of parastomal hernias is a preferred technique over the open method. This can be done in a safe and effective manner with the Sugarbaker or the modified Sugarbaker, as described in this chapter. The robotic repair is an extension of that repair and should provide similar, if not, superior results.

References

1. Goligher JC. Surgery of the anus, rectum and colon. Bailliere: Tindall; 1984.
2. Devlin HB. Management of abdominal hernias. Oxford: Butterworth-Heinemann; 1988.
3. Śmietański M, Szczepkowski M, Alexandre JA, Berger D, Bury K, Conze J, Hansson B, Janes A, Miserez M, Mandala V, Montgomery A, Morales Conde S, Muysoms F. European Hernia Society classification of parastomal hernias. Hernia. 2014;18(1):1–6.
4. Moreno-Matias J, Serra-Aracil X, Darnel-Martin A, Bombardo-Junca J, Mora-Lopez L, Alcantara-Moral M, Rebasa P, Ayguavives-Garnica I, Navarro-Soto S. The prevalence of parastomal hernia after formation of an end colostomy. A new clinic-radiological classification. Color Dis. 2009;11(2):173–7.
5. Cingi A, Cakir T, Sever A, Aktan AO. Enterostomy site hernias: a clinical and computerized tomographic evaluation. Dis Colon Rectum. 2006;49:1559–63.
6. Hino H, Yamaguchi T, Kinugasa Y, Shiomi A, Hiroyasu K, Yamakawa Y, Numata M, Furutani A, Suzuki T, Torii K. Relationship between stoma creation route for end colostomy and parastomal hernia development after laparoscopoic surgery. Surg Endosc. 2017;31:1966–73.
7. Geng HZ, Nasier D, Liu B, Gao H, Xu YK. Meta-analysis of elective surgical complications to defunctioning loop ileostomy compared with loop colostomy after low anterior resection for rectal carcinoma. Ann R Coll Surg Engl. 2015;97(7):494–501.
8. Kroese LF, de Smet GH, Jeekel J, Kleinrensink GJ, Lange GF. Systematic review and meta-analysis of extraperitoneal versus transperitoneal colostomy for preventing parastomal hernia. Dis Colon Rectum 2016:59(&):688–695.
9. Janes A, Cengiz Y, Israelsson L. Preventing parastomal hernia with a prosthetic mesh: a 5-year follow-up of a randomized study. Ann R Coll Surg Engl. 2009;93(2):118–21.
10. Tam KW, Wei PL, Kuo LJ, Wu CH. Systematic review of the use of a mesh to prevent parastomal hernia. World J Surg. 2010;34(11):2723–9.
11. Shabbir J, Chaudhary BN, Dawson R. A systematic reviw on the use of prophylactic mesh during primary stoma formation to prevent parastomal hernia formation. Color Dis. 2012;14(8):931–6.
12. Williams NS, Hotouras A, Bhan C, Murphy J, Chan CL. A case-controlled pilot study assessing the safety and efficacy of the Stapled Mesh stomA Reinforcement Technique (SMART) in reducing the incidence of parastomal herniation. Hernia. 2015;19(6):949–54.
13. Ng ZQ, Tan P, Theophilus M. Stapled Mesh stomA Reinforcement Technique (SMART) in the prevention of parastomal hernia: a single-centre experience. Hernia. 2017;21:469–75.
14. Brandsma HT, Hansson BM, Aufenacker TJ, van Geldere D, Lammeren FM, Mahabier C, Makai P, Steenvoorde P, de Vries Reilingh TS, Wiezer MJ, de Wilt JH, Bleichrodt RP, Rosman C. Prophylactic mesh placement during formation of an end-colostomy reduces the rate of parastomal hernia: short-term results of the Dutch PREVENT-trial. Ann Surg. 2017;265(4):663–9.
15. Jänes A, Cengiz Y, Israelsson LA. Preventing parastomal hernia with a prosthetic mesh: a 5-year follow-up of a randomized study. World J Surg. 2009;33(1):118–21.
16. Warwick AM, Velineni R, Smart NJ, Daniels IR. Onlay parastomal hernia repair with cross-linked porcine dermal collagen biologic mesh: long-term results. Hernia. 2016;20(2):321–5.
17. Safadi B. Laparoscopic repair of parastomal hernias: early results. Surg Endosc. 2004;18:676–80.
18. Hansson BME, Bleichrodt RP, DeHingh IHJT. Laparoscopic parastomal hernia repair using a keyhole technique results in a high recurrence rate. Surg Endosc. 2009;23:1456–9.
19. LeBlanc KA, Bellanger DE, Whitaker JM, Hausmann MG. Laparoscopic parastomal hernia repair. Hernia. 2005;9:140–4.
20. LeBlanc KA. Mesh overlap is a key determinant of hernia recurrence following laparoscopic ventral and incisional hernia repair. Hernia. 2016;20(1):85–9.
21. P W, Andersen LM. Long-term follow-up of laparoscopic repair of parastomal hernia using a bilayer mesh with a slit. Surg Endosc. 2011;25(2):526–30.
22. Muysoms F, Van De Winkel N, Ramaswamy A. The Achilles' heel of Sugarbaker. Hernia. 2017;21(3):477–9.
23. Liu F, Li J, Wang S, Yao S, Zhu Y. Effectiveness analysis of laparoscopic repair of parastomal hernia using CK Parastomal patch. Zhongguo Xiu Fu Chong Jian Wai Ke Az Zhi. 2011;25(6):681–4.
24. Mizrahi H, Bhattacharya P, Parker MC. Laparoscopic slit mesh repair of parastomal hernia using a

designated mesh: long-term results. Surg Endosc. 2012;26(1):267–70.

25. Berger D, Bientzle M. Laparoscopic repair of parastomal hernias: a single surgeon's experience in 66 cases. Dis Colon Rectum. 2007;50(10):1668–73.

26. Berger D, Bientzle M. Polyvinylidene fluoride: a suitable mesh material for incisional and parastomal hernia repair. A prospective observational study of 344 patients. Hernia. 2009;13(2):167–72.

27. Mancini GJ, McClusky DA 3rd, Khaitan L, Goldenberg EA, Heniford BT, Novitsky YW, et al. Laparoscopic parastomal hernia repair using a nonslit mesh technique. Surg Endosc. 2007;21(9):1487–91.

28. McLemore EC, Harold KL, Efron JE, Laxa BU, Young-Fadok TM, Heppell JP. Parastomal hernia: short-term outcome after laparoscopic and conventional repairs. Surg Innov. 2007;14(3):199–204.

29. Craft RO, Huguet KL, McLemore EC, Harrold KL. Laparoscopic parastomal hernia repair. Hernia. 2008;12(2):137–40.

30. Hansson BM, Slater NJ, van der Velden AS, Groenewoud HM, Buyne OR, de Hingh IH, Bleichrodt RP. Surgical techniques for parastomal hernia repair. Ann Surg. 2012;255(4):685–95.

31. DeAsis FJ, Lapin B, Gitelis ME, Ujiki MB. Current state of laparoscopic parastomal hernia repair: a meta-analysis. World J Gastroenterol. 2015;21(28):8670–7.

32. Bittner R, Bingener-Casey J, Dietz U, Fabian M, Ferzli G, Fortelny R, et al. Guidelines for laparoscopici treatment of ventral and incisional abdominal wall hernias (International Endohernia Society [IEHS])-Part III. Surg Endosc. 2014;28(2):380–404.

Shirin Towfigh and Desmond T. K. Huynh

The various incisional hernia repair techniques are essentially the same in concept, whether performed via open, laparoscopic, or robotic approaches: The defect is cleared of its content, and it is closed or patched with a mesh implant. However, with regard to postoperative management, there are specifics to the laparoscopic and robotics approaches that should be appreciated.

The enhanced recovery after surgery (ERAS) pathway applies to all approaches. Steps that may be unique to the laparoscopic vs. robotic approaches are (a) the size of the trocars, cannulas and their placement, (b) the manipulation of the abdominal wall, (c) handling of the abdominal contents, and (d) the placement options for the mesh implant. Based on these factors, postoperative management may be slightly different when handling patients who undergo laparoscopic vs. robotic repair.

Enhanced Recovery After Surgery

The enhanced recovery after surgery (ERAS) pathway for hernias is validated and should be followed to reduce postoperative morbidity and

S. Towfigh (✉)
Beverly Hills Hernia Center, Beverly Hills, CA, USA
e-mail: DRTOWFIGH@BeverlyHillsHerniaCenter.com

D. T. K. Huynh
Cedars-Sinai Medical Center, Los Angeles, CA, USA

length of stay [1]. It is a multifaceted approach aimed at reducing infections, improving pain control, and maximizing healing potential. Table 13.1 demonstrates the essential elements of the ERAS pathway for hernias. There is a more in-depth discussion on this in Chap. 3.

The ERAS pathway for hernias is most applicable to open abdominal wall reconstruction. This is especially true with regard to the diet, which is slowly advanced over a matter of days. After laparoscopic incisional hernia repair, especially with intraperitoneal mesh placement, ileus can be a significant problem. It is estimated that 20% will have a postoperative ileus beyond 24 hours and 1.3% may have it last beyond a week [2]. There seems to be no predictable risk factors for prolonged ileus, though there is a positive correlation with the amount of dissection, size of mesh, and excess use of postoperative opioids.

In contrast, for most robotic incisional hernia repairs, the patient may start on a regular diet immediately or by postoperative day 1. It is postulated that robotic repair causes a lower ileus rate because the mesh is often placed extraperitoneally, the abdominal wall and intestine are minimally manipulated, and there is overall lower postoperative pain.

The multimodal pain therapy from the ERAS pathway is excellent and should be followed for all approaches. In most situations, the robotic approach will not require IV pain medication,

© Springer International Publishing AG, part of Springer Nature 2018
K. A. LeBlanc (ed.), *Laparoscopic and Robotic Incisional Hernia Repair*,
https://doi.org/10.1007/978-3-319-90737-6_13

Table 13.1 Postoperative elements of ERAS for incisional hernias [1]

Multimodal pain control
TAP block
Patient-controlled analgesia
Acetaminophen
Oxycodone as needed
Gabapentin
Valium as needed
NSAIDs
Acceleration of intestinal recovery
Alvimopam
Early feeding
POD 0: Limited clear liquids
POD 1–2: Clear liquids
POD 3: Regular diet

ERAS enhanced recovery after surgery, *TAP* transversus abdominis plane, *PO* by mouth, *NSAIDs* nonsteroidal anti-inflammatories, *POD* postoperative day

Table 13.2 Variable width dimensions of the laparoscopic ports

Outer diameter			
5 mm trocars	11 mm trocars	12 mm trocars	15 mm trocars
≤9.7 mm	≤14.2 mm	≤15.9 mm	≤19.1 mm

Table 13.3 Width dimensions of the robotic cannulas

Outer diameter		
	8 mm cannula	12 mm and Stapler cannulas
Si	10.48 mm	13.39 mm
Xi	9.75 mm	15.20 mm

patient-controlled analgesia, or valium, as the length of stay is expected to be low (see "The Abdominal Wall" below).

Trocars and Cannulas

Laparoscopic trocars come in various diameters and insertions. Some are threaded; others have balloons tips. Insertion can be blunt, radially spreading, or sharp. The resulting fascial defect is highly variable depending on the type of trocar. We know that the typical 5, 10, 11, and 12 mm trocars have a significantly wider outer diameter than advertised (Table 13.2). Also, the fascial defect may be related to body habitus as well as the trauma inflicted on the abdominal wall at the time of operation.

The incidence of port-site hernias during laparoscopy ranges from 0.65 to 2.80% [3]. It is lower in the morbidly obese. Port-site hernias have been reported for all sizes of trocars used, though the prevalence is higher with larger port sites. One method to reduce the risk of herniation is to skive the trocar through the abdominal wall in such a way as to reduce the amount of tension during each particular operation. For example, for repair of a midline incisional hernia, one may consider entering the lateral abdominal wall at an angle toward the hernia defect, thereby reducing the amount abdominal muscle spreading at the site of the trocar during the hernia manipulation.

The da Vinci (Intuitive Surgical, Sunnyvale, CA) robotic cannula sizes used today for abdominal wall operations are typically 8 mm or 12 mm. The body of the cannulas is made of strong stiff metal. Their obturators may be blunt or sharp. Unlike most laparoscopic trocars, the robotic cannulas are introduced perpendicular to the abdominal wall; skiving is not recommended. Similar to laparoscopic trocars, the outer diameter of the robotic cannulas is wider than the noted cannula size (Table 13.3).

There have been a few articles addressing port-site hernias specifically after robotic surgery. Most are related to specimen extraction sites, which are not relevant to incisional hernia repairs.

We know from the laparoscopic literature that port-site hernias increase with increasing size of the fascial defect [3]. It is important to note that the outer diameter of almost all trocars and cannulas is greater than the purported size (Tables 13.2 and 13.3). This should lead the surgeon to be more cognizant of how he/she manages the port site. It is commonly accepted that 15 mm laparoscopic ports must be all closed. Most advocate closure of 10 and 12 mm port sites, especially if they are at higher risk for herniation, e.g., patients with thin abdominal wall. This is also the recommendation by the European Hernia Society [4]. Interestingly, port site closure has been associated with higher risk of port-site herniation in the morbidly obese undergoing bariatric surgery [5]. Port-site closure for trocars under 15 mm may not be necessary in this population.

With laparoscopy, there is a tendency to skive the trocar in the direction of the operative field. This may reduce the risk of incisional hernia. Since that is not the technique recommended with the robotic cannulas, the expectation is that there is a higher risk of incisional hernia. However, this has not yet been reported as a common complication in robotic surgery.

The reported robotic cannula-site hernia rate requiring intervention is well under 0.5% for general surgical procedures [6]. This rate may be higher in patients who have already shown a propensity for incisional hernia, though one study did not show a difference in port-site hernia whether or not one had a past history of hernia [6]. The herniations can occur at 8 and 12 mm ports, even if the port was closed at the time of surgery. The lateral vs. midline placement of the port has also not been shown to be a predictor of hernia development. Conceptually, blunt obturators may cause less tissue injury than the sharp, but there are currently no studies to correlate port-site hernia rates between the two obturator types. We know from the laparoscopic literature that bladeless and radially dilating trocars have a lower rate of port-site hernia than bladed trocars [3].

The median time to port-site hernia diagnosis is within the first 9 months [6]. We know from laparoscopic data that critical bowel obstruction due to port-site hernias occurs within 21 days of surgery, whereas symptomatic non-obstructing hernias tend to present later [5]. This is an important detail, as the differential diagnosis of any postoperative nausea, vomiting, obstructive symptoms, or port-site pain with erythema within the first 3 weeks postoperatively must include a port-site hernia.

Robotic arms may generate much more torque at the abdominal wall than that seen with laparoscopy, especially if the cannulas are not optimally positioned. In the case of incisional hernia repairs, due to the necessary angulation toward the anterior abdominal wall, one would expect the amount of torque to be higher than average.

Thus, it is possible that the abdominal wall defect caused by the robotic cannula is larger than expected, resulting in a higher rate of port-site hernia. To date, not enough data exists to support these conjectures, but it is important to understand the physics of the robot on the abdominal wall and be wary of related complications when caring for patients postoperatively.

The Abdominal Wall

The torque on the abdominal wall during laparoscopic surgery is variable, dependent mostly on the patient's body habitus. It is most taxing in the morbidly obese, with significantly lower torque and tension on the abdominal wall required for thinner patients. In general, the trauma to the abdominal wall is minimal during laparoscopic surgery. During incisional hernia repair, the angulation toward the anterior abdominal wall can be quite acute, especially in the morbidly obese. Nevertheless, the surgeon is able to feel the amount of tension he/she is exerting. This "interfering force" can often be positive feedback from the patient's abdomen, thus preventing the surgeon from applying too much force during the operation [7]. The less tension and force on the abdominal wall, the less edema, ecchymoses, and postoperative pain.

The torque on the abdominal wall during robotic surgery is variable, dependent on the operation, patient body habitus, and experience and needs of the surgeon. If the cannulas are perfectly positioned, with the rotational axis of the cannula centered at the fascia level, the expectation is that little torque will be exerted on the abdominal wall. However this amount of torque has not yet been quantified. It is important to "burp" the trocars multiple times throughout the procedure, to ensure that abnormal tension on the abdominal wall is minimized. The result will be less edema and pain at the surgical sites.

Given the stiffer robotic cannula and the mechanical power of the arms, it is conceivable that there is more transfer of force onto the patient's abdominal wall and less onto the instruments and the surgeon as compared to laparoscopic surgery. This is one of the reasons many prefer robotic approach for the morbidly obese: it is physically less taxing on the surgeon and the instruments, resulting in improved manipulation at the tissue level [8].

Laparoscopic incisional hernia repair often involves transfascial sutures with or without other fixation options, such as tackers. Transfascial sutures have been implicated as an independent risk factor for postoperative pain and prolonged length of stay after hernia repair [9]. The pain associated with these sutures is significant and can be debilitating. The key is to prevent tightly knotting these sutures, as the patient needs to be able to have a mobile abdominal wall, and thus some freedom of movement despite the placement of the mesh.

Postoperatively, patients may present with point-tenderness at a single spot, associated with the point of transfascial suture. This can be treated with local anesthetic infusion at the fascia level directly at that location. If periodic injections do not cure the chronic pain, then suture removal should be performed. This can be performed with a simple cutdown over the area of pain.

"Suture hernias" are a little known but difficult complication of transfascial sutures placed too tightly or under tension [10]. They result in a wide tear of the abdominal wall at the site of the transfascial suture. The presentation is of pain, bulging, and a new hernia, now lateral to the area of the original repair. It is often at the edge of the prior mesh repair. The patient may claim to have felt an acute pull or tear over the area, often after an activity that rapidly increases their abdominal pressure. To repair, one will need to add a second patch of mesh over this region, overlapping with the first repair. Prevention, via calculated suture placement and gentle knot tying, is key to reduce the risk of such complication.

When switching to robotic surgery, most studies show comparable or decreased postoperative abdominal wall pain, with reduction in need for opioid pain medication by as much as 30% [11, 12]. A significant difference was seen for large incisional hernias, requiring a transversus abdominis release. When performed robotically, these patients saw a significant reduction in postoperative pain and hospital length of stay [12–16]. It is no longer uncommon to see patients discharged home on the same day or on postoperative day one following a large robotic incisional hernia repair or abdominal wall reconstruction, whereas the typical postoperative length of stay may range from 3 to 5 days for patients undergoing open repair. Contributors toward reducing postoperative pain after robotic surgery may include minimizing incisions, reducing tension on the abdominal wall and minimizing use of transfascial sutures.

Though most modern studies for incisional hernias show improved outcomes and reduced pain control after robotic surgery, seromas and other surgical site occurrences remain a problem in up to half the patients [14, 16, 17]. This is a higher level than that seen in laparoscopic surgery for incisional hernias. It is possible that the reason for this is the extensive tissue plane dissection involved in the robotic approach.

The liberal use of drains can help reduce this problem, especially for the larger abdominal wall reconstructions. Many surgeons routinely use drains in the soft tissue as well as overlying the mesh. I do not place drains for the mesh, and have not had any issues with seromas at the mesh level. When placing drains, the key is to (a) skive the drain to reduce direct communication with your working space once the drain is removed, and (b) minimize the skin incision made for the drain exit. Though it is technically tricky, I use the spear that comes with such drains. It allows for easy exteriorization of the drain without digging a large tunnel.

Handling Abdominal Contents

The most dangerous risk of both laparoscopic and robotic incisional hernia repair is intestinal injury. The incidence may be up to 6% [2]. With laparoscopic surgery, we have learned that the use of electrocautery should be minimized, and many also do not advocate use of ultrasonic shears. This is also the recommendation from major surgical societies [2, 18]. In these situations, bowel injury may be occult or sealed at the time of the operation, with presentation only postoperatively.

The robotic approach adds an extra element of risk for intestinal injury. As designed today, the da Vinci robot does not offer tactile sensation. Accidentally piercing a loop of intestine can occur without any feedback from your instrument. This is most likely if the instrument is moving outside your field of view. Also, choice of instrument can affect the risk of intestinal injury. For example, the Prograsp™ instrument is inappropriate during intestinal adhesiolysis, due to its very strong grasp strength.

For both laparoscopic and robotic incisional hernia repairs, the risk of intestinal injury is real and can be missed intraoperatively. Thus, it is imperative that there be a high suspicion for missed injury with any aberrancy noted postoperatively. Similar to laparoscopic surgery, the risk of intestinal injury during robotic surgery has been associated with surgeon experience [19]. The highest rate has been reported in the gynecologic population, with 0.6% risk of intestinal injury (range 0–6.25%) [20]. These numbers are similar in the laparoscopic incisional hernia repair literature [2].

Depending on the extent of intestinal injury, most patients will present with signs and symptoms of intestinal leakage within the first 3 days postoperatively. Thus, due diligence to work up any unexpected nausea, vomiting, fever, abdominal pain, and/or hypotension, is warranted. In some cases, a return to the operating room may be the best next step, in order to minimize delay in treatment. It is well appreciated that delay in treatment of an abdominal catastrophe has a high mortality rate.

Fortunately, if noted early, some intestinal injuries may be treated with minimally invasive approach [20]. Also, since robotic incisional hernia repair is often performed with the mesh placed extraperitoneally, the risk of mesh infection is lower than with intraperitoneal mesh placement, which is more commonly seen with laparoscopic approach. However, if the mesh is intraperitoneal, removal of the mesh at the time of intestinal injury repair is mandated.

Other critical events have been reported intraoperatively which can affect the patient's outcome after robotic surgery [10]. These include malfunctions of the robotic system, inadvertent injuries to other organs and vessels. In a review of the FDA MAUDE database, between 2000 and 2013, 197 adverse events during a general surgery procedure were logged, of which 37 were during hernia repair [21]. The majority were malfunctions of the robotic system. However, 28.4% involved direct injury to the patient and 5.6% resulted in patient death.

Mesh Placement

Mesh placement during laparoscopic surgery is typically via intraperitoneal onlay mesh (IPOM). This has proven to be safe and effective for the most part, and is considered the most common laparoscopic approach. However, with time, we have noticed drawbacks to intraperitoneal mesh placement. Mesh-related complications within the first 5 years postoperatively can reach 3.7% [22]. These include mesh-related intestinal obstructions, perforations, fistulas, and infections.

With the increased penetrance of robotic surgery, we have moved away from the intraperitoneal mesh placement that was popularized with laparoscopic incisional hernia repair. Many of us agree that mesh-related complications, such as ileus, intestinal obstruction, and fistula, may be reduced with the extraperitoneal mesh placement. The data is limited for directly measuring the mesh-related complications after robotic surgery. However, it is conceivable that by reducing the risk of mesh exposure to the intestinal contents, the risk of mesh-related intestinal complications and infections may also be reduced.

References

1. Fayezizadeh M, Petro CC, Rosen MJ, Novitsky YW. Enhanced recovery after surgery pathway for abdominal wall reconstruction: pilot study and preliminary outcomes. Plast Reconstr Surg. 2014;134(4S–2):151S.

2. Earle D, Roth JS, Saber A, Haggerty S, Bradley JF, Fanelli R, et al. SAGES guidelines for laparoscopic ventral hernia repair. Surg Endosc. 2016;30(8):3163–83.

3. Tonouchi H, Ohmori Y, Kobayashi M, Kusunoki M. Trocar site hernia. Arch Surg. 2004;139(11):1248–56.

4. Muysoms FE, Antoniou SA, Bury K, et al. European Hernia Society guidelines on the closure of abdominal wall incisions. Hernia. 2015;19(1):1–24.

5. Phillips E, Santos D, Towfigh S. Working port site hernias: to close or not to close? Does it matter in the obese? Bariatric Times. 2011;8(6):24–30.

6. Comfort AL, Frey MK, Musselman K, Chern JY, Lee J, Joo L, et al. Predictors of port site hernia necessitating operative intervention in patients undergoing robotic surgery. Gynecol Oncol. 2017;145:176.

7. Picod G, Jambon AC, Vinatier D, et al. What can the operator actually feel when performing a laparoscopy? Surg Endosc. 2005;19(1):95–100.

8. Jacobsen G, Berger R, Horgan S. The role of robotic surgery in morbid obesity. J Laparoendosc Adv Surg Tech. 2003;13(4):279–83.

9. Khansa I, Koogler A, Richards J, Bryant R, Janis JE. Pain management in abdominal wall reconstruction. Plast Reconstr Surg Glob Open. 2017;5(6):e1400.

10. Muysoms FE, Cathenis KKJ, Claeys DAB. "Suture hernia": identification of a new type of hernia presenting as a recurrence after laparoscopic ventral hernia repair. Hernia. 2007;11(2):199–201.

11. Leitao MM, Malhotra V, Briscoe G, Suidan R, Dholakiya P, Santos K, et al. Postoperative pain medication requirements in patients undergoing computer-assisted ("robotic") and standard laparoscopic procedures for newly diagnosed endometrial cancer. Ann Surg Oncol. 2013;20(11):3561–7.

12. Gonzalez A, Escobar E, Romero R, Walker G, Mejias J, Gallas M, et al. Robotic-assisted ventral hernia repair: a multicenter evaluation of clinical outcomes. Surg Endosc. 2017;31(3):1342–9.

13. Bittner JG, Alrefai S, Vy M, Mabe M, Prado PARD, Clingempeel NL. Comparative analysis of open and robotic transversus abdominis release for ventral hernia repair. Surg Endosc. 2017;20:1–8.

14. Warren JA, Cobb WS, Ewing JA, Carbonell AM. Standard laparoscopic versus robotic retromuscular ventral hernia repair. Surg Endosc. 2017;31(1):324–32.

15. Martin-del-Campo LA, Weltz AS, Belyansky I, Novitsky YW. Comparative analysis of perioperative outcomes of robotic versus open transversus abdominis release. Surg Endosc. 2017;21:1–6.

16. Prabhu AS, Dickens EO, Copper CM, Mann JW, Yunis JP, Phillips S, et al. Laparoscopic vs robotic intraperitoneal mesh repair for incisional hernia: an Americas Hernia Society Quality Collaborative Analysis. J Am Coll Surg. 2017;225(2):285–93.

17. Armijo P, Pratap A, Wang Y, Shostrom V, Oleynikov D. Robotic ventral hernia repair is not superior to laparoscopic: a national database review. Surg Endosc. 2017;19:1–6.

18. Bittner R, Bingener-Casey J, Dietz U, et al. Guidelines for laparoscopic treatment of ventral and incisional abdominal wall hernias (International Endohernia Society (IEHS)—part 1). Surg Endosc. 2014;28(1):2–29.

19. Guend H, Widmar M, Patel S, Nash GM, Paty PB, Guillem JG, et al. Developing a robotic colorectal cancer surgery program: understanding institutional and individual learning curves. Surg Endosc. 2017;31(7):2820–8.

20. Picerno T, Sloan NL, Escobar P, Ramirez PT. Bowel injury in robotic gynecologic surgery: risk factors and management options. A systematic review. Am J Obstet Gynecol. 2017;216(1):10–26.

21. Alemzadeh H, Raman J, Leveson N, Kalbarczyk Z, Iyer RK. Adverse events in robotic surgery: a retrospective study of 14 years of FDA data. PLoS One. 2016;11(4):e0151470.

22. Kokotovic D, Bisgaard T, Helgstrand F. Long-term recurrence and complications associated with elective incisional hernia repair. JAMA. 2016;316(15):1575–82.

Management of Adverse Events During Laparoscopic and Robotic Hernia Repair

14

Ciara R. Huntington, Jonathan D. Bouchez, and David A. Iannitti

Introduction

Over 350,000 ventral hernia repairs are performed annually each year in the United States, accounting for more than $3.2 billion in costs [1]. However, when adverse events occur during or following hernia repair, those costs increase dramatically, and patient quality of life is directly impacted [2–4]. Meticulous surgical technique and judgment is necessary to avoid or reduce the risk of adverse events during hernia repair. Every hernia surgeon must know how to appropriately treat complications when they arise. Herein, this chapter details the management of intraoperative and perioperative adverse events for the hernia surgeon.

Intraoperative Adverse Events

Incidence and Categorization of Intraoperative Adverse Events

The incidence of intraoperative complications during laparoscopic or robotic ventral hernia repair has a direct impact on long-term patient morbidity and mortality. As experience in laparoscopic surgery and subsequently robotic surgery has increased, surgeon comfort with these advanced techniques has increased. However, intraoperative events remain a significant concern during laparoscopic procedures despite progression of techniques [5]. Intraoperative events in complex laparoscopic procedures are associated with near-doubling of local and general morbidity at 41.2 vs. 18.0% ($p < 0.001$) and 32.9% vs. 17.2% ($p < 0.001$), respectively, for colorectal resection [5]. Additionally, the occurrence of major intraoperative events is associated with a twofold increase in 30-day readmission, an important metric in the era of outcome-based reimbursement [6].

Intraoperative complications may be categorized by whether or not their occurrence is a direct consequence of a surgeon's performance. The preoperative workup may help avoid or reduce the risk of intraoperative medical adverse events, such as cardiac arrhythmia or pulmonary embolism. Additional medical concerns of operation include risks associated with anesthesia and abdominal insufflation. Of surgical intraoperative adverse events, hernia surgeons are particularly concerned with management of iatrogenic bowel injury and enterotomy. The reality is that these events can occur despite the best efforts of even the most skilled surgeon.

C. R. Huntington · J. D. Bouchez
Department of Surgery, Carolinas Medical Center, Atrium Health, Charlotte, NC, USA

D. A. Iannitti (✉)
Division of Hepatobiliary and Pancreatic Surgery, Carolinas Medical Center, Atrium Health, Charlotte, NC, USA
e-mail: David.iannitti@atriumhealth.org

© Springer International Publishing AG, part of Springer Nature 2018
K. A. LeBlanc (ed.), *Laparoscopic and Robotic Incisional Hernia Repair*,
https://doi.org/10.1007/978-3-319-90737-6_14

Nonsurgical adverse events occur frequently and require teamwork and leadership to address; one of the most common nonsurgical events is equipment malfunctions [5]. Herein, management of commonly encountered medical and surgical intraoperative complications are discussed.

Acute Medical Intraoperative Adverse Events

General Anesthesia

Though laparoscopic hernia repair under local anesthesia has been described [7], general anesthesia for all robotic and laparoscopic hernia repairs remains the current standard. Significant physiologic changes occur during induction of anesthesia and the operation itself. It is a testament to the advancement and quality of anesthetic care that complication rates related to anesthesia are quite rare [5]. However, rapid identification and appropriate interventions of intraoperative acute medical concerns are essential to safe hernia repair.

Adverse Events during Abdominal Insufflation

Abdominal insufflation is necessary during laparoscopic procedures. This, however, is not a completely benign process and may result in hemodynamic instability [8]. Adverse events such as cardiac arrhythmia and hypercapnia can occur in conjunction with insertion of carbon dioxide gas into the peritoneal space [8, 9]. Slow insufflation of gas and maintainence of intra-abdominal pressures 15 mmHg or less may help reduce the incidence of sudden cardiopulmonary changes [10].

Insufflation with carbon dioxide results in vascular compression of the low-pressure venous system (decreasing systemic vascular resistance) with a subsequent 10–30% decrease in cardiac output [10]. The pressure of insufflation causes an upward displacement of the diaphragm, which may contribute to lower lung volumes and decreased cardiac preload [9]. Using the lowest insufflation pressures, which still achieves proper

visualization for a safe operation, can help to offset these effects. In healthy patients, the hemodynamic changes of pneumoperitoneum are generally well tolerated [10]. However, patients with intravascular volume depletion or other comorbidities are at higher risk for compromised blood flow within the abdominal organs and tissues [10].

Oliguria may also result from the physiologic changes secondary to pneumoperitoneum. Though low urine output has often been a driver for increased fluid administration within the operating room, it is typically not an indicator of decreased end-organ perfusion. Intraoperative oliguria during laparoscopy is usually self-limited, has no associated hemodynamic instability, and has similar serum creatinine and blood urea nitrogen to comparable open operations with normal intraoperative urine output [11, 12]. Additionally, oliguria secondary to pneumoperitoneum is often unaffected by increased resuscitation volumes [13].

Intraoperative Fluid Overload

Intraoperative fluid resuscitation is another potential source of complications during hernia repair. The over-administration of intravenous fluid, often driven by markers such as oliguria without hemodynamic change, may increase the chance of developing pulmonary edema postoperatively. Additionally, the fluid can induce bowel edema, making the operation more technically difficult and increasing the likelihood of postoperative ileus [14]. Most importantly, excessive intraoperative intravenous fluid administration is an independent risk factor for increased hospital mortality [15]. Fluid administration in the operating room should be goal directed and take into consideration the patients' comorbidities and effects of pneumoperitoneum.

Carbon Dioxide Embolism During Laparoscopy

In the event that insufflation is initiated with a Veress needle, improper placement into a blood vessel, rather than into the peritoneal space, may lead to bleeding or direct injection of carbon dioxide into the circulatory system creating gas embolus. Needle placement into the liver can increase this likelihood [16, 17]. The risk of injury is higher in patients with significant prior abdominal operations [18].

Outside the use of the Veress needle, carbon dioxide can be injected into the vasculature through any injured vessel, including within the abdominal wall. This makes inappropriate insufflation of carbon dioxide into the preperitoneal space a potential etiology for embolism. However, intravascular embolism may occur with routine insufflation of carbon dioxide into the abdomen, even when appropriately placed within the peritoneum [17].

Should carbon dioxide embolism occur, prompt recognition is necessary. Notably, many patients may have an embolism during operation, as identified on transesophageal echocardiography, including massive embolism, without ever suffering hemodynamic collapse [19]. A rapid rise in end-tidal carbon dioxide is the earliest and most accurate clue to recognize physiologically significant embolism [20].

Once a clinically significant embolism is identified, operative procedures should be immediately ceased. The abdomen should be de-sufflated and focus shifted to addressing the embolism. The patient should be repositioned to the left lateral decubitus position and placed in Trendelenburg to prevent embolus migration into the pulmonary arteries and creating an air lock [20]. Similar to other air embolisms, the carbon dioxide can be aspirated from the right atrium via a central venous catheter in the event of life-threatening hemodynamic change [21].

Intraoperative Cardiopulmonary Arrest

Finally, the most serious acute medical intraoperative complication of laparoscopic or robotic hernia surgery is cardiopulmonary arrest. During an acute arrest, the hernia repair should immediately cease. The abdomen should be rapidly de-sufflated. The use of robotic instrumentation may interfere with access to the patient and should be undocked in a rapid and orderly fashion. Sterility should be sacrificed because access to the patient is required. Standard resuscitation efforts should occur following this with utilization of the methods prescribed by Advanced Cardiac Life Support training, led in conjunction with the anesthesia team.

Acute Surgical Intraoperative Adverse Events

Hemorrhage

Diligent hemostasis is a basic tenet of good surgical technique and is necessary for optimal outcomes. Therefore, the surgeon requires knowledge of multiple modalities of hemorrhage control. This includes preventive measures as well as management techniques once bleeding is encountered.

Often, hernia reduction is accompanied by the need for lysis of adhesions. These adhesions especially when formed by omentum are well vascularized and tend to bleed. For this reason, division should not be performed utilizing blunt avulsion alone.

While prevention is the best strategy for hemostasis, unexpected bleeding may be encountered when surgeons embark on complex and/or re-operative hernia repairs. The surgeon must identify the source of the hemorrhage to properly address it; visualization is essential to control bleeding, which may be challenging during laparoscopy. Rapid assessment of the severity of hemorrhage must be conducted to assure appropriate interventions are chosen.

Typically, the first step in hemostasis is application of direct pressure. This can be performed by pressing a blunt laparoscopic instrument directly onto the bleeding source or clamping the vessel with a grasper if well visualized and risk to surrounding tissue is low. Direct pressure alone can help induce local hemostasis through platelet aggregation and fibrin formation. Alternatively, pressure can be used as a "stop-gap" in heavy bleeding to allow for suction and proper visualization in preparation for definitive hemostasis.

In addition to their utilization to prevent bleeding, energy devices can be used to address active hemorrhage. This is dependent, however, on a low rate of bleeding as both monopolar and bipolar become increasingly inefficient in the presence of pooling blood. They are also inappropriate for management of large-vessel bleeding.

The careful utilization of robotic scissors or any other electrosurgery device can aid significantly in hemostatic adhesiolysis. Due to the risk of subjecting surrounding tissues to thermal spread utilizing a monopolar device, a robotic or laparoscopic bipolar device should be considered when adhesions are numerous or tenacious. Furthermore, ultrasonic devices are available that utilize the piezoelectric effect to generate a heated blade by vibrating at 55,500 Hz due to rapid expansion and contraction of a ceramic element [22]. This, however, comes with an increased risk of transferring this thermal energy to an unintended area of tissue. In several studies, ultrasonic devices had higher rates of rebleeding when compared to bipolar vessel sealing devices and should be avoided [23, 24]. The introduction of robotic vessel sealers approved for vessels up to 7 mm has made this an attractive option for hemostasis [25].

Mechanical hemostasis is another widely utilized technique for hemorrhage control. At its most basic, the vessel can be addressed with intracorporeal suture ligation or a pre-tied endoscopic looped suture. Intracorporeal suture ligation requires the surgeon be able to rapidly perform the ligation in the setting of ongoing hemorrhage without causing further damage to the vessel or surrounding structures. Due to the amount of time required, especially for the novice, and the technical difficulty of the maneuver, this may not be the first choice for management of hemorrhage.

Mechanical devices such as an endoscopic clip applier or linear stapling device are an excellent option for hemostasis. Multiple varieties of mechanical clips can be utilized, including both 5 and 10 mm length as well as metallic and locking nonmetallic forms. In our practice, locking nonmetallic clips are preferred for laparoscopic vessel management. This is supported by higher burst pressures when utilizing plastic laparoscopic clips in vessels ranging from 4 to 5 mm [26]. While linear stapling devices are typically utilized in bowel resection, they are valuable

tools for management of large vessels that cannot be addressed with clips.

Proximal and distal vascular control is an essential concept for adequate hemostasis. In the event of a tangential injury to a vessel, this requires ligation of both ends of an injured vessel. Should the surgeon identify a complete vessel transection, both cut ends must be addressed for bleeding to stop.

A final tool in the surgeon's armamentarium is the utilization of various hemostatic agents. Some achieve hemostasis by providing a scaffolding made from matrix materials such as cellulose, which upon which blood can coagulate. Hemostatic agents also come in the format of procoagulants such as thrombin or fibrin glues, which directly induce coagulation. While these are an acceptable adjunct to other hemostatic techniques, they are rarely sufficient as solo agents for proper control of surgical bleeding.

Enterotomy: Incidence and Identification

Incisional ventral hernia repairs are often complicated by postoperative adhesions, incarcerated bowel, and distorted postsurgical anatomy, presenting technical challenges for the hernia surgeon. An iatrogenic enterotomy may therefore result from a difficult lysis of adhesions or injury induced during trocar insertion to the abdomen. In fact, this may be an unavoidable adverse event depending on the operative conditions. Upon creation of an unintended enterotomy for any reason, the original operative plan must be reconsidered and, in some cases, modified or aborted.

The most important consideration is identification of the enterotomy. Enterotomies occur in 2.6% of patients undergoing laparoscopic ventral hernia repair [27], but goes unrecognized in 21.8% of these patients [27]. An unrecognized enterotomy is associated with considerably higher risk of mortality in laparoscopic hernia repair, with a mortality rate of 7.7% compared with 1.7% when the enterotomy was recognized [28]. This necessitates diligent and meticulous evaluation of the bowel for any evidence of unintended injury.

Following identification, the enterotomy requires repair. For the experienced laparoscopic surgeon, this can be accomplished utilizing intracorporeal repair. Most small enterotomies can be repaired using two to three interrupted Lembert-fashion sutures in transverse orientation identical to open repair to prevent stricture of the bowel at the level of the enterotomy. Larger enterotomies or bowel resections required during operation may necessitate enteric anastomoses, which can be stapled or sewn depending on the technical capabilities of the surgeon and anatomic considerations.

Intraoperative Decision-Making After Iatrogenic Enterotomy

Following creation of an enterotomy, the definitive hernia repair plan must be reevaluated. The creation of the enterotomy directly affects the choice and timing of mesh placement. There is current controversy regarding the best practice of hernia repair in a contaminated field.

One option is to plan for delayed hernia repair. In this strategy, the enterotomy is repaired or bowel resected and anastomosed during the initial operation with definitive mesh-based repair performed in 2–6 days [27, 29]. In a limited case series utilizing delayed repair, there were no early mesh infections reported [29].

Some authors advocate for synthetic mesh placement despite iatrogenic enterotomy or other known sources of contamination. Carbonell et al. studied synthetic mesh placement with clean-contaminated and contaminated cases in open ventral hernia repair. In their series of 100 patients with synthetic mesh in contaminated fields, four patients required mesh removal. A total of 7.1% of clean-contaminated cases and 19.0% of contaminated cases developed surgical site infections by 30 days [30].

Based on recommendations from the Ventral Hernia Working Group and other authors, our practice is often to proceed with definitive hernia repair with biologic mesh for high risk, complex repairs [31]. Though the research into long-term outcomes continues, a case series of 223 high-risk patients with hernia repairs in mostly contaminated cases demonstrated <1% mesh removal and recurrence rates of 31.8%—however, this varied significantly by type of biologic mesh placed with lowest rates of 14.7% achieved in an acellular porcine dermal mesh [32]. This approach obviates the need for reoperation, allows for mesh reinforcement of the hernia repair, and removes the risk of prosthetic infection requiring explanation. This has facilitated single-stage reconstruction in high-risk patients with a success rate greater than 70% after 24 months in one study [33].

When an inadvertent enterotomy is created during hernia repair, surgeons should balance the risks of reoperation, mesh infection, and hernia recurrence when choosing an approach. Risks and benefits exist to each option, and surgeons should develop their own personal algorithm prior to complex repairs and discuss this preoperatively with their high-risk patients.

Conversion to Open

When adverse intraoperative events cannot be safely managed via robotic or laparoscopic techniques, the surgeon should elect to convert to an open operation. The decision point at which this shift becomes necessary is individualized to the surgeon and their level of experience with the associated minimally invasive technique. The reported rates of conversion for adverse events has significantly decreased over time, likely secondary to increased operator comfort and experience with laparoscopy [5]. Surgeons must balance their ability to rectify the complication and maintain the benefits of laparoscopic surgery against the potential technical benefit of open exposure. During surgeons' learning curve in robotic surgery, conversion to traditional laparoscopy is also an option.

If it is unsafe to continue the operation in the current manner, conversion to an open operation should occur without delay. This can be performed through a midline incision or through a subcostal incision as has been described in bariatric literature [34]. Should the surgeon encounter an injury in which they are not experienced, they should make every effort to consult an expert in that area of surgical anatomy and join him or her in the operating room, if available.

Postoperative Adverse Events

Common Postoperative Complications After Hernia Repair

Common inguinal hernia repair postoperative adverse events include urinary retention (2.2–2.8%), urinary tract infection (0.4–1.0%), orchitis (1.1–1.4%), surgical site infection (1.0–1.4%), neuralgia and chronic pain (3.6–4.6%), seroma (3.0–9.0%), and hernia recurrence (4.9–10%), as described in randomized multicenter study from the Veteran's Affairs hospitals [35]. The incidence of these complications depends on patient risk factors, surgeon experience, and operative approach. Early in its development, laparoscopic surgery was associated with higher rates of life-threatening complications and recurrence, but more recent evidence has demonstrated equivalent long-term outcomes in experienced hands with recurrence rates of 2.7% laparoscopic and 3.1% open repair ($p = 0.2$), as described in a Cochrane Systematic Review of the topic [36].

Ventral hernia also has a range of complications, including but not limited to immediate postoperative cardiopulmonary complications, seroma, ileus, surgical site infection, mesh infection, chronic pain, and recurrence. In one study of laparoscopic ventral hernia repair, the overall rate of complications was 13.2%, including 2.2% prolonged seroma and 3.2% prolonged ileus with an average recurrence rate of 4.7% at mean 20 month follow-up [37]. Laparoscopic approaches, compared to open approach, improve rates of surgical site infection. This is especially true in diabetic and morbidly obese patients, where laparoscopic repairs have been shown to have lower rates of postoperative wound infections [38–42].

Robotic-Assisted Laparoscopic Hernia Repairs: Evidence and Outcomes

In a growing body of literature, outcomes after robotic-assisted laparoscopic ventral hernia repair have been compared to traditional laparoscopy. Robotic-assisted repair with intraperitoneal mesh placement appears to have a longer operative time than traditional laparoscopy (operative time >2 h 47% vs. 31%, $p < 0.05$), but shorter hospital length of stay (median 1 vs. 0 days; interquartile range 3.0; $p < 0.001$) and equivalent rate of wound occurrences requiring procedural intervention (0% vs. 1%, $p = 1.0$) [43].

Robotic-assisted laparoscopic hernia repair may also allow surgeons to approach more complex hernias via a minimally invasive approach. In a study examining 90-day outcomes in 102 patients who underwent transversus abdominis release in ventral hernia repair (76 open, 26 robotic), robotic-assisted had a longer mean operative time (287 ± 121 vs. 365 ± 78 min, $P < 0.01$), but lower overall morbidity (39.2 vs. 19.2%, $P = 0.09$) and median length of stay (6 days, 95% CI 5.9–8.3 vs. 3 days, 95% CI 3.2–4.3) compared to the open approach [44].

Chronic Pain After Suprapubic Ventral or Inguinal Hernia Repair

Risk Factors and Prediction

As recurrence rates stabilize, quality of life is becoming a critical marker of a successful hernia operation [45]. Except in those patients who had >10 tacks used to fix their mesh, there is no difference in long-term overall quality of life scores among patients who undergo open modified Lichtenstein, laparoscopic extraperitoneal or laparoscopic preperitoneal inguinal hernia repair in a prospective, international comparative study [46]. The presence of higher preoperative pain scores, female sex, younger age, bilateral hernias, and recurrent hernias are significant risk factors for higher rates of short- and long-term postoperative groin pain after inguinal hernia repair [45–47]. Despite advantage for bilateral and recurrent hernias, only approximately 15% of inguinal hernias are fixed via a laparoscopic approach in the United States, with even lower frequencies in Japan and the United Kingdom (4% of groin hernias repairs) [48]. However, a Cochrane meta-analysis of 41 studies demonstrated that laparoscopic inguinal hernia repair has additional quality of life advantages over an open repair, with patients reporting less narcotic usage, faster return to work and daily activities, and less postoperative pain/numbness [36].

With robotic assistance, a laparoscopic approach to inguinal hernia repair may become more accessible to surgeons. A study of 82 patients with 159 inguinal hernias examined the long-term outcomes after robotic-assisted transabdominal preperitoneal (TAPP) repair. With an average operative time of 99 min, the authors found low rates of recurrence and chronic pain in those surveyed 12–36 months after surgery [49].

Strategies for Chronic Pain Risk Mitigation and Intervention

Between 6 and 24% of patients following inguinal hernia repair report chronic postoperative pain that interferes with daily activities [50–52]. Careful preoperative consent and risk stratification can be performed with mobile apps and clinical algorithms [45]. If patients have high preoperative pain scores, surgeons must ensure that they have counseled patients appropriately that their pain may not be ameliorated despite a successful hernia operation.

During inguinal hernia, surgeons should be knowledgeable about the location of nerves in the inguinal region, though specific intraoperative nerve identification has not been shown to reduce the occurrence of postoperative neuropathic pain [53]. The ilioinguinal and iliohypogastric nerves can be identified just under the external oblique muscle, while the genital branch of the genitofemoral nerve runs with the cord structures. Nerves can be irritated or damaged by thermal injury from electrocautery or directly by suture, tacks, or placement of mesh [54]. Use of robotic-assisted techniques may have improved visualization, but these structures can still be obscured by intra-abdominal obesity or adhesions.

When fixating mesh, robotic-assisted laparoscopic surgeons have the option of suture, tack, or glue fixation. The so-called triangle of pain (defined by the iliopubic tract and spermatic vessels) should be avoided, as the lateral femoral cutaneous nerves, femoral nerve, and genitofemoral can be encountered in this region. Palpation of the anterior iliac spine and avoiding tack placement lateral to this can also aid in reducing postoperative pain.

If patients have significant, focal pain in the postoperative period, the surgeon should suspect damage or injury to one of the nerves of the groin, and immediate diagnostic laparoscopy, with potential tack removal, should be considered.

Patients who have persistent pain 3–6 months after hernia repair cause concern for the development of chronic neuropathic pain [55]. If trigger point injections with local anesthesia and medical alternatives do not improve the patient's pain score, then other interventions should be considered [56]. One approach is a combined open and laparoscopic approach, where a diagnostic laparoscopy, revisional hernia repair, explanation of previous mesh, and triple neurectomy can be utilized to address the patient's chronic pain [54].

Chronic Pain After Ventral Hernia Repair

Pain is important consideration after ventral and incisional hernia repair as well. In a study of 887 patients undergoing complex ventral hernia repair, older age was protective against chronic pain (odds ratio 0.98, $p < 0.03$), while preoperative pain, recurrent hernia repair, and female sex increased risk [57]. Notably, presence of pain at 1 month was a strong predictor of chronic pain at 1-year follow-up (OR = 2.6, $p < 0.0001$) [57].

Notably for laparoscopic approaches, laparoscopic ventral hernia may be associated with a short-term decrease in quality life, perhaps due to mesh fixation methods (such as myriads of tacks) or pain secondary to a bridged hernia defect without fascial closure [2]. However, hospital length of stay and infection rates remain lower in laparoscopic repairs than in open approaches [2].

Surgical Site and Mesh Infection: The Laparoscopic Advantage

Surgical Site Infection Risk Factors and Definition

Laparoscopic hernia surgery reduces the rate of surgical site infections (SSIs) compared to an open approach [58]. Given the cost, morbidity, and increased risk of recurrence after surgical site infection, a laparoscopic or robotic-assisted laparoscopic approach may be recommended for patients with obesity, diabetes, immunosuppression, or other significant risk factors for SSI [41, 59].

With increased focus on patient-centered outcomes and quality-based outcomes, surgical site infections have taken center stage for insurance, society, and institutional quality programs. Of the 80 million Americans undergoing a surgical procedure, almost 1.9% will be diagnosed with a surgical site infection [60]. While the use of mesh, especially in a hernia with defect size >10 cm, has been shown to be an independent risk factor for the development of wound-related complications, mesh significantly reduces the risk of hernia recurrence [61]. In today's era of hernia surgery, mesh has been shown to be superior to suture only repair and is the standard of care [62]. Yet, when mesh infection occurs a patient in a complex abdomen, the consequences can be expensive and dire. In a study from the authors' institution, wound-related complications in a complex open ventral hernia population increased mean hospital charges by more than $27,000 per patient, with follow-up charges increased from an average of $1393 for those patients without wound complications to $20,232 per wound infection and $63,389 per mesh infection [63]. These conservative estimates did not include charges related to lab tests, medications, radiologic studies, and at home nursing care over the ensuing year. Patients and their families also saw high readmission rates and a negative impact on quality of life as measured by pain and activity limitations at 6-month follow-up [63]. This study and others like it underscores the need to prevent wound infections, and for high-risk patients, choosing a laparoscopic or robotically assisted laparoscopic repair may play a role in prevention. A meta-analysis including 526 patients demonstrated that laparoscopic ventral hernia had significantly fewer wound infections and fewer mesh infections requiring removal than open ventral hernia repair [64].

Mesh Infection

One of the dreaded complications of a complex ventral hernia repair with synthetic mesh is a mesh infection. The Center for Disease Control defines surgical site infection as a soft tissue infection at the surgical site occurring within 30 days of surgery and extends that definition to 90 days for surgeries with implantable mesh [65] (Table 14.1). However, the literature demonstrates that mesh infections can present in a delayed and insidious fashion [66]. In one case series of patients with infected expanded polytetrafluoroethylene (ePTFE) mesh, patients presented with mesh infections in a range of 10–480 days after surgery, mean 70 days [66].

Mesh infections may lead to significant morbidity including reoperation, long-term antibiotics, and hernia recurrence. The diagnosis of a mesh infection may be determined by systemic signs of infection (fevers, chills, and classic signs of infection including *calor, rubor, dolor,* and induration) and/or purulent drainage from the incision. However, the diagnosis often requires a CT scan to determine the presence of deep space infection and air/fluid collection above or below the mesh. Objective tests demonstrating ongoing systemic inflammation such as a C-reactive protein (CRP) or erythrocyte sedimentation rate (ESR) can be useful to diagnosis indolent infections [67]. With hundreds of biologic, bioabsorbable, absorbable synthetic, and permanent synthetic mesh available, considerable debate continues as the best position and type of mesh to utilize for hernia repairs. Once infected, the type of implanted mesh will partly determine the optimal treatment. Depending on the type of mesh, complexity of the hernia repair, type of bacterial infection, and patient risk factors, nonoperative treatment—mesh salvage—may be possible [68]. In most cases, mesh salvage will require long-term suppressive antibiotics and percutaneous

Table 14.1 CDC strategies for prevention of surgical site infection

Timing of strategy	Strength of recommendation
Preoperative	
Shower with soap or antiseptic night before surgery	Category IB—strong recommendation
Preoperative smoking cessation before surgery (>3 weeks before surgery suggested)	Category IA—strong recommendation
Intraoperative	
Use alcohol-based antiseptic agent	Category IA—strong recommendation
Maintain normothermia	Category IA—strong recommendation
For patients with normal pulmonary function, administer increased F_{IO_2} during surgery and in the immediate postoperative period	Category IA—strong recommendation
Administer preoperative antibiotics specific to case and recommendation, so that a bactericidal tissue level is achieved prior to incision	Category IB—strong recommendation
Perioperative	
Target glucose levels <200 mg/dL in patients with and without diabetes	Category IA—strong recommendation
Do not apply antimicrobial ointments to incision	Category IB—strong recommendation
Do not continue preoperative antibiotics after incisions is closed	Category IA—strong recommendation

Data from:
Centers for Disease Control (CDC) and Prevention Guideline for the Prevention of Surgical Site Infection, 2017. *JAMA Surg. Published March 3, 2017*
The clinical impact of smoking and smoking cessation: a systematic review and meta-analysis. Archive of Surgery. 2012;147(4):373–83

drainage of any residual fluid collection via CT-guided drain. Cultures are paramount to guide antibiotic selection. In the authors' experience, particularly tenacious infections, such as fungal infections or methicillin-resistant *Staphylococcus aureus* (MRSA), may require mesh excision. Early infectious disease consultation is recommended. Biofilm formation may prevent the penetration of antibiotics, and there-fore mesh salvage may not be possible with mesh with construction conducive to allowing formation of biofilms or trapping infection, including mesh with small pores, woven threads such as PTFE, or unhelpful coatings [67, 69, 70]. The use of antibiotic coated meshes has an unclear role in reducing the incidence of mesh infection [71]. Infection may have a greater chance of clearance when meshes are wide-pore, monofilament, polypropylene, and lighter-weight compared to other meshes [67, 69, 70].

While biologic meshes can become infected with the same frequency that synthetic meshes, mesh excision is usually not required. Most biologic meshes, as a result of their intrinsic properties, are more able to clear infection with antibiotics alone. Though there is no Level 1 evidence to guide decision-making, a body of literature supports the use of biologic mesh in complex, contaminated cases [72]. In one large case series of >230 complex, contaminated open ventral hernia repairs utilizing biologic mesh, the rate of mesh infection requiring excision was less than 1% [32]. Recurrence rates are higher with biologic mesh compared with synthetic. However, when mesh infection occurs in synthetic mesh, the chances of mesh infection and required excision is high, and this risk/benefit analysis must be strongly considered preoperatively. Previous research from our institution has demonstrated the average cost of a mesh infection is more than $100,000 with a year follow-up [25, 26], and a patient with a synthetic mesh infection after ventral hernia repair has an 9.9% mesh salvage rate at 36 months with the remainder requiring mesh explantation [23, 27].

Laparoscopy, as with robotic-assisted surgery, decreases the risk of mesh infection substantially compared with an open approach; nonetheless, prevention of infection is critical.

Hernia Recurrence

Risk Factors for Recurrence
Surgeons are aware of the many risk factors for wound dehiscence and hernia recurrence. These include: surgical technique, chronic steroid use,

obesity, chronic cough, connective tissue disorders, emergent surgery, hematoma, protein deficiency, and perhaps mostly important to hernia surgeons: wound infection. Wound infection is particularly important to the hernia surgeon. Tobacco use, obesity, diabetes, surgical technique, and intraoperative contamination are important risk factors for infection leading to recurrence [3, 4, 35, 39, 59, 61, 64, 68, 69, 73–77].

While infection is a significant risk for hernia recurrence, even in clean cases, diabetic patients have higher rates of recurrence compared to nondiabetic patients [63, 75, 78]. In one multicenter study, matched diabetic patients had 12% rate of hernia recurrence compared to less than 7% for nondiabetic patients [40]. Tobacco use and higher body mass index (BMI) have also been linked to hernia recurrence. Preoperative modification of comorbidities is paramount, before leading to costly infection and recurrence [3].

Evaluation for Recurrence

Recurrence can be challenging to diagnose in the immediate postoperative setting for patients who have undergone a robotic-assisted laparoscopic hernia repair, as many patients will naturally develop a seroma that fills the potential space previously filled by their hernia sac. To many patients, this bulge may feel like a recurrent hernia. Patients should be warned of this common postoperative finding; over time, most postoperative seromas disappear without intervention [42].

However, recurrence may occur at any time point postoperatively. Patients are often the first to correctly make the diagnosis. In one study of patients with average follow-up of 46 months after incisional hernia repair, a patient-reported postoperative "bulge" had 81% sensitivity and 85% specificity for hernia recurrence [79]. Imaging can confirm the diagnosis, and a CT scan may be needed if re-repair is contemplated. Timing of repair depends on the presence of infection, obstruction, and patient preference. In the face of recurrent repair, surgeons should obtain previous operative notes, partner with patients to address modifiable preoperative risk factors, and plan an approach that takes into con-

sideration the altered tissue planes and previous mesh that may exist intra-abdominally.

Conclusion

Managing Adverse Events: An Ounce of Prevention

"The only surgeon without complications is the one who does not operate" states the surgical adage. While many adverse events cannot be avoided, many hernia centers are realizing the importance of preoperative optimization to mitigate the risk of postoperative complication. While risk factors may be easily identified and listed, the next step requires adequately and comprehensively *modifying* those risk factors. To do this, surgeons, patients, perioperative medicine specialists, and primary care providers should form partnerships for better surgical outcomes. When a surgeon prioritizes preoperative preparation, patients are motivated to complete preoperative goals such as smoking cessation and hyperglycemia management in order to undergo elective hernia repair. Preoperative optimization is necessary and is worth the upfront investment of resources.

Wound-related complications increased mean hospital charges by more than $27,000 per patient, with follow-up charges increased from an average of $1393 for those patients without wound complications to $20,232 per wound infection and $63,389 per mesh infection [63]. These conservative estimates do not include additional charges for blood work, medications, radiologic studies, and nursing care over the ensuing year. Not surprisingly, wound-related complications had a significant negative impact on quality of life as measured by pain and activity limitations at 6-month follow-up [63].

Managing adverse events begins in the preoperative clinic visit. Patients should undergo systematic needs assessment and coordinated interventions to reduce postoperative complications including evidence-based inventions such as preoperative nutritional support, improved glucose control, smoking cessation, preoperative skin cleaning, nasal decolonization of MRSA, and weight loss [40, 75, 80–85]. Except in cases of emergency, surgeons should not offer elective hernia repairs to patients with uncontrolled diabetes (a goal would be HbA1c < 7.5), active tobacco use, or morbid obesity without demonstration of some weight loss. Diabetic patients undergoing general and hernia surgery have delayed wound healing, increased complications, and prolonged hospital stays [31, 75, 76, 78, 85, 86]. Modest weight loss impacts health status and postoperative outcomes; for each kilogram of excess body fat lost, patients in one study had 16% reduction in their risk of developing diabetes [87]. Obesity, smoking, and controlling diabetes represent a comorbidity that can be optimized with subsequent improvement in postoperative outcomes [63, 88]. Surgery is a "teachable moment" for some preventable comorbidities—as shown in one study, where more than 8% of smokers reported quitting smoking due to a surgeon's intervention [89].

With careful surgical planning, surgeons may rarely have to turn to the techniques addressed in this chapter. However, when intraoperative or postoperative adverse events occur, the techniques discussed herein may guide the next steps forward to recovery.

References

1. Poulose BK, Shelton J, Phillips S, Moore D, Nealon W, Penson D, Beck W, Holzman MD. Epidemiology and cost of ventral hernia repair: making the case for hernia research. Hernia. 2012;16:179–83.
2. Colavita PD, Tsirline VB, Belyansky I, Walters AL, Lincourt AE, Sing RF, Heniford BT. Prospective, long-term comparison of quality of life in laparoscopic versus open ventral hernia repair. Ann Surg. 2012;256:714–23.
3. Cox TC, Blair LJ, Huntington CR, Colavita PD, Prasad T, Lincourt AE, Heniford BT, Augenstein VA. The cost of preventable comorbidities on wound complications in open ventral hernia repair. J Surg Res. 2016;206:214–22.
4. Plymale MA, Ragulojan R, Davenport DL, Roth JS. Ventral and incisional hernia: the cost of comorbidities and complications. Surg Endosc. 2017;31:341–51.
5. Kambakamba P, Dindo D, Nocito A, Clavien PA, Seifert B, Schäfer M, Hahnloser D. Intraoperative

adverse events during laparoscopic colorectal resection—better laparoscopic treatment but unchanged incidence. Lessons learnt from a Swiss multi-institutional analysis of 3,928 patients. Langenbeck's Arch Surg. 2014;399:297–305.
6. Nandan AR, Bohnen JD, Chang DC, Yeh DD, Lee J, Velmahos GC, Kaafarani HMA. The impact of major intraoperative adverse events on hospital readmissions. Am J Surg. 2017;213:10–7.
7. Ferzli G, Sayad P, Vasisht B. The feasibility of laparoscopic extraperitoneal hernia repair under local anesthesia. Surg Endosc. 1999;13:588–90.
8. O'Malley C, Cunningham AJ. Physiologic changes during laparoscopy. Anesthesiol Clin North Am. 2001;19:1–19.
9. Srivastava A, Niranjan A. Secrets of safe laparoscopic surgery: anaesthetic and surgical considerations. J Minim Access Surg. 2010;6:91–4.
10. Gutt CN, Oniu T, Mehrabi A, Schemmer P, Kashfi A, Kraus T, Büchler MW. Circulatory and respiratory complications of carbon dioxide insufflation. Dig Surg. 2004;21:95–105.
11. Chang DT, Kirsch AJ, Sawczuk IS. Oliguria during laparoscopic surgery. J Endourol. 1994;8:349–52.
12. Nguyen NT, Perez RV, Fleming N, Rivers R, Wolfe BM. Effect of prolonged pneumoperitoneum on intraoperative urine output during laparoscopic gastric bypass. J Am Coll Surg. 2002;195:476–83.
13. Matot I, Paskaleva R, Eid L, Cohen K, Khalaileh A, Elazary R, Keidar A. Effect of the volume of fluids administered on intraoperative oliguria in laparoscopic bariatric surgery: a randomized controlled trial. Arch Surg. 2012;147:228–34.
14. Thacker JKMM, Mountford WK, Ernst FR, Krukas MR, Mythen M (Monty) GMG. Perioperative fluid utilization variability and association with outcomes: considerations for enhanced recovery efforts in sample US surgical populations. Ann Surg. 2016;263:502–10.
15. Silva JM, de Oliveira AMRR, Nogueira FAM, et al. The effect of excess fluid balance on the mortality rate of surgical patients: a multicenter prospective study. Crit Care. 2013;17:R288.
16. Yuval JB, Chapchay K, Mazeh H. Carbon dioxide embolism following veress needle laparoscopic adrenalectomy. https://doi.org/10.4293/CRSLS.2014.00236.
17. Park EY, Kwon JY, Kim KJ. Carbon dioxide embolism during laparoscopic surgery. Yonsei Med J. 2012;53:459–66.
18. Azevedo JLMC, Azevedo OC, Miyahira SA, et al. Injuries caused by Veress needle insertion for creation of pneumoperitoneum: a systematic literature review. Surg Endosc. 2009;23:1428–32.
19. Kim CS, Kim JY, Kwon J-Y, Choi SH, Na S, An J, Kim KJ. Venous air embolism during total laparoscopic hysterectomy: comparison to total abdominal hysterectomy. Anesthesiology. 2009;111:50–4.
20. Mirski MA, Lele AV, Fitzsimmons L, Toung TJ, Warltier DC, Mirski MA, Lele AV. Diagnosis and

treatment of vascular air embolism. Anesthesiology. 2007;106:164–77.

21. Prasad Upadhyay S. Near fatal carbon dioxide embolism during laparoscopy and its successful aspiration using ultrasound guided catheter. J Anesth Intensive Care Med. 2016;1:1–4.

22. Bittner JG, Varela E, Herron D. Ultrasonic energy systems. In: Feldman LS, Fuchshuber P, Jones DB, editors. The SAGES manual on the fundamental use of surgical energy (FUSE). New York: Springer; 2012. p. 123–32.

23. Takada M, Ichihara T, Kuroda Y. Comparative study of electrothermal bipolar vessel sealer and ultrasonic coagulating shears in laparoscopic colectomy. Surg Endosc. 2005;19:226–8.

24. Campagnacci R, De Sanctis A, Baldarelli M, Rimini M, Lezoche G, Guerrieri M. Electrothermal bipolar vessel sealing device vs. ultrasonic coagulating shears in laparoscopic colectomies: a comparative study. Surg Endosc. 2007;21:1526–31.

25. Lambrou N, Diaz RE, Hinoul P, Parris D, Shoemaker K, Yoo A, Schwiers M. Strategies to optimize the performance of robotic-assisted laparoscopic hysterectomy. Facts Views Vis Obgyn. 2014;6:133–42.

26. Harold KL, Pollinger H, Matthews BD, Kercher KW, Sing RF, Heniford BT. Comparison of ultrasonic energy, bipolar thermal energy, and vascular clips for the hemostasis of small-, medium-, and large-sized arteries. Surg Endosc. 2003;17:1228–30.

27. Tintinu AJ, Asonganyi WA, Turner PL. Staged laparoscopic ventral and incisional hernia repair when faced with enterotomy or suspicion of an enterotomy. J Natl Med Assoc. 2012;104:202–10.

28. LeBlanc KA, Elieson MJ, Corder JM. Enterotomy and mortality rates of laparoscopic incisional and ventral hernia repair: a review of the literature. JSLS. 2007;11:408–14.

29. Lederman AB, Ramshaw BJ. A short-term delayed approach to laparoscopic ventral hernia when injury is suspected. Surg Innov. 2005;12:31–5.

30. Carbonell AM, Criss CN, Cobb WS, Novitsky YW, Rosen MJ. Outcomes of synthetic mesh in contaminated ventral hernia repairs. J Am Coll Surg. 2013;217:991–8.

31. Krpata DM, Blatnik JA, Novitsky YW, Rosen MJ. Evaluation of high-risk, comorbid patients undergoing open ventral hernia repair with synthetic mesh. Surgery. 2013;153:120–5.

32. Huntington CR, Cox TC, Blair LJ, Schell S, Randolph D, Prasad T, Lincourt A, Heniford BT, Augenstein VA. Biologic mesh in ventral hernia repair: outcomes, recurrence, and charge analysis. Surgery. 2016;160:1517–27.

33. Itani KMF, Rosen M, Vargo D, Awad SS, Denoto G, Butler CE. Prospective study of single-stage repair of contaminated hernias using a biologic porcine tissue matrix: the RICH study. Surgery. 2012;152:498–505.

34. Jones KB. When and how to "open" in laparoscopic or robotic surgery. Obes Surg. 2016;26:891–5.

35. Neumayer L, Giobbie-Hurder A, Jonasson O, Fitzgibbons R, Dunlop D, Gibbs J, Reda D, Henderson W, Veterans Affairs Cooperative Studies Program 456 Investigators. Open mesh versus laparoscopic mesh repair of inguinal hernia. N Engl J Med. 2004;350:1819–27.

36. McCormack K, Scott NW, Go PM, Ross S, Grant AM. Laparoscopic techniques versus open techniques for inguinal hernia repair. Cochrane Database Syst Rev. 2003;(1):CD001785.

37. Heniford BT, Park A, Ramshaw BJ, Voeller G. Laparoscopic ventral and incisional hernia repair in 407 patients. J Am Coll Surg. 2000;190:645–50.

38. Arita NA, Nguyen MT, Nguyen DH, Berger RL, Lew DF, Suliburk JT, Askenasy EP, Kao LS, Liang MK. Laparoscopic repair reduces incidence of surgical site infections for all ventral hernias. Surg Endosc. 2015;29:1769–80.

39. Finan KR, Vick CC, Kiefe CI, Neumayer L, Hawn MT. Predictors of wound infection in ventral hernia repair. Am J Surg. 2005;190:676–81.

40. Brahmbhatt R, Carter SA, Hicks SC, Berger DH, Liang MK. Identifying risk factors for surgical site complications after laparoscopic ventral hernia repair: evaluation of the ventral hernia working group grading system. Surg Infect. 2014;15:187–93.

41. Huntington C, Gamble J, Blair L, Cox T, Prasad T, Lincourt A, Augenstein V, Heniford BT. Quantification of the effect of diabetes mellitus on ventral hernia repair: results from two national registries. Am Surg. 2016;82:661–71.

42. Heniford BT, Park A, Ramshaw BJ, Voeller G. Laparoscopic repair of ventral hernias: nine years' experience with 850 consecutive hernias. Ann Surg. 2003;238:391–9; discussion 399–400

43. Prabhu AS, Dickens EO, Copper CM, Mann JW, Yunis JP, Phillips S, Huang L-C, Poulose BK, Rosen MJ. Laparoscopic vs robotic intraperitoneal mesh repair for incisional hernia: an Americas Hernia Society Quality Collaborative Analysis. J Am Coll Surg. 2017;225:285. https://doi.org/10.1016/j.jamcollsurg.2017.04.011.

44. Bittner JG, Alrefai S, Vy M, Mabe M, Del Prado PAR, Clingempeel NL. Comparative analysis of open and robotic transversus abdominis release for ventral hernia repair. Surg Endosc. 2017;32:727. https://doi.org/10.1007/s00464-017-5729-0.

45. Belyansky I, Tsirline VB, Walters AL, Colavita PD, Zemlyak AY, Lincourt AE, Heniford BT. Algorithmic prediction of chronic pain after an inguinal hernia repair. New York: International Hernia Congress; 2012.

46. Belyansky I, Tsirline VB, Klima DA, Walters AL, Lincourt AE, Heniford TB. Prospective, comparative study of postoperative quality of life in TEP, TAPP, and modified lichtenstein repairs. Ann Surg. 2011;254:709–15.

47. Tsirline VB, Colavita PD, Belyansky I, Zemlyak AY, Lincourt AE, Heniford BT. Preoperative pain is the strongest predictor of postoperative pain and

diminished quality of life after ventral hernia repair. Am Surg. 2013;79:829–36.

48. Kulacoglu H. Current options in inguinal hernia repair in adult patients. Hippokratia. 2011;15:223–31.

49. Iraniha A, Peloquin J. Long-term quality of life and outcomes following robotic assisted TAPP inguinal hernia repair. J Robot Surg. 2017. https://doi.org/10.1007/s11701-017-0727-8.

50. Rosenberg J, Bisgaard T, Kehlet H, Wara P, Asmussen T, Juul P, Strand L, Andersen FH, Bay-Nielsen M, Danish Hernia Database. Danish hernia database recommendations for the management of inguinal and femoral hernia in adults. Dan Med Bull. 2011;58:C4243.

51. Jenkins JT, O'Dwyer PJ. Inguinal hernias. BMJ. 2008;336:269–72.

52. Fränneby U, Sandblom G, Nordin P, Nyrén O, Gunnarsson U. Risk factors for long-term pain after hernia surgery. Ann Surg. 2006;244:212–9.

53. Bischoff JM, Aasvang EK, Kehlet H, Werner MU. Does nerve identification during open inguinal herniorrhaphy reduce the risk of nerve damage and persistent pain? Hernia. 2012;16:573–7.

54. Keller JE, Stefanidis D, Dolce CJ, Iannitti DA, Kercher KW, Heniford BT. Combined open and laparoscopic approach to chronic pain after inguinal hernia repair. Am Surg. 2008;74:695–700; discussion 700–1

55. Reddi D, Curran N. Chronic pain after surgery: pathophysiology, risk factors and prevention. Postgrad Med J. 2014;90:222–7. quiz 226

56. Callesen T. Inguinal hernia repair: anaesthesia, pain and convalescence. Dan Med Bull. 2003;50:203–18.

57. Cox TC, Huntington CR, Blair LJ, Prasad T, Lincourt AE, Heniford BT, Augenstein VA. Predictive modeling for chronic pain after ventral hernia repair. Am J Surg. 2016;212:501–10.

58. Al Chalabi H, Larkin J, Mehigan B, McCormick P. A systematic review of laparoscopic versus open abdominal incisional hernia repair, with meta-analysis of randomized controlled trials. Int J Surg. 2015;20:65–74.

59. Novitsky YW, Cobb WS, Kercher KW, Matthews BD, Sing RF, Heniford BT. Laparoscopic ventral hernia repair in obese patients. Arch Surg. 2006;141:57.

60. Berríos-Torres SI, Umscheid CA, Bratzler DW, et al. Centers for disease control and prevention guideline for the prevention of surgical site infection, 2017. JAMA Surg. 2017;468:45–51.

61. Ejaz A, Schmidt C, Johnston FM, Frank SM, Pawlik TM. Risk factors and prediction model for inpatient surgical site infection after major abdominal surgery. J Surg Res. 2017;217:153. https://doi.org/10.1016/j.jss.2017.05.018.

62. Luijendijk RW, Hop WCJ, van den Tol MP, et al. A comparison of suture repair with mesh repair for incisional hernia. N Engl J Med. 2000;343:392–8.

63. Colavita PD, Zemlyak AY, Burton PV, Dacey KT, Walters AL, Lincourt AE, Tsirline VE, Kercher KW, Heniford B. The expansive cost of wound complica-

tions after ventral hernia repair. In: American College of Surgeons 2013 Clinical Congress, Washington DC, October 7th; 2013.

64. Forbes SS, Eskicioglu C, McLeod RS, Okrainec A. Meta-analysis of randomized controlled trials comparing open and laparoscopic ventral and incisional hernia repair with mesh. Br J Surg. 2009;96:851–8.

65. Horan TC, Gaynes RP, Martone WJ, Jarvis WR, Emori TG. CDC definitions of nosocomial surgical site infections, 1992: a modification of CDC definitions of surgical wound infections. Infect Control Hosp Epidemiol. 1992;13:606–8.

66. Paton BL, Novitsky YW, Zerey M, Sing RF, Kercher KW, Heniford BT. Management of infections of polytetrafluoroethylene-based mesh. Surg Infect. 2007;8:337–41.

67. Narkhede R, Shah NM, Dalal PR, Mangukia C, Dholaria S. Postoperative mesh infection-still a concern in laparoscopic era. Indian J Surg. 2015;77:322–6.

68. Sanchez VM, Abi-Haidar YE, Itani KMF. Mesh infection in ventral incisional hernia repair: incidence, contributing factors, and treatment. Surg Infect. 2011;12:205–10.

69. Leber GE, Garb JL, Alexander AI, Reed WP. Long-term complications associated with prosthetic repair of incisional hernias. Arch Surg. 1998;133:378–82.

70. Robinson TN, Clarke JH, Schoen J, Walsh MD. Major mesh-related complications following hernia repair. Surg Endosc. 2005;19:1556–60.

71. Yabanoğlu H, Arer İM, Çalıskan K. The effect of the use of synthetic mesh soaked in antibiotic solution on the rate of graft infection in ventral hernias: a prospective randomized study. Int Surg. 2015;100:1040–7.

72. Darehzereshki A, Goldfarb M, Zehetner J, Moazzez A, Lipham JC, Mason RJ, Katkhouda N. Biologic versus nonbiologic mesh in ventral hernia repair: a systematic review and meta-analysis. World J Surg. 2014;38:40–50.

73. Sørensen LT. Wound healing and infection in surgery: the clinical impact of smoking and smoking cessation: a systematic review and meta-analysis. Arch Surg. 2012;147:373.

74. Olsen MA, Nickel KB, Wallace AE, Mines D, Fraser VJ, Warren DK. Stratification of surgical site infection by operative factors and comparison of infection rates after hernia repair. Infect Control Hosp Epidemiol. 2015;36:329–35.

75. Novitsky YW, Orenstein SB. Effect of patient and hospital characteristics on outcomes of elective ventral hernia repair in the United States. Hernia. 2013;17:639–45.

76. Qin C, Souza J, Aggarwal A, Kim JYS. Insulin dependence as an independent predictor of perioperative morbidity after ventral hernia repair: a National Surgical Quality Improvement Program analysis of 45,759 patients. Am J Surg. 2016;211:11–7.

77. Falagas ME, Kasiakou SK. Mesh-related infections after hernia repair surgery. Clin Microbiol Infect. 2005;11:3–8.

78. Hornby ST, McDermott FD, Coleman M, et al. Female gender and diabetes mellitus increase the risk of recurrence after laparoscopic incisional hernia repair. Ann R Coll Surg Engl. 2015;97:115–9.

79. Baucom RB, Ousley J, Feurer ID, Beveridge GB, Pierce RA, Holzman MD, Sharp KW, Poulose BK. Patient reported outcomes after incisional hernia repair-establishing the ventral hernia recurrence inventory. Am J Surg. 2016;212:81–8.

80. Benowitz NL. Cotinine as a biomarker of environmental tobacco smoke exposure. Epidemiol Rev. 1996;18:188–204.

81. Hawn MT, Houston TK, Campagna EJ, Graham LA, Singh J, Bishop M, Henderson WG. The attributable risk of smoking on surgical complications. Ann Surg. 2011;254:914–20.

82. Waitzberg DL, Saito H, Plank LD, Jamieson GG, Jagannath P, Hwang T-L, Mijares JM, Bihari D. Postsurgical infections are reduced with specialized nutrition support. World J Surg. 2006;30:1592–604.

83. Cerantola Y, Grass F, Cristaudi A, Demartines N, Schäfer M, Hübner M. Perioperative nutrition in abdominal surgery: recommendations and reality. Gastroenterol Res Pract. 2011;2011:739347.

84. Bode LGM, Kluytmans JAJW, Wertheim HFL, et al. Preventing surgical-site infections in nasal carriers of Staphylococcus aureus. N Engl J Med. 2010;362:9–17.

85. Won EJ, Lehman EB, Geletzke AK, Tangel MR, Matsushima K, Brunke-Reese D, Pichardo-Lowden AR, Pauli EM, Soybel DI. Association of postoperative hyperglycemia with outcomes among patients with complex ventral hernia repair. JAMA Surg. 2015;150:433–40.

86. Ata A, Lee J, Bestle SL, Desemone J, Stain SC. Postoperative hyperglycemia and surgical site infection in general surgery patients. Arch Surg. 2010;145:858–64.

87. Hamman RF, Wing RR, Edelstein SL, et al. Effect of weight loss with lifestyle intervention on risk of diabetes. Diabetes Care. 2006;29:2102–7.

88. Heniford BT. CeDAR Mobile Application.

89. Shi Y, Warner DO. Surgery as a teachable moment for smoking cessation. Anesthesiology. 2010;112:102–7.

Index

© Springer International Publishing AG, part of Springer Nature 2018
K. A. LeBlanc (ed.), *Laparoscopic and Robotic Incisional Hernia Repair*,
https://doi.org/10.1007/978-3-319-90737-6